Cooking for Halflings & Monsters: Volume 2

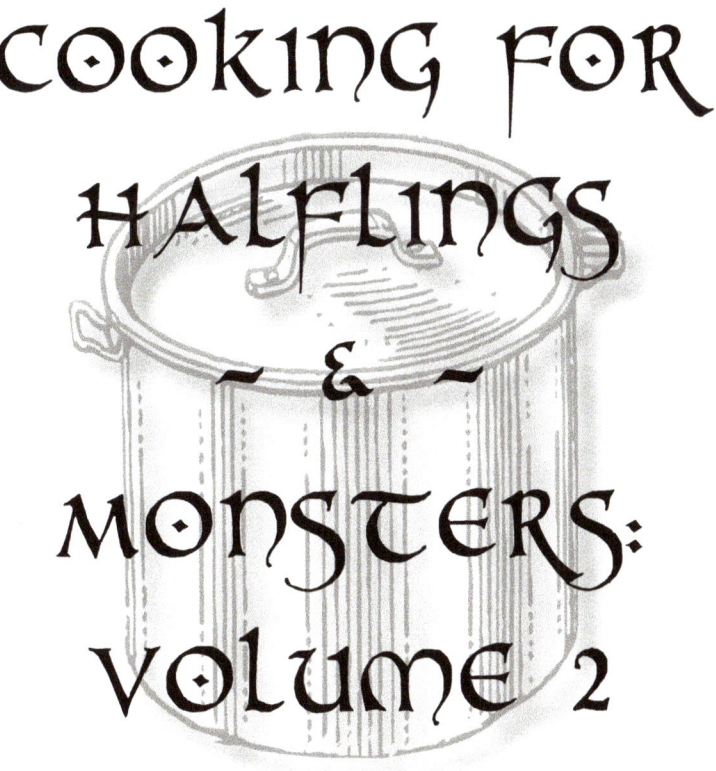

A Year of Comfy, Cozy Soups, Stews, and Chilis

Astrid Tuttle Winegar

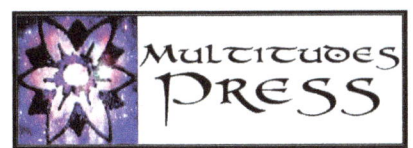

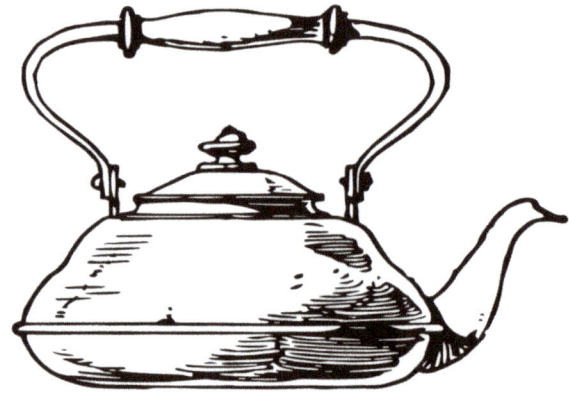

A Year of Comfy, Cozy Soups, Stews, and Chilis: Cooking for Halflings & Monsters, Volume 2

Copyright © 2019 Astrid Tuttle Winegar

All rights reserved. No part of this book may be used or reproduced in any manner whatsoever, including Internet usage, without written permission from the author, except in the case of brief quotations embodied in critical articles and reviews.

First edition © 2019
First printing

Paperback edition: ISBN 978-0-9994179-1-1
Ebook edition: ISBN 978-0-9994179-3-5

Printed in U.S.A.
Graphics © 2019 Graphic Goods | Design Cuts
Graphics © 2019 Shutterstock
Photographs © 2019 Astrid Tuttle Winegar
Cover Design © 2019 Astrid Tuttle Winegar
Author Photo © 2017 Kate the Photographer

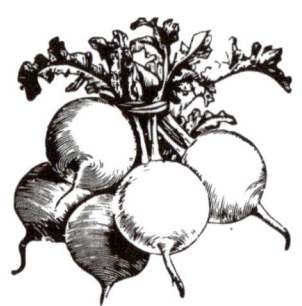

For more information, please see: www.astridwinegar.com

DEDICATION

To all of my cutie-patootie grandchildren,
who keep me on my toes.

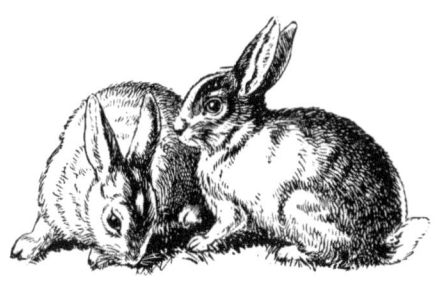

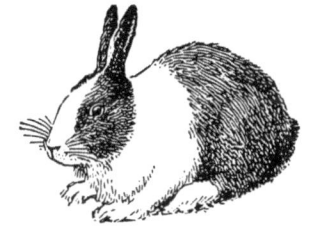
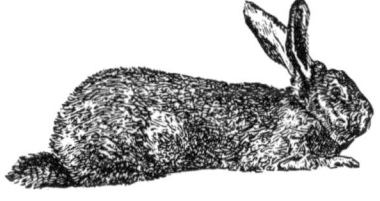

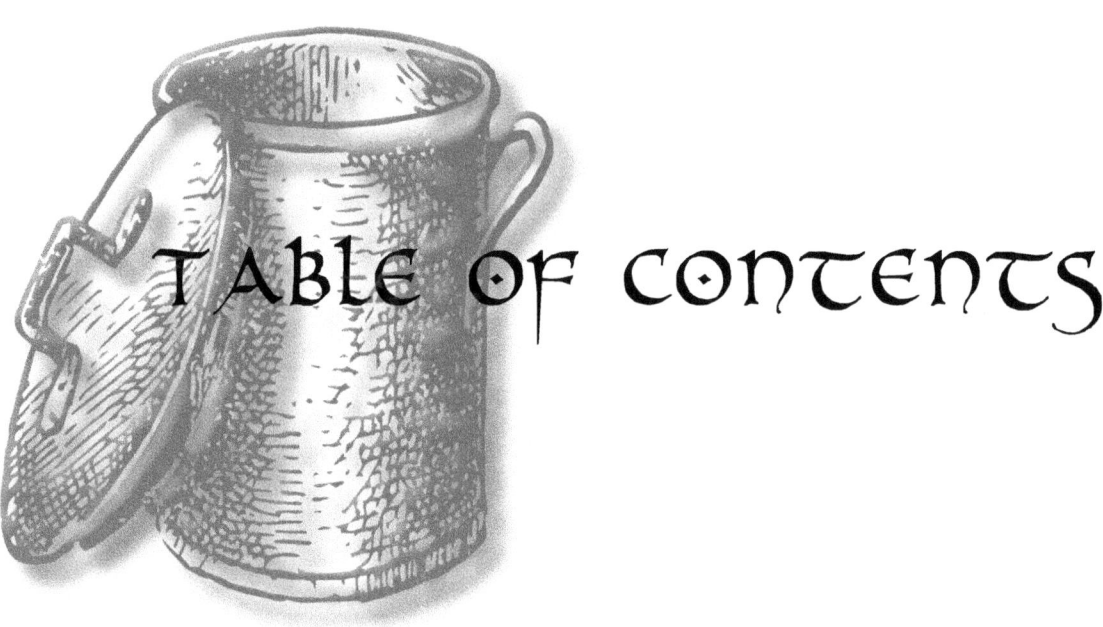

TABLE OF CONTENTS

INTRODUCTION | I

    Is Soup the Perfect Food? | i
    Soup Semantics | ii
    Breads, Carbs, and Pot Pie Conversion Tactics | iii
    Garnishes & Photography | iv
        Nice New Mexican & Mexican Garnishes | iv
        Charming Chili Garnishes | v
    Quantities | vi
    Quickie Versions, Substitutions, and Ingredient Quantities | vi
    Vegetarian & Meat-Lovers | viii
    Green Chiles & Other Hot Stuff | viii
    Seasoning, Salt, and Butter | ix
    Leftovers | xi
    Miscellaneous Idiosyncrasies | xi
    Sort of a Philosophical Mission Statement | xiii
    Hey… Where's the Fantasy? | xiv

SOME ESSENTIALS FOR SOUPS, STEWS, AND CHILIS | XVII

    Mirepoix (or that which is known by dozens of other names…) | xvii
    Crème Fraîche & Other Creamy Options | xviii
    Cooked Hominy | xx
    Stocks and/or Broths | xxii

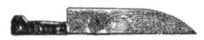

CHAPTER ONE—BEEF | 1

CHAPTER TWO—CHICKEN | 33

CHAPTER THREE—PORK & SEAFOOD | 73

CHAPTER FOUR—VEGETABLES | 113

CHAPTER FIVE—BREADS | 147

CONCLUSION | 183

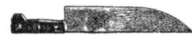

LIST OF KITCHEN UTENSILS | 185

    Cooking Utensils & Miscellaneous Items | 185
    Small & Large Appliances | 186
    Pots & Pans | 186
    Baking Essentials | 187

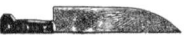

CONVERSION CHARTS | 189

    Dry Ingredients by Weight | 189
    Liquid Ingredients by Volume | 190
    Lengths & Widths | 191
    Temperatures | 191

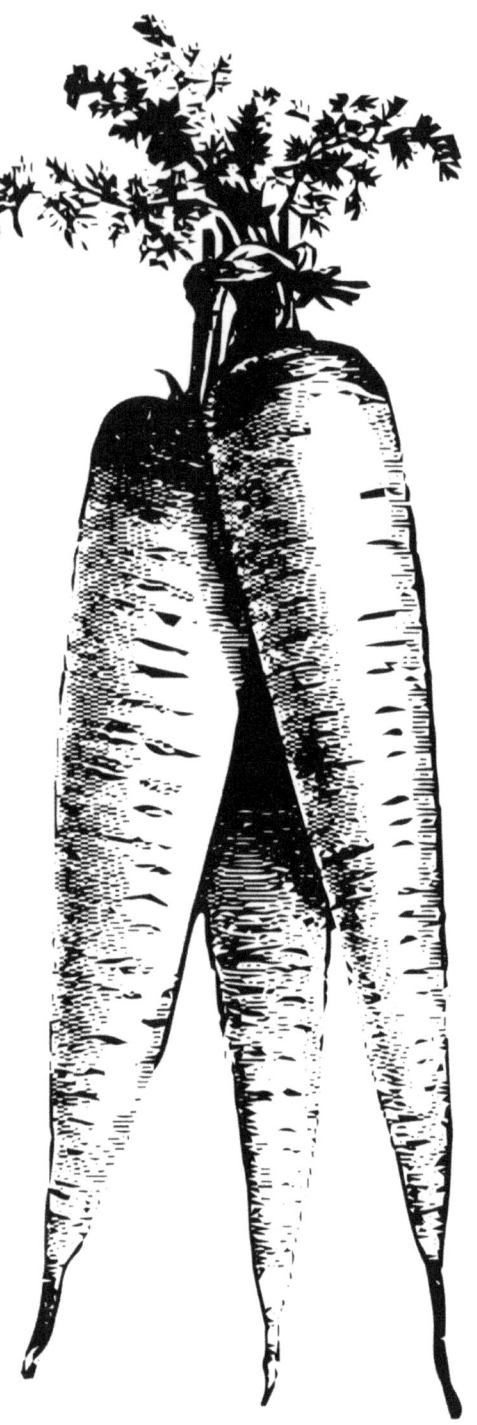

ACKNOWLEDGMENTS | 193

THE FELLOWSHIP OF THE RECIPE TESTERS | 195

WORKS CITED & SOURCED | 197

MISCELLANEOUS NEW MEXICO ITEMS | 201

SHOPPING SOURCES | 203

INDEX | 205

AUTHOR'S BIOGRAPHY | 215

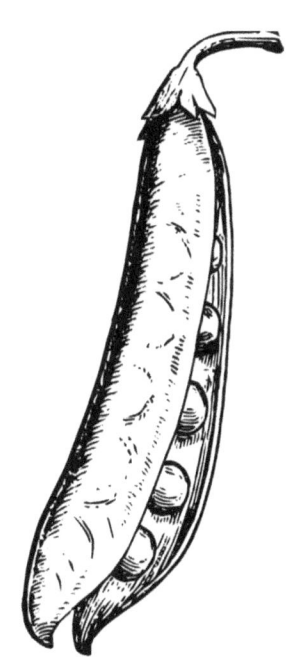

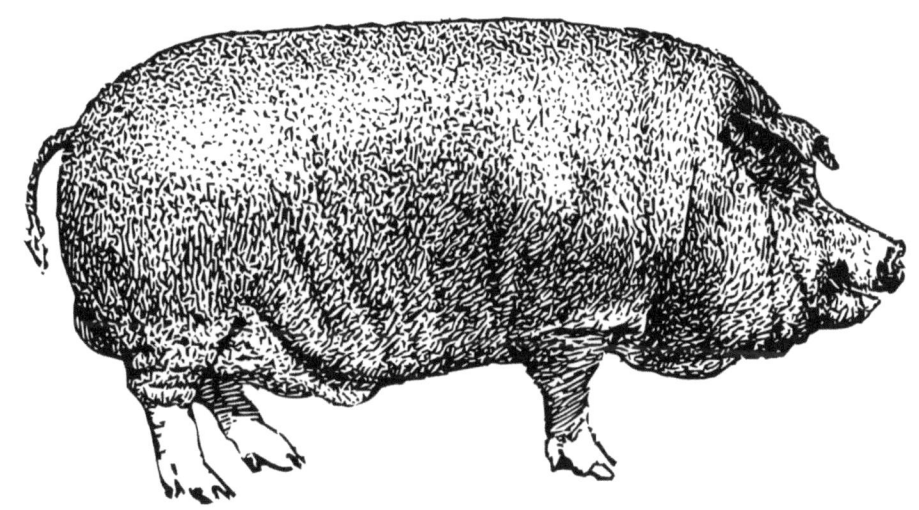

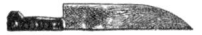

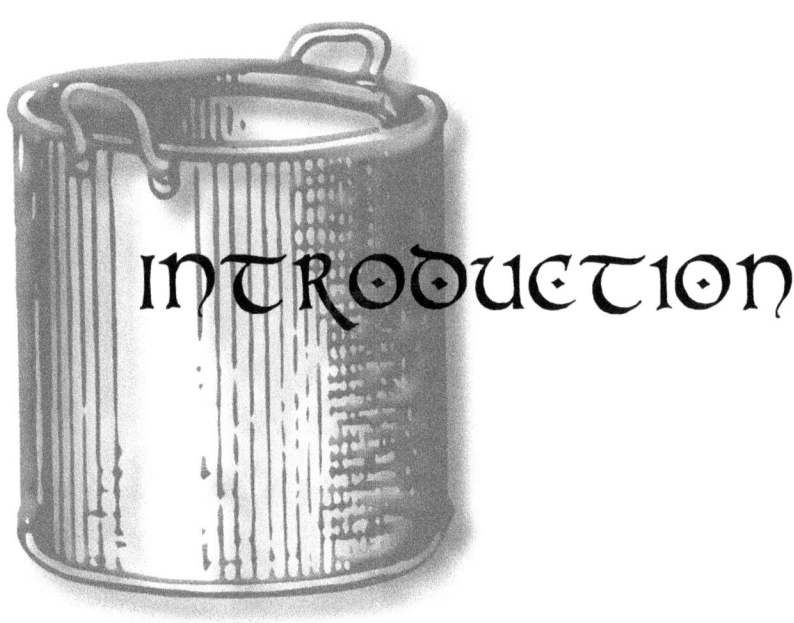

INTRODUCTION

Is Soup the Perfect Food?

It seems that people are always debating about the "perfect food." One day it's kale, another day it's blueberries. Two bananas each day will supposedly keep you going strong, which is fine until the banana supply runs out. An apple a day keeps the doctor away. The debate seems to imply that one should consume mass (meaning daily) quantities of a particular "perfect food" and one's health problems would magically disappear.

But food trends come and go, and relying on a few food items for optimal health is unhealthy at worst and boring at best. I would make an argument for soup (and its extended iterations of stew and chili) as a more nutritious, versatile, and fulfilling perfect food. Soup is perfect because all of your nutrients are contained within a single pot. It is perfect because most recipes are manageable even by absolute beginners. It is perfect because your vegetables are cooked, either a little or a lot, and they will not wreak havoc with your digestive system as much as raw vegetables sometimes will.

It is perfect because nothing is more satisfying than a steamy bowl of gumbo on a blustery day in January or a spicy bowl of posole on a blistering day in July.

Soup is (generally) unfussy; it is the ultimate comfort food. It (generally) combines carbohydrates, proteins, and vegetable nutrition in pleasing dishes that satisfy friends and family. It is (generally) conducive to substitutions, so it can be flexible. It can be pureed and served to picky toddlers. It usually keeps well for awhile, it often freezes well, and it is economical. You can serve it at your table or hunker down with a bowl on the couch or even on the floor.

Once upon a time I was reminiscing about my single life, back when I lived alone as a poor college undergraduate. My diet seemed to consist mainly of raisins, Cheddar cheese, and packages of ramen soup. This was when I was about 20 years old—I figured I was cheaply hitting some major food groups. I only did this for a few months before I gave up on my poverty and decided to move back in with mom and dad. A few years later, a husband and children eventually took over my life. Now, young grandchildren completely and pleasantly dominate many of our days.

In hindsight, as a single person who was busy in school, I wished I had spent maybe one day a week making a pot of soup to live on. Two quarts of soup would make four two-cup portions—or four perfect (and filling!) dinners. Or those two quarts could make two dinners and three or four smaller lunch portions. I suppose this might seem to be a problem if you tend to get bored with food easily. However—if you had 52 delicious choices all in one cookbook, how could you become bored?

I'm an extremely organized person. My grown-up daughters, Chloë and Callista, would say I am an annoying (yet endearing, perhaps…?) control freak. I find menu planning to be a soothing pastime and essential to my sanity, at least at this stage in my life. You could compare it to coloring, I suppose. Planning a menu is probably a reaction to my late mother, who was rather obese for most of her adult life. She hardly ever planned for basic meals and usually seemed to regard a trip to the grocery store as her version of an amusement park ride: "Let's go here and buy this! Now, over here! This looks good!" It just never made sense to me.

Now, menu planning has (usually) not made me inflexible; life routines and menus change frequently around my household, and we also have plenty of spontaneous and impulsive events. This means that I have occasionally refrozen meats. But those unpredictable moments give routines meaning. I have noticed I tend to feel better, not only emotionally but also physically, when I (mostly) stick to my routines. Fortunately, my husband Bob is also a creature of habit. We have made it past 31 years of marriage, so something must be working. Maybe it's all those soups, stews, and chilis I keep making? Could be.

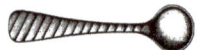

Soup Semantics

I suppose we can define a "soup" as a specific food which is made from cooking a specific quantity of other foods in a relatively large amount of a specific liquid. All of the "specifics" can vary, of course. A "stew" is almost the same, except the cooked foods are usually cut into bigger chunks and you use less liquid. A "chili" can end up soupy or stewy, and often utilizes ground meats and beans; however, sometimes it does not. There can be myriad variations on all three of these products. What do they have in common? They are served in a bowl with a spoon.

We have many terms for soup. A *consommé* is the thinnest soup you can possibly imagine, so why isn't it considered merely a beverage? A *potage* is a thick soup, so shouldn't it be considered a stew? A soup might be called a bisque or a chowder, though a bisque should be a puree, which might have meats and/or vegetables added after the puree. A chowder is more specific, being made usually with seafood or pork, with various vegetables such as onions, tomatoes, and potatoes. However, the word "chowder" can also apply to other soups that simply resemble a traditional chowder, such as a corn chowder. Thus, chowder equals chunky and bisque equals blended. Technically, any soup, stew, or chili could be turned into a bisque just by pureeing it, but you probably would not want to bother doing that, especially if you have gone to the effort of cutting your vegetables and meats into lovely bits. And obviously, you can never turn a bisque into a chowder, because doing so would defy the laws of physics. If you possess a time-traveling device, then that would be another story.

Breads, Carbs, and Pot Pie Conversion Tactics

Sometimes you want to bake up some sort of bready accompaniment to round out your meal. Bob is keen on crumbled-up saltines in many soupy dishes, but I'll have to pass on that. So, I have invented 13 carbohydrate-type items that can be mixed and matched accordingly—one recipe for every four weeks. Sometimes the soup, stew, or chili is enough; other times, you might feel that strong desire to whip up some biscuits or cornbread. Then there are those busy occasions when you might only have time to purchase a nice artisan loaf, or some ciabatta bread, or a can of crescent rolls. Do what you have time and energy for, if it isn't too stressful. I have made some good soup-pairing suggestions for each bread recipe.

  I live in Albuquerque, New Mexico, the high altitude home of the Sandia Mountains in all their purple majesty. Therefore, your baked goods might need slight adjustments. They might not; you will have to experiment. My own baking time is always right in the middle, if I give a range of times. All dry ingredients should be level, unless specified otherwise. Your oven's baking rack should be in the middle, unless specified otherwise. I have a conventional oven; if you are using a convection type, you might have to adjust your timing or your temperature.

  Some of the stews and chilis within the cookbook can be cleverly converted into pot pies; then you don't have to bother making a separate carbohydrate. You could divide your stew into, say, one-cup ramekins (coat each with cooking spray first or grease lightly). Place them on a large (18" by 13") baking sheet. Cut items like purchased pie crust, either single or even double, and place on top of each ramekin. Cut a small X in the center of each, then pinch around the edge and bake at 375° for about 15-20 minutes.

  Or cut circles from a thawed sheet of puff pastry. You could even purchase those Pepperidge Farm puff pastry cups and place them upside-down on your ramekins. You would want to bake these for about ten minutes at 450°.

  If a stew or chili is thick enough, you could do a double-crust pie, either with purchased pie crusts or your own favorite recipe. Bake a double-crust pie for 46-50 minutes at 375°. Scraps of dough can be cut into small designs with cookie cutters and attached with an egg wash or a bit of melted butter. Well now, aren't you a fancy dish, you humble stew?

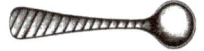

Garnishes & Photography

I took all of the photos with my Samsung Galaxy phone, without flash, on my backyard patio. I am not a professional, obviously, and I do not have a design team working for me. Nevertheless, I tried to represent each item well and in an appetizing way, thematically by chapter. All the bowls were purchased (on clearance!) from Pier One Imports. All the bread dishes and other various display items were from Bed Bath and Beyond. All the utensils, napkins, and small props were either family antiques or found objects.

All the soups were photographed in substantial two-cup portions along with some sort of garnish. Each soup, stew, and chili recipe has garnishing suggestions. Sometimes the garnish is more integral to the dish (see Onion Soup C'est Magnifique on page 116), but many other recipes can fit into what I am going to call the Nice New Mexican & Mexican Garnishes category. As you can see, these would be too numerous to list on every single recipe, so I am listing them all here. When I took photographs, I would usually pick out two or three of these to garnish a dish, depending on what I had around. If you were planning to have a chili buffet, however, it would be great to put out a dozen garnishing options or so, then guests could decorate their own bowls. In addition to the New Mexican & Mexican list, I have added a Charming Chili Garnishes list for kicks. These lists are by no means exhaustive. Perhaps you like jelly beans on your soup, or chocolate-covered ants... feel free to add whatever gives you joy.

Again, all of these garnishing suggestions are completely optional and you can certainly omit them. But maybe you want to dress up a soup for company or add some nutritional components for variety. The main point is—don't stress about the garnish!

NICE NEW MEXICAN & MEXICAN GARNISHES

- ANY sort of onion, chopped or diced finely or coarsely
- Radishes, sliced thinly, or chopped finely or coarsely
- Fresh cabbage, chopped or diced finely or shredded
- Avocado, sliced or diced; a scoop of guacamole can also serve as a garnish
- Iceberg lettuce or other greenery, chopped coarsely or shredded
- Tomatoes, chopped or diced coarsely
- Green or black olives, sliced (regular canned variety, not kalamatas)
- Sliced fresh jalapeños
- Sliced jalapeños, from a jar or can, drained; however spicy you can endure
- Other pickled chili peppers
- Any other assorted chopped vegetables you might like
- Sour cream (I use the light kind; you have to save calories somewhere, right?)

- Mexican Crema or Crème fraîche (often available for purchase—if you would like to dabble in making your own, please see the *Some Essentials for Soups, Stews, and Chilis* section starting on page xviii)
- Cheeses such as Cheddar, Monterey Jack, Pepper Jack; shredded
- Cheeses such as Cotija, queso Fresco or Panela; crumbled
- Fresh cilantro, minced or chopped coarsely
- Jicama, peeled and shredded; minced, diced, or chopped coarsely
- Lime wedges
- Hot sauce, whatever is your favorite variety
- Salsa—ANY variety you like, a tablespoon or two over the top (a half-cup if you're Bob)
- Red chile sauce and/or green chile sauce, same as above (see *Shopping Sources* on page 203)
- Fried eggs (These are generally reserved for things like enchiladas, but you might want to throw an egg on top of your posole. I wouldn't, but you might. In New Mexico, usually an egg garnish is fried over medium with a runny yolk.)
- Tortilla chips, broken up (Fritos will also work… Oh, let's face it, any chip you like will work as a crunchy garnish)
- Thin strips of crispy tortillas

CHARMING CHILI GARNISHES

- Anything listed above in the NICE NEW MEXICAN & MEXICAN GARNISHES section
- Crumbled cornbread or cornbread croutons
- Other types of croutons, any flavor
- Fried onions in a can or a bag (such as French's)
- Fried ANYTHING in a can or a bag (other assorted vegetables; again, French's)
- Pickled vegetables or other pickles, sweet or dill; chopped or sliced
- Chow mein noodles or crispy rice sticks
- Crumbling cheeses such as Goat, Feta, or Bleu varieties
- Baked tater tots or other frozen potato products, such as fries or curly fries
- Roasted garlic cloves
- Cooked spaghetti (or the following items), with chili served on top
- Cooked small-shaped pasta
- Cooked rice, white or brown
- Cooked couscous, any variety
- Cooked grits, any variety
- Cooked barley
- Seasoned mashed potatoes

Quantities

I have designed the majority of the recipes to serve either three to four, four to six, or six to eight, as rather substantial main courses. A few recipes serve eight to ten, but they are usually easy to cut in half. If a recipe serves three to four, it is most likely because Bob is not too crazy about a recipe, so I end up being the only one who eats it. I have figured that each serving would be one and a half to two cups. Two cups is a large bowl of soup, and you might be stuffed after you eat it, which is fine; then you don't really need to make anything else. If you happen to use a soup as an appetizer serving of half- to three-quarters of a cup, then your two quarts of soup could serve more like 12.

There are light soups here, medium ones, and thicker, heartier ones. If you are going to double a recipe, you might need to add more cooking time. Conversely, now that it is just the two of us in our empty nest, I often cut recipes in half. Then my cooking time might be reduced somewhat. I don't mind having a couple of leftover meals, but we really don't want to eat one soup six separate times. I am actually not in the habit of freezing foods very much because freezing sometimes changes the textures of certain items.

I was originally thinking of writing a series of "Empty Nest" cookbooks, which would be geared to couples or individuals who wanted to "cook small." Research led me to abandon that idea; namely, it seemed there were already quite a few cookbooks catering to that niche, and sometimes it is annoying to use ingredients in such a minimal way. I mean using, say, a quarter-cup of canned, diced tomatoes. Now I have three-quarters of a can of tomatoes leftover. A book reviewer also mentioned that she didn't like to bother going to all the trouble of making a dish just for one meal. In other words—*please* leave me some leftovers. I figured it was better to compromise by writing a recipe to feed (usually) four to six people and the reader can increase or decrease according to his/her particular needs.

Quickie Versions, Substitutions, and Ingredient Quantities

When appropriate, I have included suggestions for making a soup, stew, or chili in a speedier way. Let's face it—you're not always up for cooking a whole chicken for stock, removing the meat, then cooking the soup. Please consult the recipe's introductory text or the anecdotal material after the recipe for time-saving suggestions or other variations when you're feeling extra busy.

This brings us to the subject of substitutions. Thus, instead of using a whole chicken, water, and seasonings, you might substitute some precooked chicken and pre-made stock. You should feel free to change various vegetables, but you might have to adjust your cooking times. Perhaps you hate broccoli and would like to substitute cauliflower. Perhaps you hate basil and would like to substitute tarragon. Perhaps you hate garlic and simply want to omit it completely. These changes will work out fine. Actual structural changes are more tricky—you should not use milk if the recipe calls for cream.

When it comes to the measurements of various purchased ingredients, you should strive to come as close as you can. If I call for a can of beans that measures 15.5 ounces and your favorite brand is a can that measures 15 ounces, that will be fine. I had no idea that inventing recipes would be so dependent on the timely vicissitudes of marketing. But then, who would ever have suspected that a famous ice cream manufacturer would suddenly decide that a 14-ounce container should be an acceptable substitute for a true pint? Or soft drink, beer, or coffee manufacturers who have now determined that 11.5 ounces is the new 12 ounces? The price remained the same (or increased, more likely), yet the consumer is now getting less. Who knows how small cans of beans will become in the future? I revisited a cake recipe printed in 2004 that started with an 18.25-ounce box of German Chocolate cake mix. When I made it in 2019, the cake mix measured 15.25 ounces. Over the course of 15 years, Betty Crocker cut three ounces out of their mix. I have a feeling the price probably went up by a dollar, though I can't prove that. The cake turned out fine; nevertheless, as consumers, we can complain about these changes, but it won't matter to the manufacturers.

If you prefer not to use any type of alcoholic product in your recipe, simply use the same quantity of whatever broth the recipe has specified instead of the beer or wine. Generally, the recipes are cooked for a long enough time to eliminate any alcoholic content, but if there is any concern, you are free to substitute broth. Non-alcoholic beer can be a perfect substitute.

You might also want to use a fresh ingredient where I have called for a canned variety. This will often work out well; for example, you might want to cook your own beans or you might have a bumper crop of tomatoes in your garden. The only time this might affect a recipe is when the recipe calls for using the liquid that comes with the product in the can. For example, if a recipe calls for a can of stewed tomatoes, but you only want to use fresh ones, you would need to recreate that sort of product. All that means is you would want to add a bit of liquid and a bit of herbs. It's not a big deal obviously. You might want to make a soup in wintertime and might not have access to fresh garden tomatoes, so you shouldn't feel bad about using a canned product. Frozen corn is sometimes fine, sometimes canned corn is fine, sometimes you have easy access to fresh. This can apply to many of the ingredients within. With our busy lives, sometimes convenience is important; I can assure you that a soup can be a wondrously forgiving dish, much of the time.

Vegetarian & Meat Lovers

Though I am not a vegetarian (and definitely not a vegan), I have made sure to give you options to convert each recipe. Therefore, every single soup recipe within this cookbook could be vegetarian, if you prefer. If you are vegan, you are probably used to switching oil for butter and that might be the only adjustment you need to make. However, some of the vegetable soups do start with a meat-based broth (the classic example being Onion Soup C'est Magnifique). These options will be represented by this lovely squash on the right.

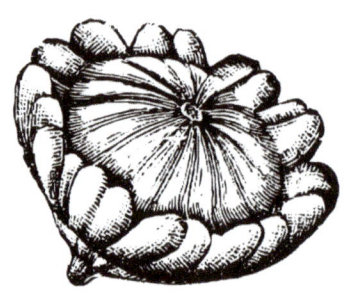

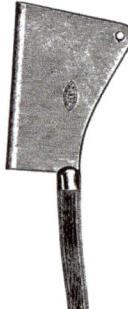

And if you must have meat in everything you eat, all the vegetarian recipes have protein suggestions. Occasionally, a particular meat recipe will also offer a different option for your protein. All of these options will be represented by this wicked cleaver on the left.

Green Chiles & Other Hot Stuff

My first cookbook, *Cooking for Halflings & Monsters: 111 Comfy, Cozy Recipes for Fantasy-Loving Souls,* was filled with green chile suggestions to perk up all of the Middle-earth inspired comfort food. Here, I felt free to use chile quite liberally. Some items within were not designed to be spicy; however, you would be pleasantly surprised at how delicious an Italian wedding soup can be with green chile or salsa. Please consult the chili pepper icon at the right for helpful spice suggestions. And if you have a shy stomach, be sure to reduce any spicy ingredients right from the start. You can always add more as you cook, but you can't take it out once it's there.

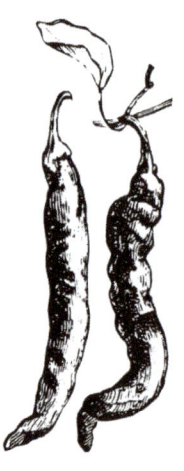

In case you were wondering—to differentiate between the two items, I always spell the dish "chili" but the New Mexican pepper is always spelled "chile" in the singular and "chiles" in the plural. Other spellings might be more erratic; such as when referencing items such as "chili powder" or "sweet chili sauce," which can also be known as "chilli powder" and "sweet chilli sauce." Plural spellings can also be unpredictable. It might not seem important to mention, but I'm going to aim for consistency wherever possible. Thus, there are a few chilis in this cookbook, and all of them are made with green chiles.

Seasoning, Salt, and Butter

I strive to be moderate with seasonings. Plenty of the soups within the cookbook are meant to be spicy, others are not. Plus, food is (in my humble opinion) the most subjective thing in the entire world. Every person has different tastes. If you have concerns about salt or spices, be sure to adjust the ingredients according to your needs. As I said in the previous section, you can always add more seasoning as you cook, but you can't remove it once it's in the pot. So, season judiciously and remember you (probably) have salt and pepper shakers on your table for good reason. All the recipes call for low-sodium broths or stocks. By "low-sodium" I mean a product that has somewhere between 400-600 milligrams of sodium per serving.

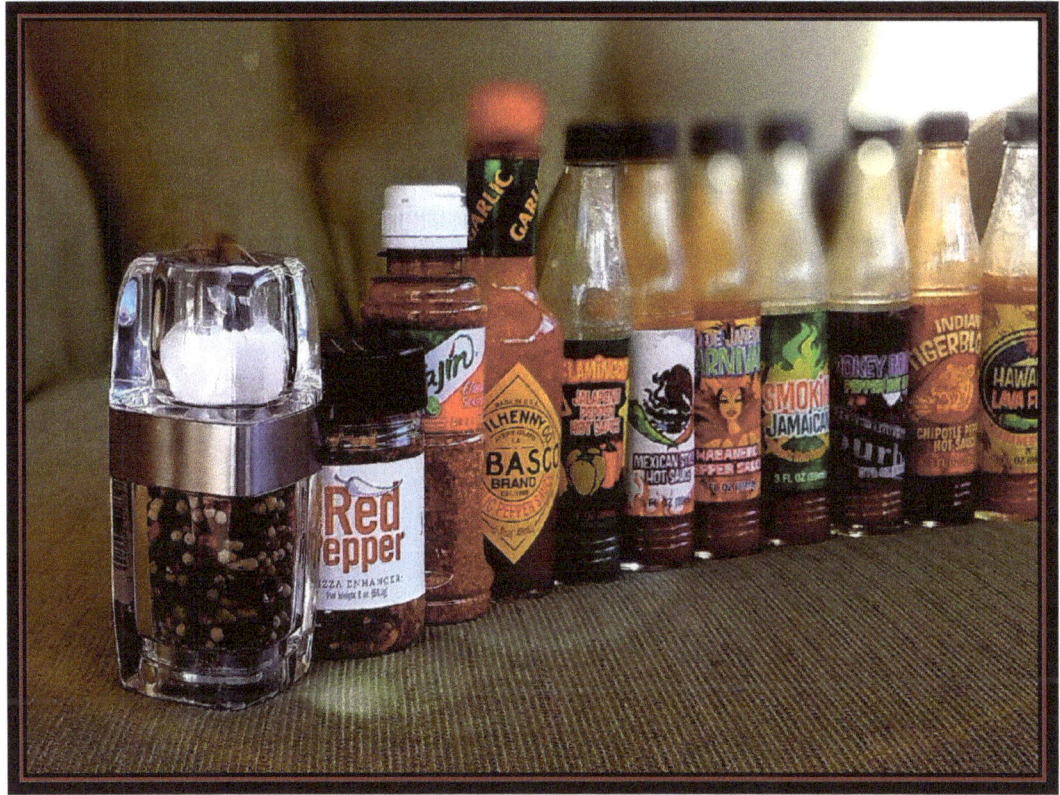

    I am using salted sweet cream butter (from Costco) throughout—you can certainly use an unsalted variety. I know that every cook or chef has his or her own opinion on butter and its sodium content, but I've used salted forever. Therefore, these recipes have been designed and tested with that particular product. If you only use unsalted butter, your recipe might turn out to be fine; but if not, that's what the final seasoning is for, right?

I have listed specific varieties of pepper, such as black, white, cayenne, or crushed red pepper flakes. You may grind your pepper if you prefer. Sometimes that is hard to measure, but you might prefer absolutely fresh pepper flavor for your dish. I like to use a coarse ground black pepper, but a finer grind will also work. Mixed-color peppercorns are fine to use.

When it comes to herbs and spices, I have listed both dry and fresh varieties. I'm not snobby about herbs, so fresh is not always required. Sometimes the season is wrong for fresh herbs, so a dried variety will be fine. You can usually assume that every teaspoon of a dried herb is equal to about two or three tablespoons of a minced fresh herb. All of these flavorings should be guidelines for you and you can adjust accordingly.

When it comes to other ingredients, I generally use a regularly-salted version. This includes items such as canned beans or tomato products. If you prefer to use organic products, sometimes they might have a reduced sodium content. This only means you might have to season more at the end of cooking. If I do use a reduced-type of product, I'll specify that in the list of ingredients; however, if you only use full-fat sour cream or whole milk, that will turn out fine.

Salt can be tricky, since you cannot always predict how salty your broth might be. You can't always predict just how much flavor ingredients such as potatoes, rice, or pasta will soak up in the cooking. To top it all off, dishes can sometimes become saltier after they have been refrigerated. Salt substitutes will be fine to use. When I list salt, I merely refer to common table salt; however, different salt varieties will also be fine, if you happen to prefer kosher, sea, or pink Himalayan. If the recipe requires a special salt, the ingredient will be listed more specifically.

If you have severe sodium restrictions on your diet, I would recommend using unsalted butter, only using sodium-free versions of stock or broth (you could even substitute water all around), and substituting the low-sodium versions of all other ingredients that you might encounter in this cookbook (such as canned goods, salt, soy sauce, or Worcestershire sauce, etc.). Then you could season accordingly after cooking. It's hard to imagine a chicken noodle soup made with water, but if you have to do it, then you have to do it. Bone broths are often prepared without salt, while still having the taste of chicken; this might be a good option to try.

Leftovers

Most soups, stews, and chilis will last a week or so in your refrigerator as long as they are stored in an airtight container. For convenience, I will often cook my soup in a six-quart pot, serve it for dinner, then transfer the leftovers into a three-quart pot, covered, for heating up the next day or the second day after the original meal. Many recipes improve with age, as their flavors have more time to develop. I know nutritional experts would prefer all of us to trash our leftovers after two or three days tops, but besides the obvious disregard for the food waste dilemma, I am not going to toss a soup that still smells good on day six. We haven't died yet.

Not every item in this cookbook should be frozen, mostly those recipes with potatoes because they can become mushy. I will let you know if a recipe should NOT be frozen. But most of the recipes can be frozen and thawed for later use, which is good to do if you would rather double recipes to save time later.

Some soups become much thicker after being refrigerated, which is usually due to carbohydrate absorption. In other words, your pasta or rice, though initially cooked, has taken on even more moisture. When you reheat, either on the stove or in a microwave, try not to add additional water, broth, or cream until your soup has heated up a bit. Then add a little extra liquid to help loosen it up. Don't open up your soup (which now seems as firm and thick as a mass of wet concrete) and add half a cup of water immediately. Heat slowly and add new liquid sparingly—this way you won't dilute the flavors too much as the soup loosens up.

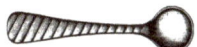

Miscellaneous Idiosyncrasies

Cooks and chefs have many idiosyncrasies, but ultimately, we all want to produce a dish that tastes good. Sometimes I might mention techniques that are second nature to me, but might not seem that intuitive to another cook. Take chopping techniques, for example: I believe that finely chopping implies cutting vegetables into approximately ¼" bits. Mincing should be even smaller. A dice should be about ½" and should be as neatly cut as possible; whereas, a coarse chop should also be around ½" but ends up being more of a casual cut (if that makes any sense… I hope it does…). Other items are cut into ¾" or 1" chunks. I've tried to be relatively specific regarding the cutting of vegetables and meats in the recipes.

I often (not always, but often) start my saucepan with a coating of cooking spray on the bottom, even if I've got butter and/or oil going on; this is mostly to ensure easier cleanup. I haven't yet joined the modern world and upgraded my cookware to non-stick technology, unfortunately. Maybe one day, but it is not this day. I think I also use a bit of spray to cut down on the amount of fat used in a recipe, mainly because the medical community has convinced us that fat is so bad, though it tastes so good. I only mention this because cooking spray has apparently generated some controversy in the culinary world.

All of the chili recipes included happen to have beans in them. To amuse myself and conduct legitimate (though completely unscientific) research, I ran polling on various social media platforms to gauge whether beans are popular in chili or not. I concluded that roughly 75% of poll participants either liked/preferred beans in chili, or they could go either way. Only about 25% preferred NO beans. I was concerned that I didn't have any non-bean chili recipes, but I felt better after seeing the results from these polls. Perhaps that doesn't seem like an idiosyncrasy, but this section seemed to be a good place to discuss the matter. Beans are a great addition to chilis; they are full of fiber and they can reduce the overall quantity of meat you consume, which is beneficial to your health and the health of our planet.

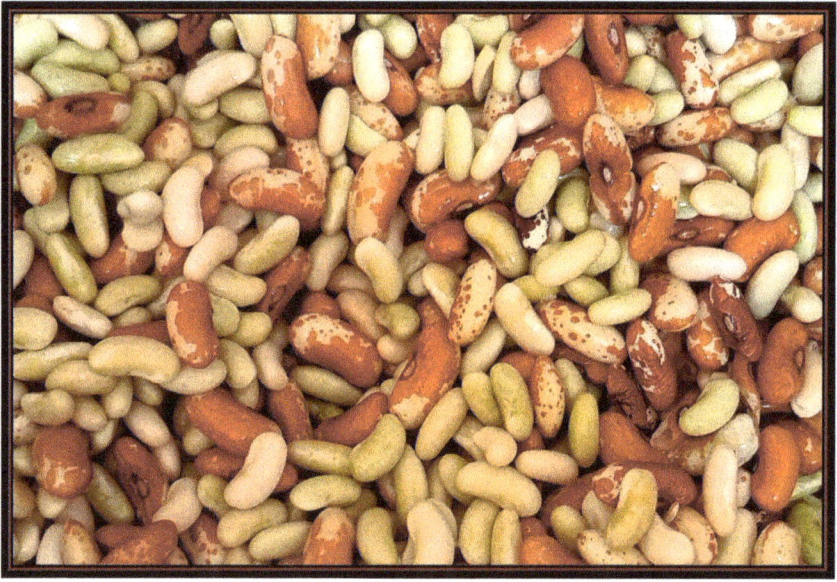

Sometimes I write a measurement as ounces, as opposed to cups. When this happens, be sure to measure your ingredients specifically as directed (I have also included *Conversion Charts,* starting on page 189). When I was in cooking school, my teacher stressed that there were times when you need a weight for accuracy. Various other ingredients are more casual; often you can skimp on measurements such as "1 cup coarsely chopped onion," or make it a heaping cup full of onion. I usually like to list measurements as opposed to specific items, usually; not all celery stalks or cloves of garlic are equal in mass.

I try to create as little waste—not only with actual objects, but also with time—as possible in the kitchen. Not that I'm a fanatic about it, but, if there is a way to save some time on doing dishes, I'm all for that. If I can make a soup with one saucepan and one measuring cup and one measuring spoon, I'm also all for that. I'm not keen on my kitchen looking like a cyclone went through it after I've cooked a meal, but that's just one of my idiosyncrasies. We all have them; I'm hopeful you'll be able to accept mine during the course of this quirky cookbook.

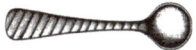

Sort of a Philosophical Mission Statement

I had worked with hundreds (thousands? Maybe…) of other people's recipes over the years before I ever started inventing my own. A long while ago, I remember trying out a chocolate chip cookie recipe. The cookbook implied it was a fantastic recipe, but alas! It really wasn't. I started to think about what would be the ultimate chocolate chip cookie. What would represent the very essence of chocolate-chipness in a cookie? That led me to start thinking about all sorts of other recipes in all sorts of other types of foods, and for better or worse, it is often the way I approach recipe development—I'm seeking a sort of culinary Platonic ideal. Many of those thoughts have manifested here. Of course, all of these thoughts are my own and you might disagree with them. Plato would probably have disagreed with them. But then you hold the power to improvise on my thoughts, if you wish, and create your own essential and ultimate dish which will reflect your own tastes. We can all be wizards in the kitchen!

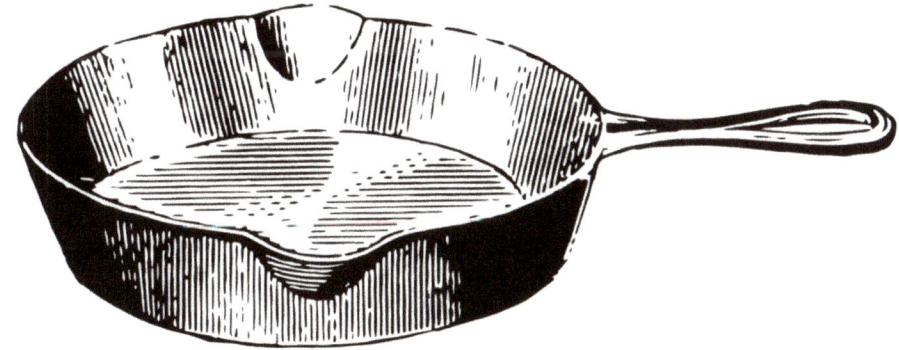

Hey... Where's the Fantasy?

Pretty much every recipe I invent ends up being comfort food for hobbits, even if it's Italian or Chinese or Mexican. Fantasy, science fiction, pop culture, and mythology (which is merely ancient fantasy and science fiction) constantly permeate my consciousness and probably always will. So, even though I have ostensibly left part of my heart in the fantasy world of my first cookbook, you will still see inklings of fantasy here. I'm not going to try to compete with unauthorized cookbooks from various fantasy franchises; in other words, I'm (probably) not going to invent a recipe for Butterbeer. I also do not want to risk any sort of legal issues (which I originally encountered with my first cookbook). Some recipes included within, however, were specifically invented for my Internet writings on subjects such as Narnia and Star Wars.

Will I miss writing at length about Middle-earth and Narnia? Maybe, but writing about New Mexico occasionally has its own rewards. I once had a boyfriend who moved here from Chicago in the early 1980s. I asked him why exactly did he decide on a cross-country move to the Land of Enchantment? He said New Mexico held a compelling sort of exotic vision in his mind; it was a strangely romantic notion based on childhood fantasies, to live in a weird and magical place filled with cowboys. The milder weather also influenced his decision, of course. So, in a way, I'm actually still writing about a fantasy land, even though it is one of the United States of America. Some Americans still think they need a passport to travel here, which proves that geography is obviously not a well-taught subject in our modern schools.

Let's do some Fantastic Cooking!

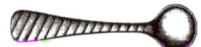

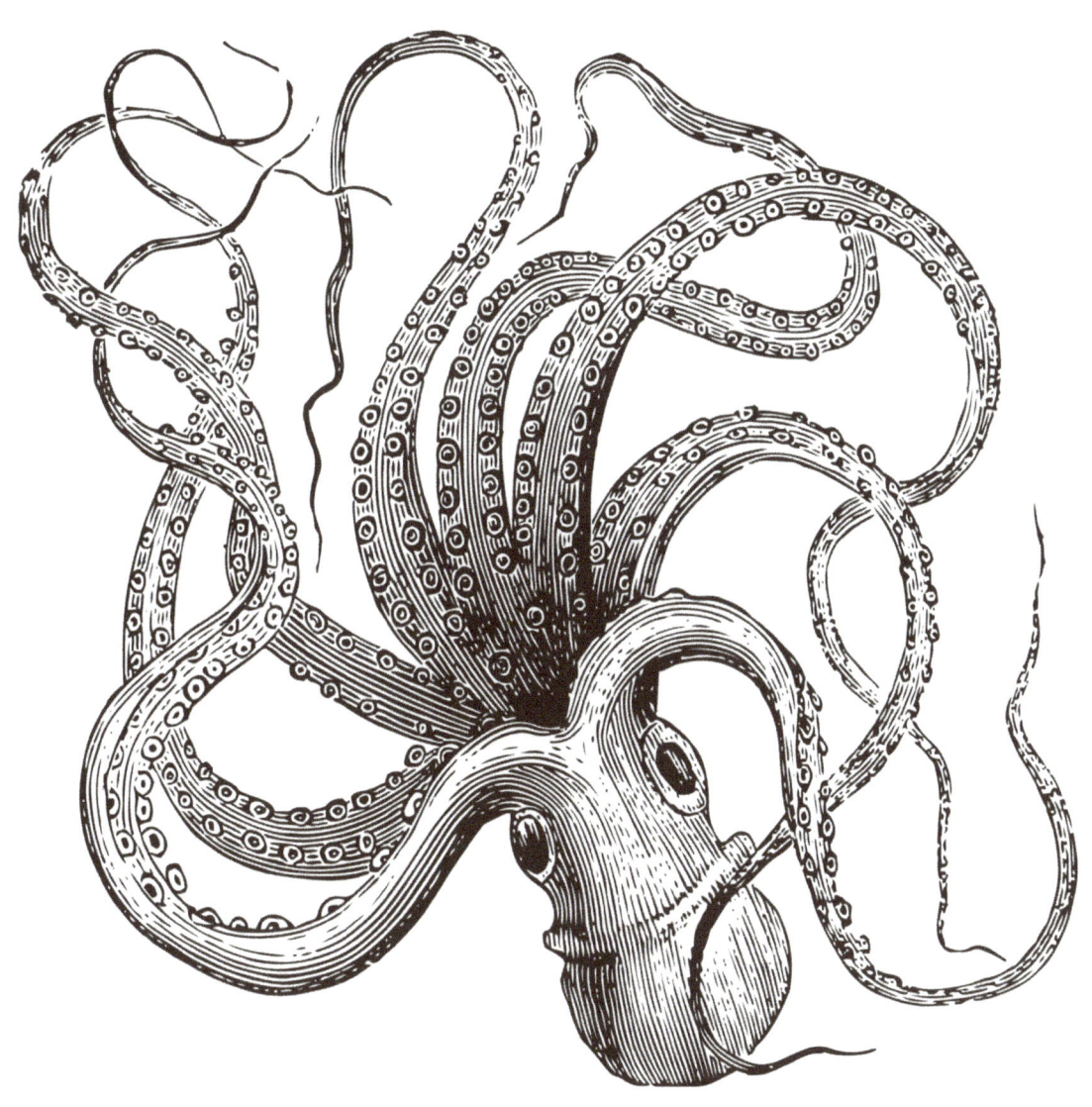

RELEASE THE

KITCHEN KRAKEN!

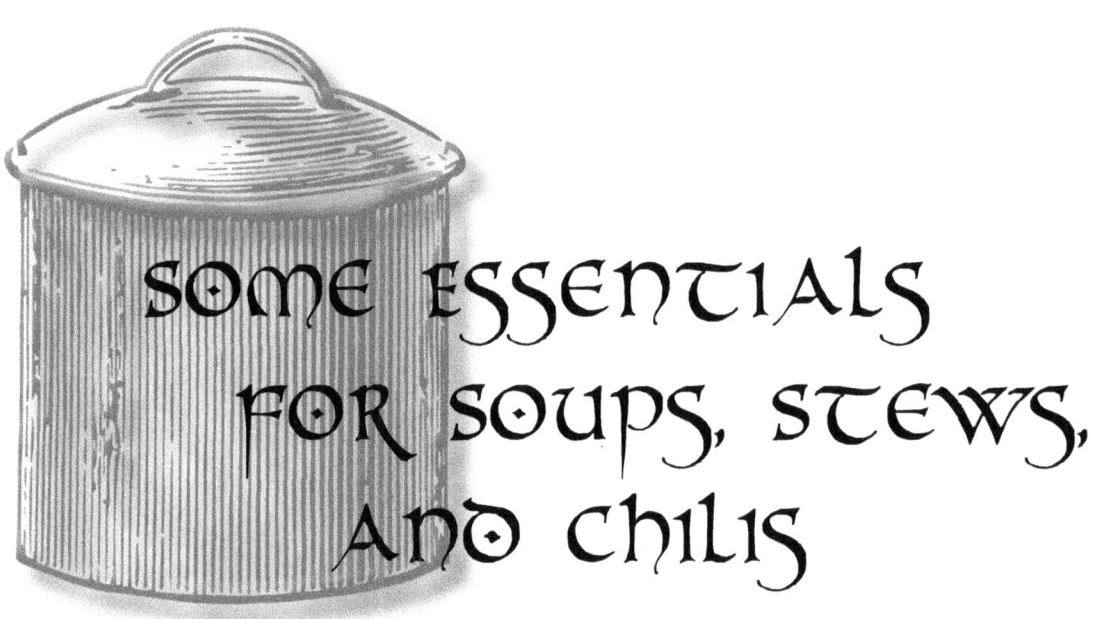

Some Essentials for Soups, Stews, and Chilis

Mirepoix
(or that which is known by dozens of other names...)

A *mirepoix* (mir-pwä) is often used to start your dish. But don't be put off by the fancy French word—a *mirepoix* is simply a combination of humble chopped vegetables sautéed for awhile in some butter or oil, or a mixture of both butter and oil. Traditionally, the vegetables are carrots, onions, and celery. There are variations on the theme, such as the "holy trinity" of Cajun and Creole cuisine, which uses yellow onions, celery, and (green) bell peppers.

In the photo below, I've cut my vegetables into a rather uniform ½" dice so they will look pretty. Sometimes your *mirepoix* vegetables will be finely chopped (a rather uniform ¼" dice); sometimes they will be coarsely chopped (which I take to mean a less regular cut of around ½"); sometimes they will be sliced (either thinly or cut into ¼" slices). They might even be minced, which I take to mean something more like ⅛". None of these measurements require you to get out a ruler, however; that's why I'm writing "rather uniform."

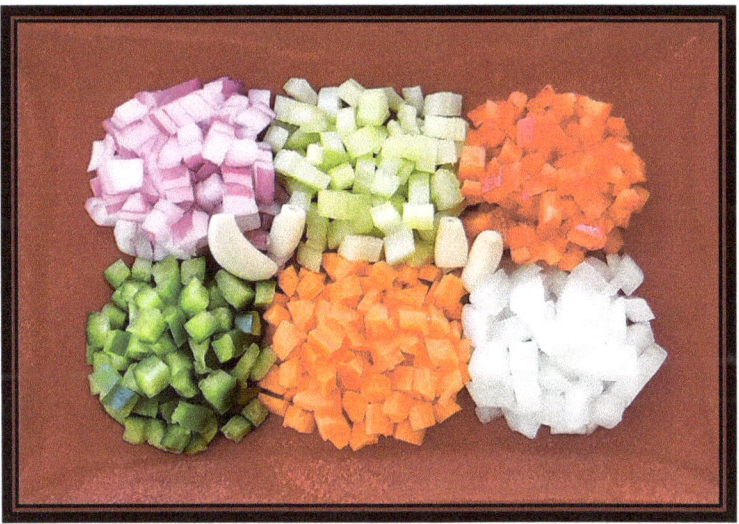

You are welcome to research all the myriad cultural varieties of *mirepoix* (and there are many!). It is the subtle background that imparts flavor to your dish right from the start. If you skip it, you will miss it.

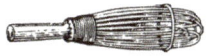

Some Essentials for Soups, Stews, and Chilis

Crème Fraîche & Other Creamy Options

I am including a few options for making creamy toppings here. Sometimes you might like to dollop something creamy on your dish, or you can be fancy and drizzle it all over, like a mad chef with a plastic squirt bottle. You might have to thin your crème with a bit of heavy cream or half-and-half to make it drizzle more easily, and it does take practice to make your crème look fairly nice on your plate. Some of these products are readily available in markets, but sometimes you don't want to commit to buying a whole jar of Mexican table cream, or you might find that the crème fraîche in the container is really much thicker than you would like it to be. Here are a few quick versions to make these products (or mock versions) in your home. Sour cream is often the right consistency and taste, but sometimes it can't take the heat and starts to break down. This is still edible, but might be unattractive in your bowl. Crème fraîche is much more stable, and still has a sour bite to it. Instead of curdling next to heat, it will melt.

How long will these types of items keep in your refrigerator? It is hard to generalize your storage times for each product; I've had crème fraîche sitting in the fridge for a month or two, and it was actually still good. You'll have to give it the sensory test: If it smells funny, it's bad; if it has mold on it, it's really bad. It might even be considered evil. Please discard it immediately upon discovery. I'm not going to supply a photograph for any of these creamy options, since they will all look like a dollop of white cream in a bowl.

Crème de la Crème Fraîche

Incredibly simple to make, but you do have to give it adequate time to thicken. In the summer, this will most likely happen in 24 hours; however, if the weather is cooler, your crème might not thicken adequately in only one day. It is okay to let it sit on your counter even up to 48 hours or so. When you notice it has the consistency and appearance of sour cream, just place it in the refrigerator.

1 cup heavy cream
2 tablespoons fresh buttermilk

AT LEAST 24 hours before using, combine with a whisk in a 2-cup glass container. Cover and let stand undisturbed at room temperature at least 24 hours. Stir and use, then keep covered in the refrigerator. Stir before using again. Makes 1 cup.

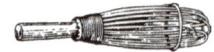

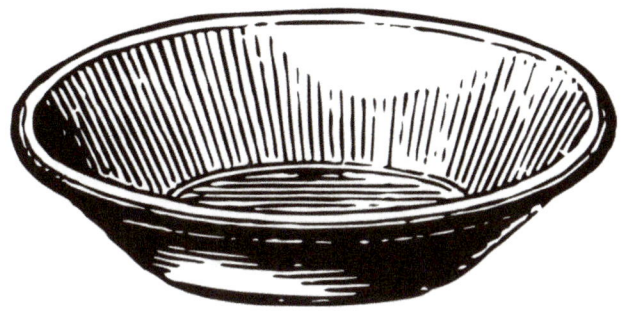

Crème Fraîche Mimic

For times when you really don't have time to let your cream thicken.

1 cup light sour cream
2 tablespoons heavy cream

WHISK both ingredients well in a medium bowl. Cover and chill leftovers; stir before using again. Makes 1 cup.

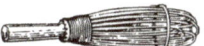

Mexican Crème

A tasty finishing touch to any sort of New Mexican or Mexican recipes included here, as well as other recipes, such as enchiladas. Thin it with a bit of cream to make a sauce to drizzle over fish tacos.

1 cup prepared Crème de la Crème Fraîche (see recipe above)
1½ teaspoons lime juice
½ teaspoon salt

WHISK the 3 ingredients well in a 2-cup glass container. Cover and chill 2-3 hours. Stir before using again. Makes 1 cup.

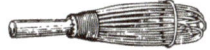

Sweet Crème Dream

As the name implies, this is simply a sweetened version of Mexican Crème. It will work well on savory dishes, if you would like a sweeter way to cut down on spice. But try it on other dessert products and especially on the final soup recipe in the cookbook, Elfryda's Strawberry Soup (a.k.a. Elfryda's Söt Suppe), on page 142.

1 cup prepared Crème de la Crème Fraîche (see recipe above)
1½ teaspoons lime juice
½ teaspoon salt
2 tablespoons honey (or you may use ¼ cup powdered sugar)

WHISK all ingredients well in a 2-cup glass container. Cover and chill 2-3 hours. Stir before using again. Makes 1 cup.

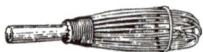

Cooked Hominy

I have five wonderful recipes for posoles in this cookbook. What exactly is posole? It merely refers to a soup/stew/chili that has hominy in it. Posole (sometimes spelled pozole) is hominy, which is made from soaking corn kernels in an alkali solution such as the mineral lime or lye. This softens the corn hulls and they are now ready to be used in posole or ground into *masa* for corn tortillas (these softened kernels are called *nixtamal*). You're probably never going to make your own hominy; you're just going to buy it canned, packaged in your freezer, or perhaps in a dry form. All of my posole recipes call for canned hominy because it is easy to obtain year round.

However, you might prefer to cook your own; it produces a chewier, almost meatier, version of hominy. It is usually more economical to cook your own from the frozen variety, although I suppose one could make an argument that you are using your own gas or electricity and that would add cost to your hominy. I haven't bothered to figure out the actual costs of cooking your own hominy as opposed to buying it in cans. They are definitely different in texture, however. Try both and see which one you prefer; Bob absolutely prefers the canned variety. The advantage with the canned option, of course, is that your hominy is always consistent and predictable. Hominy is generally available in white or yellow, though usually the white is more common. They taste the same; you might choose one color over another simply because the yellow kind looks better with your red chile. Two (15.5-ounce) cans of drained hominy yield between 2½ to 3 cups of hominy, but for simplicity's sake, I am writing 3 cups in all of the posole recipes. It is not the type of ingredient that needs to be measured exactly, though 4 cups would definitely be too much and 2 cups would definitely be too little.

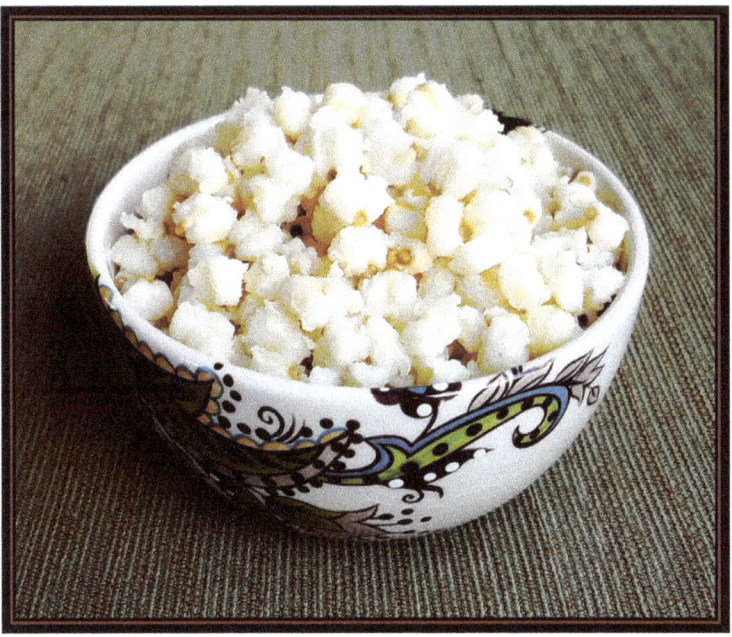

If you happen to start with a pound of dry hominy, soak it overnight in water to cover by a couple of inches (use a 6-quart saucepan, which you can then use again to cook it). Drain this, then follow the recipe below. If you would like to cook this in a slow cooker, please read the anecdotal material following the recipe.

2 pounds frozen uncooked hominy, thawed overnight in the refrigerator
1 tablespoon salt
3 quarts water

PLACE thawed hominy in a 6-quart saucepan. Add the salt and water and combine; break up any hominy that is still a bit frozen. Bring to boil, then cook on a low, rolling simmer, covered, 60-70 minutes. Stir a couple of times. It will become starchy in the pot. Let stand covered 1 hour, undisturbed. Drain in a large colander, then give it a good rinse with cool water. Drain well. You may use immediately or freeze in 3-cup portions. Makes at least 9 cups, or roughly the equivalent to 6 (15.5-ounce) cans, drained.

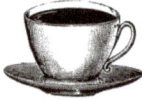

You can cook hominy in a slow cooker that has a minimum capacity of five quarts. Combine the hominy, salt, and water in the slow cooker; cover and cook on high for one hour. Then cook on low for four hours. Drain and rinse as directed above.

If you cook two pounds of posole and divide it into three (three-cup) portions, you will have enough hominy to make three pots of posole (and perhaps some leftover). Any kernels that are still rather chewy will be cooked more in your particular recipe.

If you do end up with a cup or two leftover, do a quick sauté in a medium skillet with a generous amount of salted butter. Season it liberally with items such as salt, pepper, onion powder, and garlic powder. You can add other herbs or green chile and serve this as a hearty side dish; top it with some shredded Cheddar cheese as a garnish.

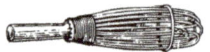

Stocks and/or Broths

I have included some basic stocks in this section. Is it stock? Is it broth? Tomato, to-mah-to. Yes, there are supposedly differences between the two, but I use the terms interchangeably. I'm beginning to believe that the debate over stock and broth is simply a device to write magazine copy or blog posts. Why get bogged down with picayune details? It is basically cooked, flavored water. What about bone broth? Now we are treading into a trendy designation, and you know I am not one to follow trends very often. Unless they are fantastically delicious, of course. I was comparing prices at my local Costco and discovered that the same quantity of bone broth will cost you about $6.00 more than your plain old stock/broth; plus, it had no sodium added and produced an exceptionally bland soup. I know this because I bought it by accident once. My regular grocery store did not reflect such an extreme difference in price, however, which just proves that Costco is not always the cheapest source for your foods. Trends; sheesh…

I am not a stock snob. Cans, boxes, cubes, jars, granules, powders, and base concentrates are all perfectly acceptable. I know you are busy—so am I. The recipes specify low-sodium versions of whatever stock/broth is listed. As I mentioned in the sodium section above, this means that each serving should have around 400-600 milligrams of sodium. Currently, I have some powdered beef base in my kitchen spice cabinet. The sodium content for this product is 950 milligrams per serving. So, I simply use half the amount that is required; instead of using two teaspoons per cup of water, I use one teaspoon to achieve 475 milligrams sodium per serving. Easy, peasy. Regardless of which option you end up using, you will always want to do a final check on seasoning at the end of cooking.

Be sure to taste first. And remember you have salt and pepper shakers on your table for precisely those pesky people (like my perpetually-teased-in-my-cookbooks-husband Bob) who sometimes feel compelled to add flavor to your creation.

To paraphrase Julia Child, do not apologize for your cooking. Do not feel inadequate if you are using a box of Swanson's (or Pacific Foods, or Emeril's, or Progresso, or Knorr, or Campbell's, or Kitchen Basics, or even your basic generic store brand, etc.) low-sodium beef broth in your dish. I have used all the stock/broth options listed above and, you know what? In the end, they are ALL fine. You might prefer one brand over another, or canned or boxed. When you have energy, time, freezer space, and adequate containers, then that's the right time to make homemade stock. So, here are some basics. Most make fairly large quantities, but stock freezes extremely well. You can even freeze stock in plastic ice cube trays or single-cup containers for those times when you need smaller quantities for various recipes. If you have issues with the mysterious ingredients and shenanigans inherent in the corporate food industry, then you will undoubtedly want to make your own. You will probably want to buy organic meats and vegetables to make these stocks. When it comes to food, you really have to follow your belief systems and do what feels right. I'm also not including photos of the finished products here, because they will all look like a portion of liquid in a bowl.

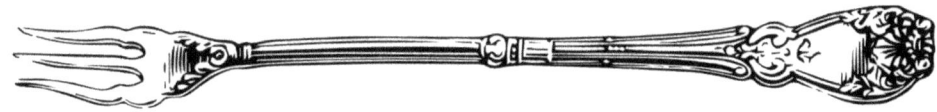

Finally, when it comes to making your own stock/broth, you might have to deal with foam, fat, and straining issues. Sometimes stock develops excessive foam or fat on top of the liquid; you might want to skim this off, if it becomes bothersome. You just have to play it by ear, depending on the ingredients you are using. After chilling or freezing, fat deposits might float to the top. When you thaw out your stock, you can easily pick off the fat and discard it.

The other issue is straining your broth after cooking. Depending on your sieve or colander, you might want to line it with cheesecloth to catch tiny particles (which might be more crucial if you make the seafood broth). This is handy because you can simply gather up your leavings and dispose of them with the cloth. However, I rarely do either of these things; foam and fat are usually minimal, and I usually use a fine strainer which catches pretty much all of the debris. Again, these steps are something to attend to only if your stock seems to need this attention.

Roasted Beef Bone Broth

(MAY ALSO SUBSTITUTE PORK, LAMB, OR VENISON)

3 pounds meaty beef bones (such as shank, neck, or back ribs)
A large onion
A large carrot
A large stalk of celery
6 quarts water
2 tablespoons coarse kosher salt
2 tablespoons whole peppercorns, black or mixed
1 tablespoon Kitchen Bouquet (a browning sauce;
    soy sauce or Worcestershire sauce will also work)

PREHEAT oven to 450°. Coat a 13" by 9" baking dish with cooking spray or grease lightly. Place the bones in a single layer in the prepared dish. Roast 45 minutes; turn all bones over halfway. Place in a 12-quart saucepan. Discard any fat that accumulated in the baking dish. Leave the peel and stems on the 3 vegetables. Wash them, then cut each into chunky quarters and place in the pot. Add the remaining ingredients and bring to a boil. Set on lowest heat and simmer 3 hours, uncovered. Stir a couple of times. Turn off heat, cover, and let stand 1 hour. Skim if necessary. Strain into a very large bowl (you might need to do this in stages). When cool enough to handle, pick off any extra meat you can find, which can be used in other dishes. Discard all the remaining solids. Portion off broth in covered containers and refrigerate or freeze. Makes about 5 quarts, depending on your reduction.

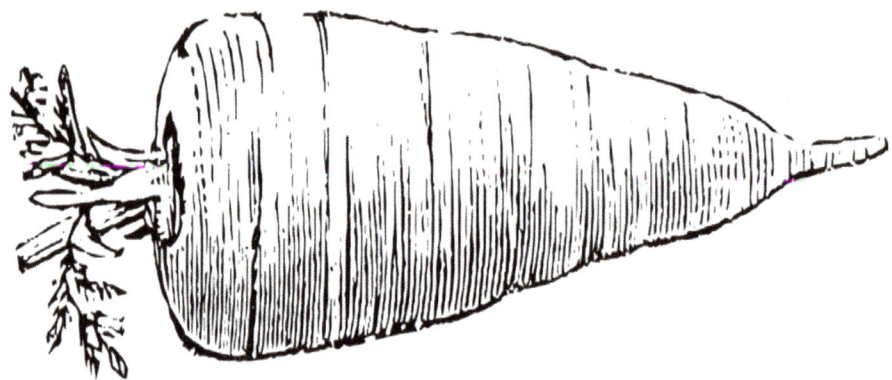

Roasted Chicken Stock

(MAY ALSO SUBSTITUTE OTHER POULTRY)

If you're pinched for time, just skip the entire preliminary roasting process; it'll still taste fine. Honor the bird which has given its life to this broth by removing every single morsel of meat from its frame; you'd be surprised how much meat you will find after you've cooked it for awhile.

A carcass plus any other leavings from a good-sized roasted or rotisserie chicken (bones, skin; everything—hmm, am I referring to a Costco-sized chicken here? Yes, I am; but you can use a chicken you have roasted yourself, of course.)

PREHEAT oven to 375°. Coat an 11" by 7" baking dish with cooking spray or grease lightly. Place the chicken frame and any frame leftovers in the pan and roast 45 minutes.

A large onion
A large carrot
A large stalk of celery
4 quarts water
1 tablespoon coarse kosher salt
2 teaspoons whole peppercorns,
 black or mixed

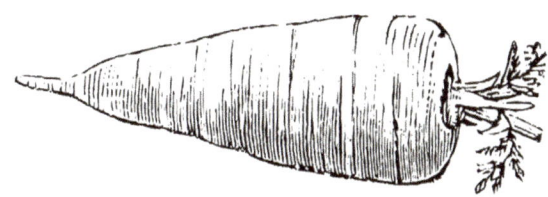

LEAVE the peel and stems on the 3 vegetables. Wash them, then cut each into chunky quarters and place in an 8-quart saucepan. Add water, salt, peppercorns, and chicken frame (either roasted or not). Bring to a boil. Set on lowest heat and simmer 2 hours, uncovered. Halfway through cooking, turn the chicken frame over and continue to simmer. Turn off heat, cover, and let stand 1 hour. Skim if necessary. Strain into a very large bowl and cool. Pick off any extra meat you can find, which can be used in other dishes. Discard all the remaining solids. Portion off broth in covered containers and refrigerate or freeze. Makes about 3 quarts, depending on your reduction.

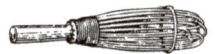

Some Essentials for Soups, Stews, and Chilis

Turkey Frame Broth

I've gotten to the point where I prefer to use a boneless, skinless turkey breast for our Thanksgiving meals, mainly because that seems to be the meat most people want. When you roast a whole bird, then you're stuck with legs and wings and a frame. For many years, I cooked a turkey frame soup from an old *Better Homes and Gardens* cookbook, but we grew immensely tired of that. However, I know many people still cook a whole bird, so here is a recipe that simply uses the leftovers from a turkey. Now that I have completed this recipe, I will never cook a whole bird again (well, most likely never; though you hate to say never, because you just never know, do you…).

A carcass plus any other leavings
    from a whole roasted turkey
    that weighed between 16-20
    pounds (bones, skin; everything)
3 tablespoons coarse kosher salt
3 tablespoons whole peppercorns,
    black or mixed
A large onion
2 large carrots
2 large stalks of celery
8 quarts water

PLACE turkey carcass in a 16-quart pot. Add salt and peppercorns. Leave the peel and stems on the 3 vegetables. Wash them, then cut into chunky quarters and place in the pot. Pour the water over all. Bring to a boil, then cook on low 2 hours, covered. Raise heat to medium and cook on a rolling simmer 1 hour, uncovered. Cover and let stand 1 hour. Skim if necessary. Strain into a very large bowl (you might need to do this in stages). When cool enough to handle, pick off any extra meat you can find, which can be used in other dishes. Discard all the remaining solids. Portion off broth in covered containers and refrigerate or freeze. Makes about 6-7 quarts, depending on your reduction.

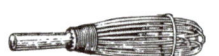

Seafood Stock

This will substitute for bottled clam juice, which is generally readily available in many grocery stores. It's a handy recipe if your household happens to end up with lots of shellfish tails and other leavings. You can store these items in a plastic Ziploc bag or a covered container in your freezer until you are ready to use them. Thaw overnight in the refrigerator. I've made this a rather small quantity, but it is easy to double.

12 ounces frozen shellfish tails and shells (such as from shrimp, crab, lobster, clams, and mussels; these can be raw and/or cooked)
A medium onion
A medium carrot
A medium stalk of celery
2 teaspoons salt
2 teaspoons whole peppercorns, black or mixed
2 teaspoons Old Bay seasoning
2 tablespoons lemon juice
½ cup dry white wine, such as Chardonnay
3 quarts water

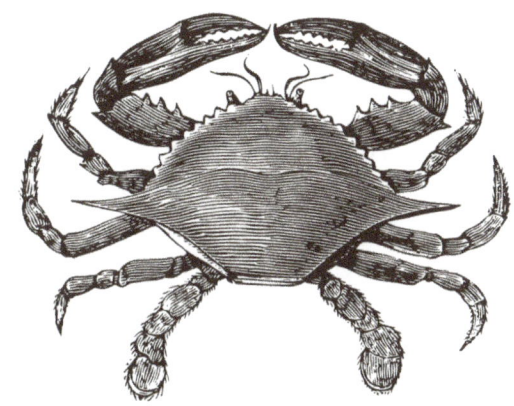

THAW tails/shells overnight in refrigerator. Rinse in cold water and drain. Preheat oven to 375°. Coat an 11" by 7" baking dish with cooking spray. Place shells in pan. Bake 30 minutes; stir halfway through. Place in a 6-quart saucepan. Leave the peel and stems on the 3 vegetables. Wash them, then cut each into chunky quarters and place in the pot. Add the remaining ingredients and bring to a boil. Set on lowest heat and simmer 2 hours, uncovered. Stir a couple times. Turn off heat, cover, and let stand 1 hour. Skim if necessary. Strain into a large bowl; when it cools, you may pick off any bits of meat that are left in the shells and use them in your soup recipe, if desired. Discard the remaining solids. Portion off broth in covered containers and refrigerate or freeze. Makes about 2½ quarts, depending on your reduction.

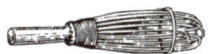

Some Essentials for Soups, Stews, and Chilis

Slow-Roasted Herbed Vegetable Stock

If you're organized and industrious, you can also save all sorts of vegetable scraps in a large container or a gallon-size plastic bag. Peelings, ends, and the cores of harder-textured vegetables can all be saved for stock. Soft vegetables, such as tomatoes or cucumbers, are not appropriate for this purpose. But carrots, onions, celery, garlic, herbs, bell peppers, cauliflower, broccoli, and the ends of summer squashes can all work here. Save the washing for when you want to prepare the stock, place your scraps in your designated container, and seal it well. Keep this in the freezer and add to it for a few weeks or so. My bag was full in about five to six weeks' time. When you're ready to use your collection, thaw it overnight in the refrigerator, then follow the recipe.

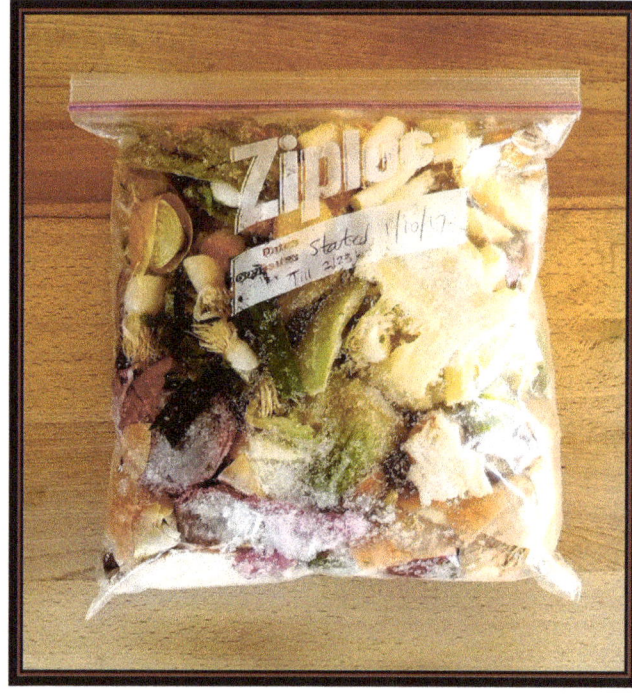

If you are including fresh herb trimmings with your vegetables, you can skip using the dry ones, if you like. I'm including my Easy Herbes de Provence recipe from my first cookbook, if you'd like to whip some up. It's a handy dry mix to have around, and it does appear here, as well as in a few of the recipes in the cookbook.

2-3 pounds of frozen vegetable scraps, thawed overnight in refrigerator
    (total weight will depend on many factors)
1 tablespoon coarse kosher salt
1 tablespoon Easy Herbes de Provence (see recipe below), or other dry herb
5 quarts water

PREHEAT oven to 350°. Coat a 13" by 9" baking dish with cooking spray. Rinse all of the vegetable scraps well in a large colander and shake off excess water. Place in the prepared pan. Roast 1 hour; stir a couple times. Pour the vegetables into an 8-quart saucepan; add the remaining ingredients. Bring to a boil; then cook, uncovered, on a low heat 3 hours. Stir a couple times. Strain into a very large bowl; discard solids. Place portions into covered containers and refrigerate or freeze. Makes about 3-4 quarts, depending on your reduction.

Easy Herbes de Provence

This incredibly versatile dry herb mix is readily available in many grocery stores, and some versions even come with non-traditional additions such as salt and pepper. I really prefer to limit this mix just to herbs. The lavender is a completely optional ingredient. I often whip this up to sell at our local lavender festival. Lavender can be hard to find sometimes, so don't feel bad if you omit it. You could replace it with a different herb, such as basil, oregano, or tarragon. Try it on any sort of meat, but especially chicken and fish, sauté some vegetables with salted butter and add a teaspoon or so, or scramble some eggs with cream cheese and add a generous sprinkling of the herb mix.

1 teaspoon each, all in dried form:

- parsley
- rubbed sage
- crushed rosemary
- thyme
- summer savory
- marjoram
- lavender

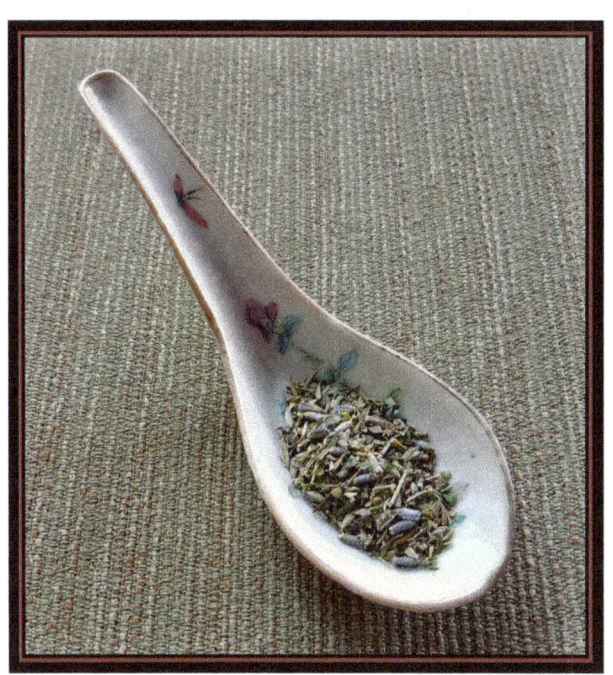

COMBINE all ingredients in a small bowl. If you like, you may use a mortar and pestle if you want the herbs to be a finer consistency, or you can simply crush it a little with your fingers. Keep in an airtight container in your pantry. Makes about 2 tablespoons.

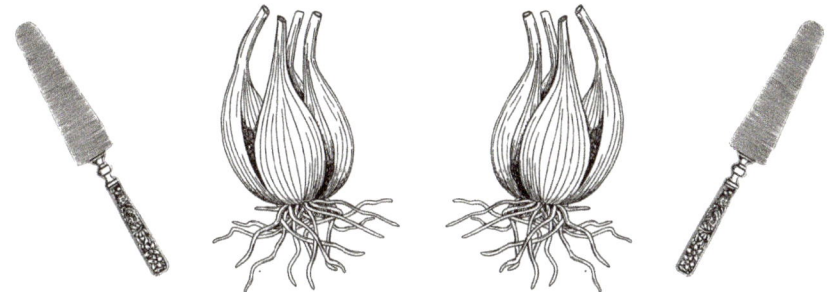

Some Essentials for Soups, Stews, and Chilis

CHAPTER ONE
BEEF

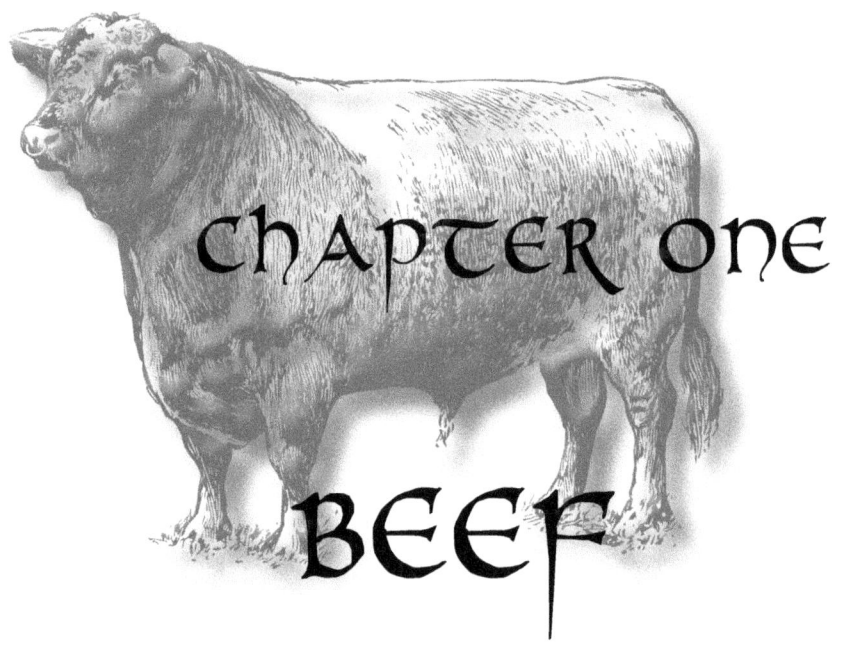

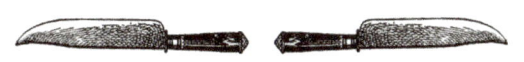

Holy Beef Posole, Batman!

Happy Medium Ramen

Bob's Old-Fashioned Beef Stew

It's a Nice Day for a Wedding Soup

Pepper Pot Chili

Bodacious Brisket Soup

Pasta e Fagioli

Cheeseburger Soup

Dragon Fire Chili

Coconut Beef Stew

Oodle Noodle Soup

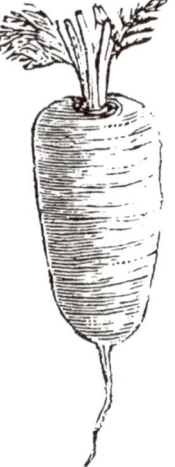

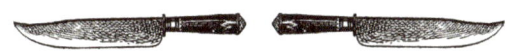

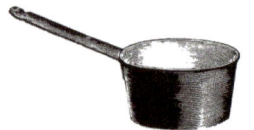 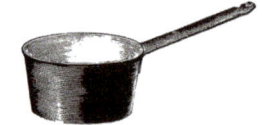

Chapter One—Beef
(VEAL, LAMB, AND VENISON)

Though I have only used beef in this chapter's recipes, I'm confident you can substitute the other meats listed. Probably other game could fit into this chapter, but I am not conversant in exotic game. If you happen to obtain some elk or buffalo, it should fit nicely into these recipes. I could list rabbit here as well, but we never eat rabbit at our house (please see my first cookbook for the reasons why we never do). How about goat? If you like it, go for it; I'm afraid I have a severe distaste for goat products which stems from my childhood.

Why exactly do I hate goat products? Well, it's nothing traumatic; I guess it's just the way I'm made. My first experience around goats happened when I was around seven, when my parents would take occasional trips down to the old mining town of Silver City, New Mexico, to visit the Bear Mountain Guest Ranch (now known as the Bear Mountain Lodge; it has obviously changed quite a bit from my last visit, which was in 1980, when I was 18). This was mainly in the late 1960s and early 1970s, when my parents were avid birdwatchers, and the ranch was well known for attracting many varieties of birds. At the time, Myra McCormick was the owner of this rustic ranch, which is located just south of the Gila Wilderness. She kept a few rooms available for rent, and guests would share meals in a common room. It was certainly not an immersive ranching experience such as you see depicted in the film *City Slickers;* however, guests could help feed the goats and chickens.

The moment I walked out to the goat pen, my first reaction was, "EEEWWW!!! What's that SMELL???" Goats do have a particular odor, as do all animals, obviously. Myra would serve up some goat's milk, and I just could not stand it. Now, don't get me wrong; I have nothing against goats. I love screaming Internet goats, and, when Chloë was in

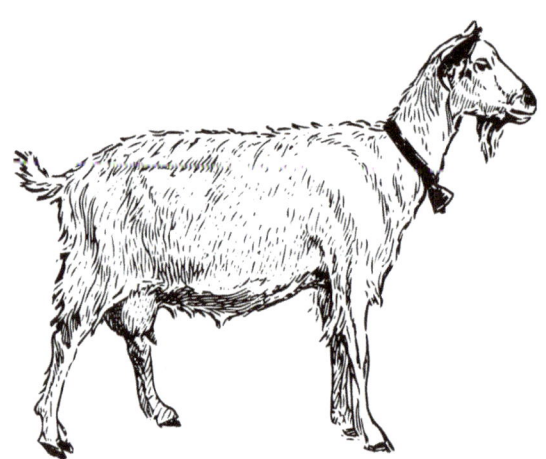

kindergarten, I took her and her little sister Callista on a field trip out to The Old Windmill Dairy, a goat farm which operated in nearby Estancia (sadly, it closed in 2018). It was a fabulous time; the keepers let the children feed these crazily energetic baby goats from a bucket equipped with multiple nipples, and the whole experience was hysterical, with bleating baby goats and screaming kindergarteners. Oddly enough, my kids (har, har…) apparently don't remember this day, which is a shame; it was a joyful experience.

I gave up drinking any and all types of milk when I was around ten (I mean as a beverage; I use milk in lots of recipes, of course). As an adult, I've tried goat meat in a couple of dishes, and I can perhaps tolerate the taste if it is highly seasoned, such as in Indian food. But then there is the CHEESE…

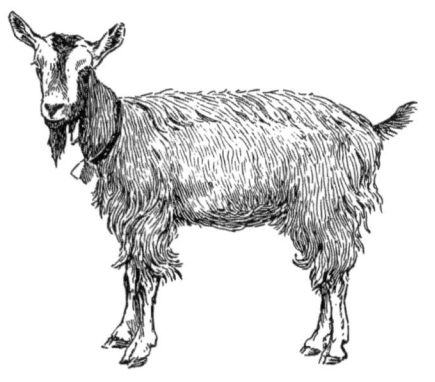

As an adult foodie, I have occasionally forced myself to try various versions of goat cheese, from plain varieties to ones seasoned with all sorts of exotic flavors. I just cannot acquire a taste for it. But… but… but… everybody loves goat cheese! It's on everything! Finally, when I was around 50, I told myself I had had enough. I was done sampling goat cheese. And I have made peace with that decision. There is only one kind of goat-based cheese that I can endure, but I definitely do not go out of my way to eat it. It is called Gjetost, and my late Norwegian mother would buy the Ski Queen variety, which was a blend of goat and cow's milk; yet even that is pretty intense. She would slice it thinly with her ostehøvel (is this cheese slicer the greatest Norwegian invention known to the entire world? Yes, it is!) and place it on buttered toast. I believe the cow's milk and the caramelized flavor make it almost tolerable; but again, it's not something I ever buy.

You know, it's funny when and where grief will hit you, and how often food is evocative of loved ones. One day I was looking for something weird at Whole Foods, when I saw that bright red block of Ski Queen Gjetost cheese in their deli area. I hadn't cried about my mom for at least six months, but there I was, weeping at cheese in Whole Foods and wishing I could buy it for her to enjoy. Then I thought about my dad, who died four years before she did, and how he would have appreciated some fancy cookies from the bakery (though Pepperidge Farm was also just as good, in his opinion). Thoughts constantly mingle with memories. Moms and dads never really leave you, do they?

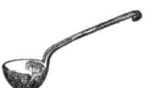

Well, I feel better now, since I've gotten that out in the open.

Chapter One: Beef   3

Holy Beef Posole, Batman!

I'm going to start each soup chapter with a posole. Why? Because my family LOVES posole! It is (almost without fail) served on Christmas Eve at my house, but we also enjoy it throughout the whole year. All five posole recipes included in the cookbook call for canned hominy, but you may cook your own. Sometimes I call for yellow hominy, but you can certainly use white; the flavors are the same. Please see the recipe for Cooked Hominy on page xx in the *Some Essentials for Soups, Stews, and Chilis* section. You might also prefer to use the entire can of hominy and not bother to drain or rinse it—my daughter Chloë always does this. Try it both ways and see which one you prefer; the extra bit of salty liquid shouldn't make too much of a difference in the entire recipe.

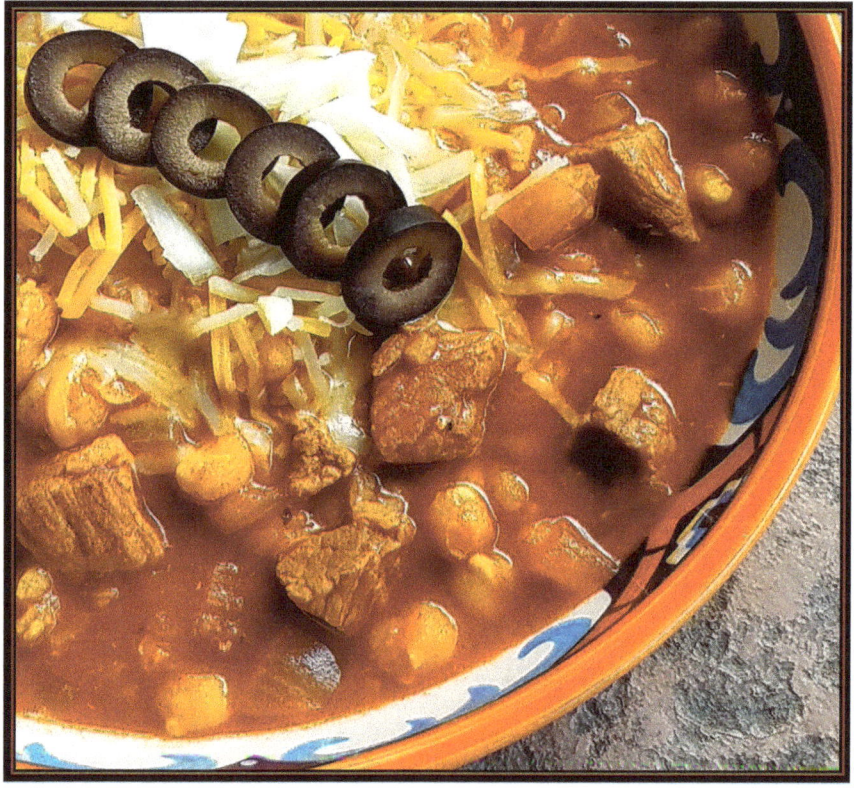

1 quart low-sodium beef broth
2 cups water
1 pound beef stew meat, cut into ¾" chunks
16-ounce jar red chile sauce (or any variety of salsa)
2 tablespoons fresh garlic, sliced paper thin
2 cups onion, coarsely chopped

2 (15.5-ounce) cans yellow hominy, drained and rinsed (if you like, or 3 cups
    cooked hominy; white hominy is also fine)
2 teaspoons dry oregano (3-4 tablespoons fresh, minced)
1 teaspoon salt
½ teaspoon black pepper
¼ cup short grain rice

OPTIONAL GARNISH:

Sliced black olives
Finely chopped white onion
Finely shredded Fiesta blend cheese
Any of the **NICE NEW MEXICAN & MEXICAN GARNISHES** will work with this dish.

COAT a 6-quart saucepan with cooking spray. Combine the broth, water, beef, red chile, garlic, onion, hominy, oregano, salt, and pepper in the pot and bring to a boil. Lower heat to medium and cook on a rolling simmer, uncovered, 1 hour. Stir a few times. Add the rice, then cook 30 minutes, covered, on a low heat. Stir a few times. Season, if desired. Garnish, as desired. Cover and chill leftovers. Serves 4-6.

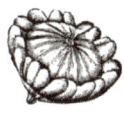

Try a pound of carrots or parsnips, peeled and cut into ¾" chunks instead. A pound or so of chunky summer squash would work well, peeled or not. You can reduce the initial cooking time by about 30 minutes. You could also try a pound of peeled winter squash, such as butternut, acorn, or even pumpkin; these will probably need to cook the entire hour.

Other meats such as chicken (breasts or thighs) and pork (sirloin or tenderloin) will be fine in this posole.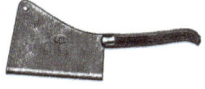

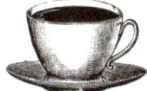
This ended up being Bob's favorite posole. If you can't find red chile sauce, you may certainly use a jar of your favorite salsa. You may use the salsa as is, or you might puree it if you would like a smoother sauce.

You might be wondering why I chose this particular name for this recipe. Well, I posted this photo on my Instagram account and, for some inexplicable reason, I captioned it, "Holy Beef Posole, Batman!" It got 23 likes (as of May 7, 2017). Would Batman eat this posole? Tough question to answer. In one movie he appeared in, all he ate was Lobster Thermidor, but it was of the LEGO variety.

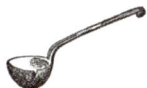

Chapter One: Beef

Happy Medium Ramen

This recipe requires quite a bit of exposition first, so I hope you'll bear with me. I developed it as a compromise between the practically instant version of ramen (meaning, less than five minutes of preparation) and the ultra-complicated and time-consuming version of an authentic ramen (meaning, more like five days worth of preparation); hence, the title "Happy Medium Ramen." With this recipe, you can get a great ramen in less than an hour.

    I know a few people who consider a box of macaroni and cheese the perfect comfort food (meaning my two daughters, and now my grandchildren). For me, however, comfort food is usually a packet of ramen. Inevitably it's either beef or chicken, and it used to be sold in a box of 48 packets at one of my favorite stores, Costco, but now they only seem to carry it in Styrofoam cups, which I prefer not to buy. Other stores carry this packaged variety, which I make with one and three-quarters cups of water, as opposed to the two cups the package calls for; plus, I like to break up the noodles before cooking them. Yes, we all have our ridiculous rituals. I discovered ramen in my poor college student days, as I suppose many of us do.

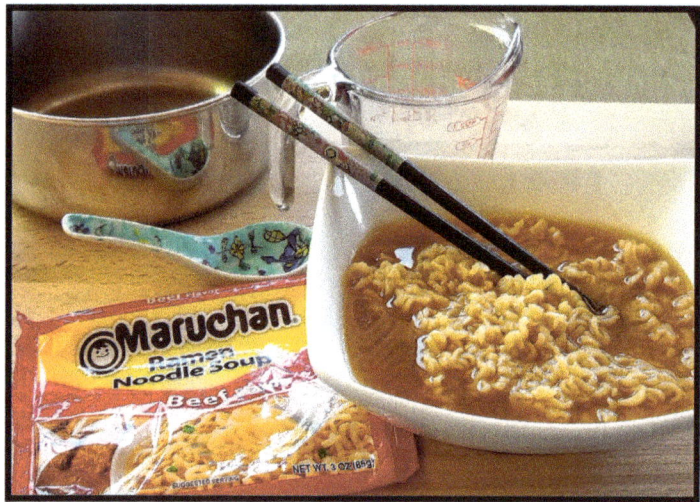

    This is my go-to meal when I've had surgery, or when there's nothing much around the house. This doesn't happen too often, maybe three or four times a year (not surgery, obviously, just the "not having much around the house" bit). So, a box of 48 ramen packets used to last a long while. Sometimes I would go nuts and cook two packages, then I'd share it with Bob. Or there were the absolutely crazy times when I would add meat and/or vegetables to it for a more substantial meal. But this really doesn't happen much anymore, since, as you might have guessed, I spend a lot of time cooking regular food, and I try not to open packages too often.

For some bizarre reason, my BFF from elementary school sent me a copy of David Chang's *Momofuku* for my 50th birthday. I don't know why, since we hadn't exchanged gifts since mid-school, but I really appreciated it since I had been messing around with developing all my hobbity comfort food around that time, and I was glad to look at some upscale Asian recipes for a change. It was also refreshing to read about Chang's struggles getting all of his business ventures off the ground.

The first recipe is actually "Momofuku Ramen." Finally, I could make some REAL RAMEN!!!

And then you start reading the recipe—always a good policy before you dash off to the grocery store, half-cocked and desperate for oodles of noodles. The recipe on page 39 starts with the fateful words, "First, get everything ready."

ALL RIGHT THEN—what needs to be ready?

Well, Chang goes on to list 11 ingredients which, in my calculations, would probably amount to a generous and filling quart of soup. This supposedly serves **ONE** person.

Out of these 11 ingredients, eight require you to follow other recipes on other pages. I'm not going to list the recipe here, because that would require me to seek permission from Chang's publisher and I'm really not up for that particular challenge. But you can probably get the gist with this exhaustive description of me going back and forth within his cookbook for the details:

> As I look at page 40, I see Ramen Broth. The recipe makes five quarts. It has its own list of preparations; one of the items requiring advance preparation is something called Taré. This item pops up again in the actual ramen recipe, so that should save some time; though I see that you can substitute some other sort of sodium product for the Taré, such as kosher salt, soy sauce, or mirin. Can't I just buy some thin noodles? Okay, yes I can. Oh dear (I used a different word in real life), I see that the five pounds of meaty pork bones alone will require simmering for six to seven hours, or "as much time as your schedule allows." Fortunately, you can freeze this stock, although I'm not sure if I have enough containers or even room in my freezer for all of this stock. Chang strongly suggests using Benton's smoky bacon for this stock, so that entails a trip to page 147 to read about the curing process for this fabulous bacon. In the end, I am not interested in having to order a pound of bacon that will most likely arrive in Styrofoam and/or dry ice. So, my ramen broth might be inferior if I end up using Hormel and I'll just have to be content with that. I have to poach an egg! Oh dear (again, I used a different word in real life…)! What exactly can I just purchase at a grocery store? Nori, scallions, and fish cakes; okay. Now I have to pickle some additional vegetables and roast some pork… and there is also some pork belly… I'm so tired…

I read the entire book and found many recipes that sounded great and just a few that didn't sound so great. At one time, I thought I might make it a long-term goal/project to try most everything and occasionally blog about the experience. That was about five years ago and never amounted to anything. I'm okay with that. I know that making ramen can be a time-consuming process. I've intended this ramen to be pleasantly spicy and salty enough, because some ramen can be incredibly salty. My ramen will probably not satisfy David Chang. I'm also okay with that, since it is likely we will never meet. Nevertheless, I present to you a simplified version of ramen that is salty enough for my own family's taste. You can always add more salt, if you like.

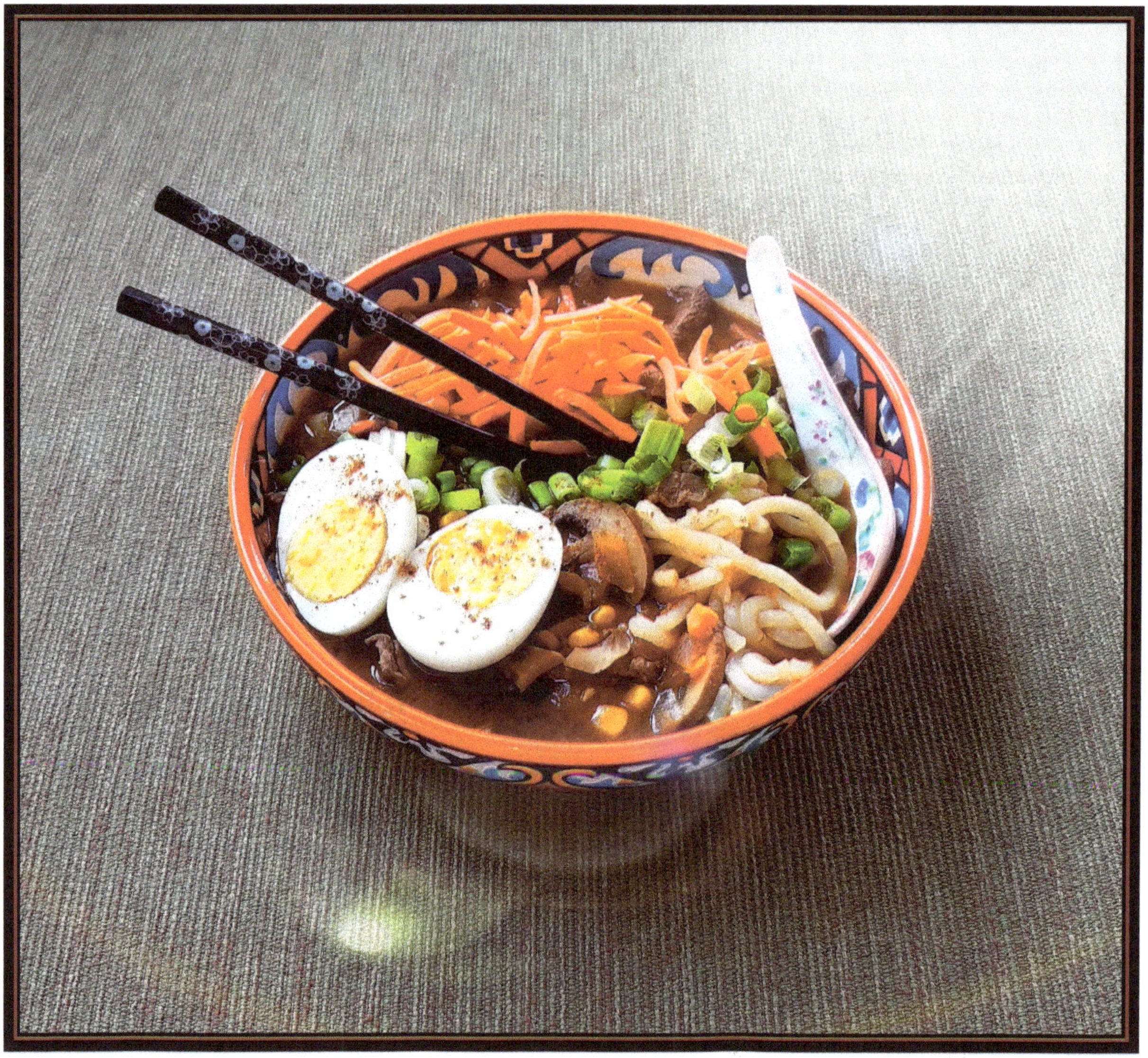

8 quarts water
2 tablespoons salt
1½ pounds Japanese udon noodles
2 tablespoons toasted sesame oil
2 tablespoons minced garlic
2 tablespoons crushed ginger
2 cups onion, coarsely chopped
¼ cup soy bean paste
¼ cup white miso (yellow is also fine;
    use red if you want to start off
    with a stronger and saltier flavor)
2 tablespoons chili garlic sauce
2 teaspoons 5-spice powder
2 quarts low-sodium beef broth
¼ cup aji-mirin (sweet cooking rice wine)
2 tablespoons soy sauce
8 ounces fresh mushrooms, thinly sliced
1½ cups corn (either cut off the cob, frozen, or drain a 15.25-ounce can)
1 pound beef sirloin; partially frozen, then cut into very thin strips,
    approximately 3" by ½"

OPTIONAL GARNISH:

Shredded or matchstick carrots
Chopped scallions
Fresh bean sprouts
Finely chopped or shredded cabbage
A sprinkling of 5-spice powder
A softly boiled large egg is a lovely addition—poach for around 7 minutes; you want the white to be cooked, and the yolk to be slightly creamy if you can manage it. Peel it if you have prepared it in the shell, then cut it in half to serve on the side in your bowl.

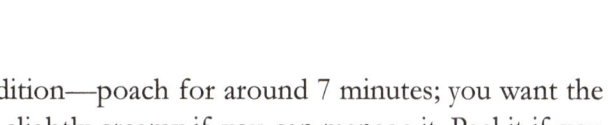

BRING water to boil in a 12-quart saucepan. Add salt and noodles. Bring to another boil, then cook as directed on the package until desired doneness; stir a few times. Drain; return to the pot and cover to keep warm.

Chapter One: Beef   9

MEANWHILE, sauté the oil, garlic, ginger, onion, soy bean paste, miso, chili garlic sauce, and 5-spice powder in a 6-quart saucepan over rather high heat 5 minutes, stirring frequently. Add the broth, aji-mirin, soy sauce, mushrooms, and corn and bring to a boil. Cook at a moderate boil 10 minutes, uncovered. Stir a few times. Add beef and cook 1 minute. Season, if desired. Place desired portion of noodles in big soup bowls and ladle soup over. Garnish, as desired. Cover and chill leftovers; you can mix the noodles with the soup, if you like, or store them separately. Serves 6-8.

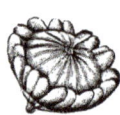
Change your broth to vegetable and substitute a pound of thinly sliced zucchini or other summer squash. Or you could use a combination of other thinly sliced vegetables—carrots, snow peas, bamboo shoots; whatever you like. You can also add 2-3 cups of finely chopped cabbage, if you have some hanging around. I often do, because my husband's favorite dish in the entire world is my own version of coleslaw (included in my first cookbook). Add the cabbage with the mushrooms and corn.

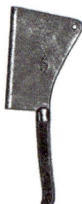
You might prefer a chicken ramen; change your broth to low-sodium chicken and substitute a pound of thinly sliced cooked chicken. Or you could try a pound of thinly sliced breaded, boneless pork chops; beef or chicken broth will work with pork. Change your broth to seafood or clam juice and substitute peeled, raw shrimp (cook anywhere from 2-4 minutes at the end, depending on the size of your shrimp; tail on or off).

You won't go wrong with a tablespoon (or more) of Sriracha or additional chili garlic sauce, though it might be best to let diners add this on their own at the table.
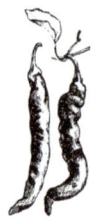

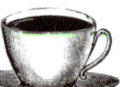
Serve your ramen with chopsticks and a large spoon; it's a slurpy kind of soup, and apparently that is part of the joy of eating it. Wear something washable, because inevitably you will spatter some soup on your shirt!

If you have trouble locating udon, *you may substitute other flour-type noodles, such as fettuccine or linguine. You are also welcome to use fresh noodles (though you might need more like three pounds worth), and prepare them as directed on the package; either on your stove top or in your microwave.*

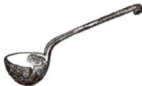

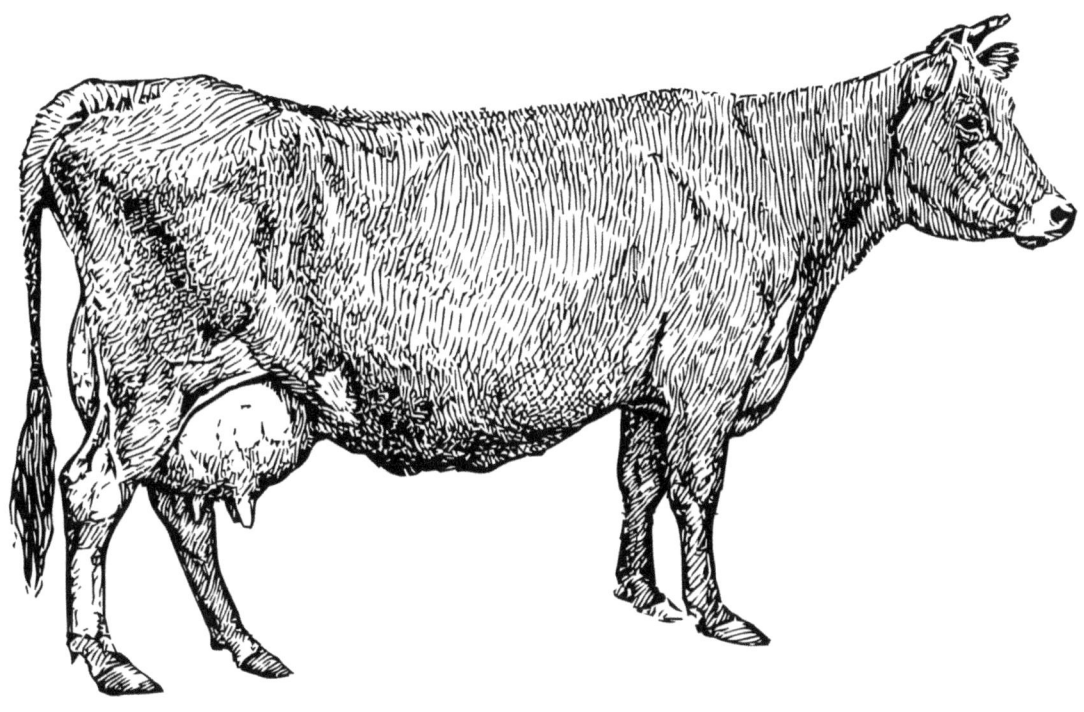

Bob's Old-Fashioned Beef Stew

Bob is your typical meat-and-potatoes kind of guy. This is a traditional, thick beef stew with a little bit of unusual spice added for kicks. If you use regular carrots, peel them and cut into 1" chunks. You can use fingerlings, unpeeled, or regular potatoes, peeled. Cut all into 1" chunks. If you happen to find some of those adorable grape-sized potatoes, just use them whole.

2 tablespoons olive oil
1 tablespoon minced garlic
2 cups onion, coarsely chopped
2¾ pounds beef stew meat,
    cut into 1" chunks
2½ cups water
1 tablespoon sugar
1 tablespoon lemon juice
2 tablespoons Worcestershire sauce
2 teaspoons salt
1½ teaspoons black pepper
1 teaspoon smoked paprika
1 teaspoon nutmeg
1 teaspoon allspice
1 pound medium-sized baby carrots
1½ pounds baby gold potatoes;
    unpeeled (cut larger ones in half)
8 ounces frozen lima beans (or peas)
1 cup low-sodium beef broth
½ cup all-purpose flour

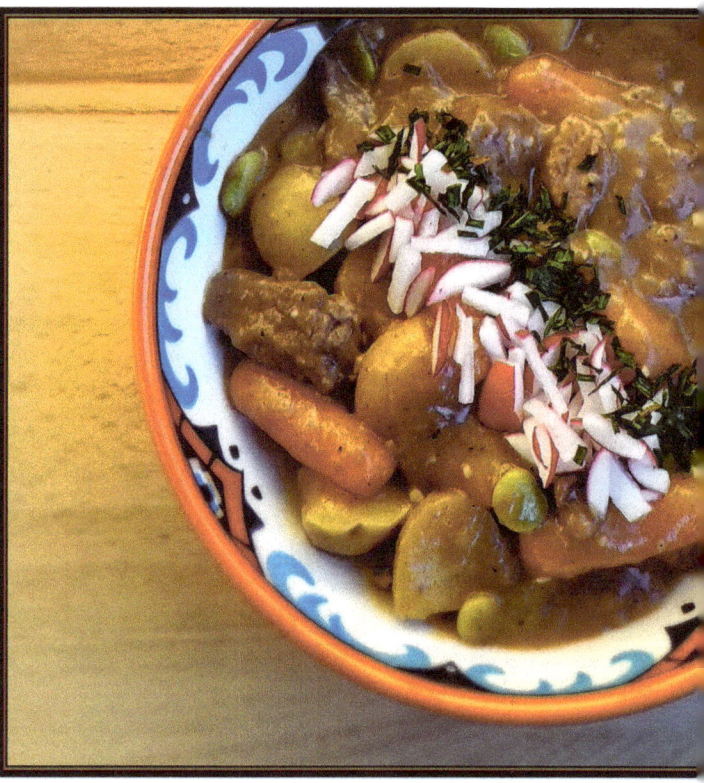

OPTIONAL GARNISH:

Minced fresh chives
Coarsely chopped radishes

LIBERALLY coat a 6-quart saucepan with cooking spray. Over rather high heat, sauté the oil, garlic, onion, and beef 6-8 minutes, until most of the pink is gone, stirring frequently. Add the water, sugar, lemon juice, Worcestershire sauce, salt, pepper, paprika, nutmeg, and allspice and bring to a boil. Cover and simmer on lowest heat 1½ hours. Stir a few times.

Add carrots and potatoes; bring to another boil. Cover and cook on a rolling simmer 30 minutes. Stir a few times. Add the lima beans and continue cooking 10 more minutes. In a 2-cup glass measuring cup, combine the broth and flour well with a whisk. Raise heat to medium and stir in the flour mixture. Cook on a rather low heat until the stew thickens nicely, uncovered, about 5-10 minutes or so; your vegetables should be tender. Season, if desired. Garnish, as desired. Cover and chill leftovers; do not freeze. Serves 6-8.

You could substitute vegetable broth for the beef broth and soy sauce for the Worcestershire. Then you could cut up a pound or so of zucchini, a pound or so of cauliflower, plus a pound of fresh mushrooms. Cut your mushrooms according to their relative size. Your other vegetables could be peeled or not, depending on your preference, and you could cut them into about 1" chunks. You could just give your onions and garlic a sauté for 5 minutes or so, and your total initial cooking time would be reduced somewhat.

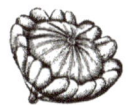

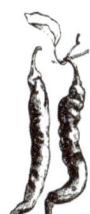

Green chile? Yes, please! Add 4-8 ounces roasted and chopped, with juice, near the end of cooking, or anytime you like.

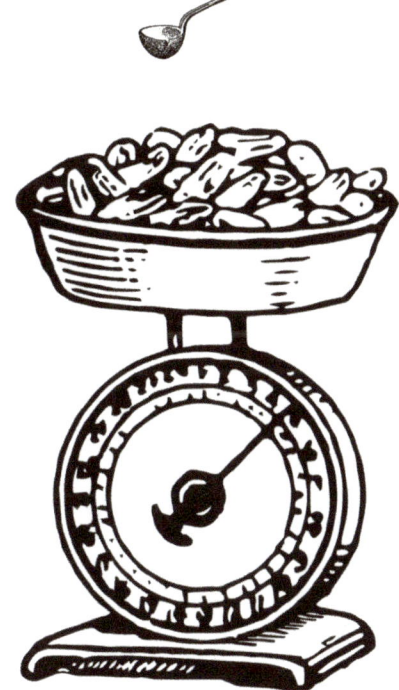

It's a Nice Day for a Wedding Soup

This is one of my all-time favorites, so it is always a nice day for it. The most vital part of this soup is the teeny, tiny meatballs. I'm sorry; but you have to have teeny, tiny meatballs—otherwise, just don't bother.

Well, if you must have bigger meatballs, you'll have to cook them a little longer.

I'm really not kidding you, however; teeny, tiny meatballs are the best. Be glad I have consistently added the word 'meat' to the word 'balls.' I figure you're probably snickering about all of this, anyway…

You might think, how can I possibly stand around making 111 or maybe even 144 meatballs? Usually, I put myself in a Zen-like trance while I watch the news, and it generally takes me about 15 to 20 minutes to make them all. And it's worth the time. Use just this meatball recipe and make 8 or 12 larger meatballs to add to your favorite spaghetti sauce.

8 ounces ground beef sirloin
8 ounces mild Italian sausage
1 tablespoon dry parsley
    (2-3 tablespoons fresh, minced)
2 tablespoons dry Parmesan cheese
    (Parmesan and/or Romano is fine)
2 tablespoons seasoned bread crumbs
¼ cup 1% milk
1 teaspoon dry oregano
    (2-3 tablespoons fresh, minced)
1 teaspoon onion powder
1 teaspoon garlic powder
½ teaspoon salt
½ teaspoon black pepper

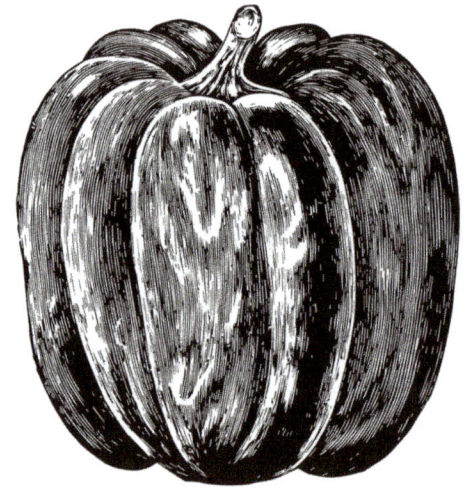

USING just your hands, combine the above ingredients in a medium bowl. Pinch off small pieces and roll into ¾" meatballs (½" will work, too). You can moisten your hands and fingertips with a bit of water if the mixture seems too sticky. Place on a large (18" by 13") baking sheet in a single layer. You'll probably end up making at least 111 meatballs, or maybe even twelve dozen, or 144. Place in the refrigerator while you prepare the rest of the soup.

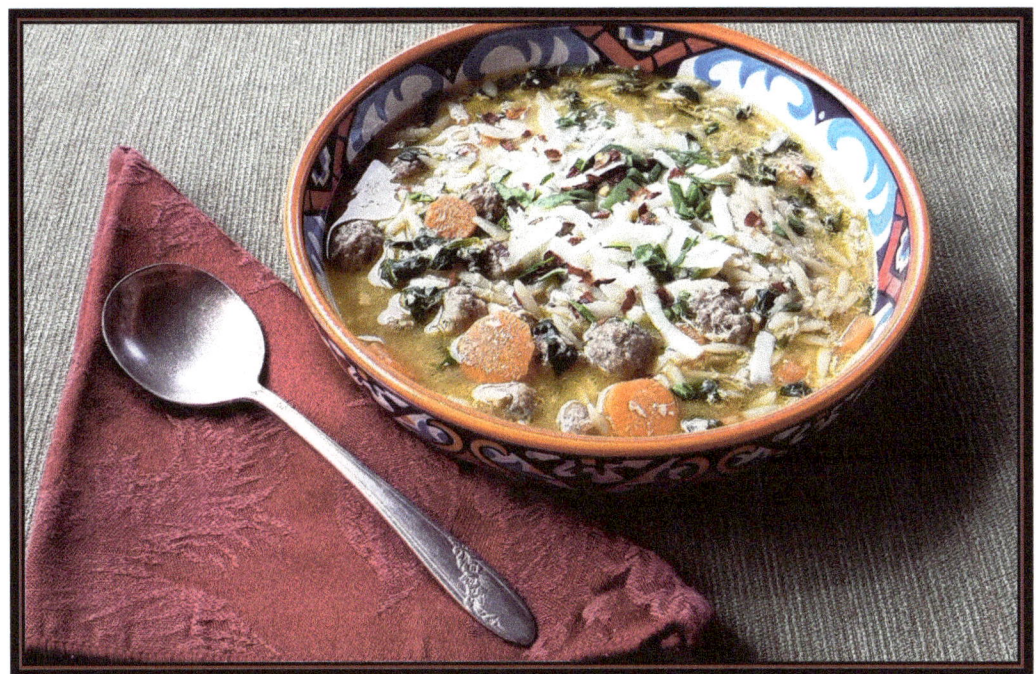

2 tablespoons olive oil
1 cup onion, coarsely chopped
1 cup carrot, peeled and thinly sliced
1 tablespoon minced garlic
½ teaspoon salt
½ teaspoon black pepper
1 quart low-sodium chicken broth
1 quart low-sodium beef broth
1 cup orzo (or other very small pasta)
2 large eggs
5-6 ounces fresh baby spinach, coarsely chopped

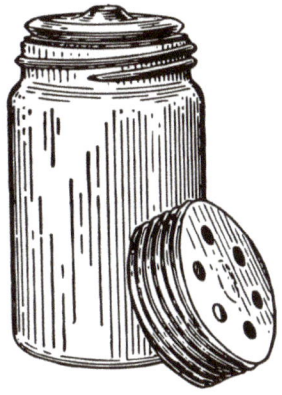

OPTIONAL GARNISH:

Extra chopped baby spinach leaves and/or fresh parsley
Shredded fresh Parmesan and/or Romano cheese
Crushed red pepper flakes

HEAT the olive oil in a 6-quart saucepan over moderately high heat. Add the onion, carrot, garlic, salt, and pepper and sauté for 5 minutes. Add both broths and bring to a boil. Add orzo and boil, then cook on medium heat 15 minutes, uncovered. Stir a few times. Whisk the eggs well in a 2-cup glass measuring cup. Turn the heat down to low and slowly pour the eggs into the soup, using the whisk in a back and forth motion to make the eggs thready. Add the spinach and cook on low 2 minutes. Raise heat to a rolling simmer and carefully add the meatballs. Cook 5 minutes, stirring a few times. Season, if desired. Garnish, as desired. Cover and chill leftovers. Serves 6-8.

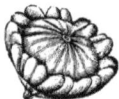
Change your broth to vegetable; you wouldn't want to use water here. A pound of coarsely chopped cremini mushrooms would be your best substitute for the meatballs.

Other ground meats will be fine; how about mixing turkey sausage and ground pork? Maybe a bit of ground lamb?

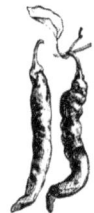
Long ago in the introduction, I mentioned you would be surprised how delicious a cup of green chile or salsa would be in this soup. So try it for a change, and see if you are, indeed, pleasantly surprised.

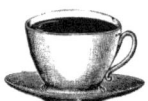
Some wedding soups are rather thin and skimp on the meatballs, but I've designed this one to be quite hearty. Is this traditionally served at weddings? Apparently not; the recipe was originally called "married soup," from the Italian phrase, minestra maritata, *which merely indicates the happy and fortuitous marriage between greenery and meat.*

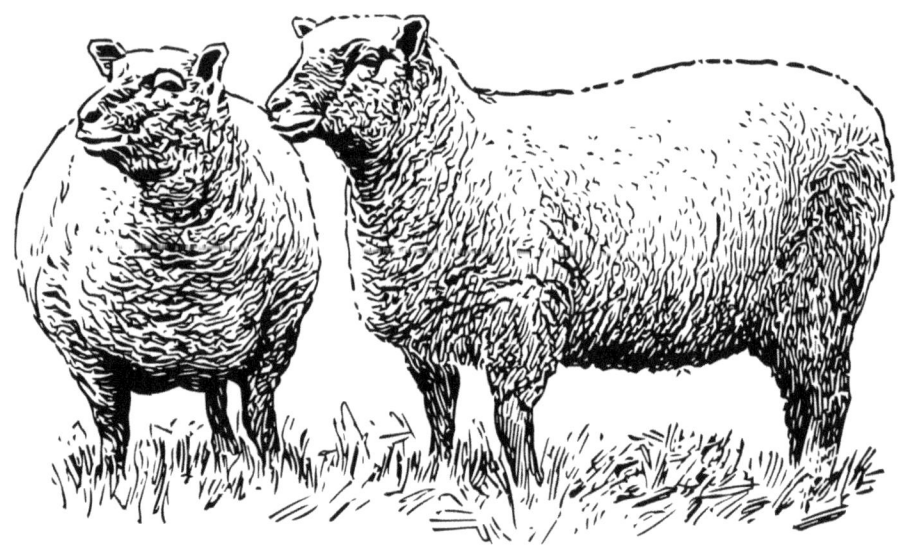

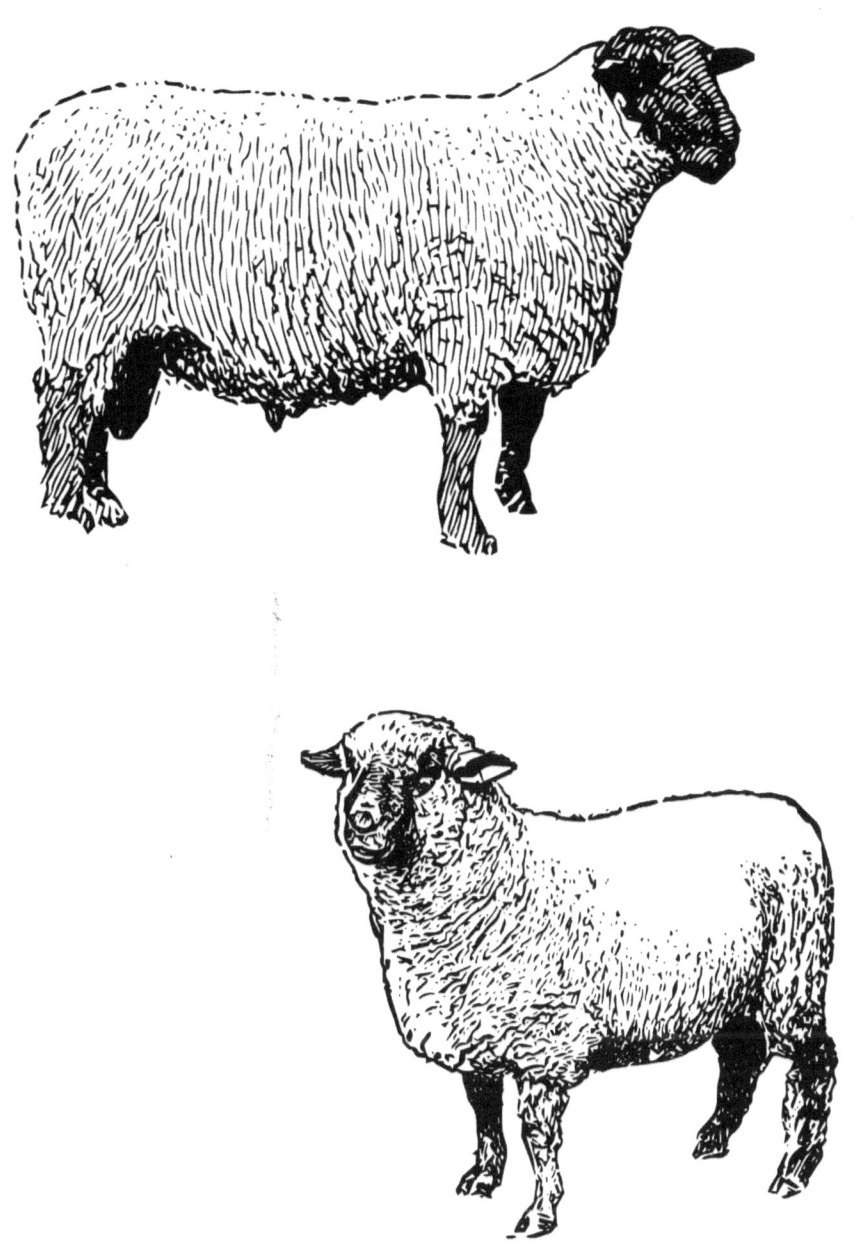

Pepper Pot Chili

While it's not mandatory, it will make a colorful chili if you use three different colors for your bell peppers and your beans. I like to use a red, yellow, and orange pepper. For the beans, I like to use pinto, black, and cannellini. For the hot sauce, any variety is fine; a chipotle Tabasco sauce will impart a delicious smoky flavor.

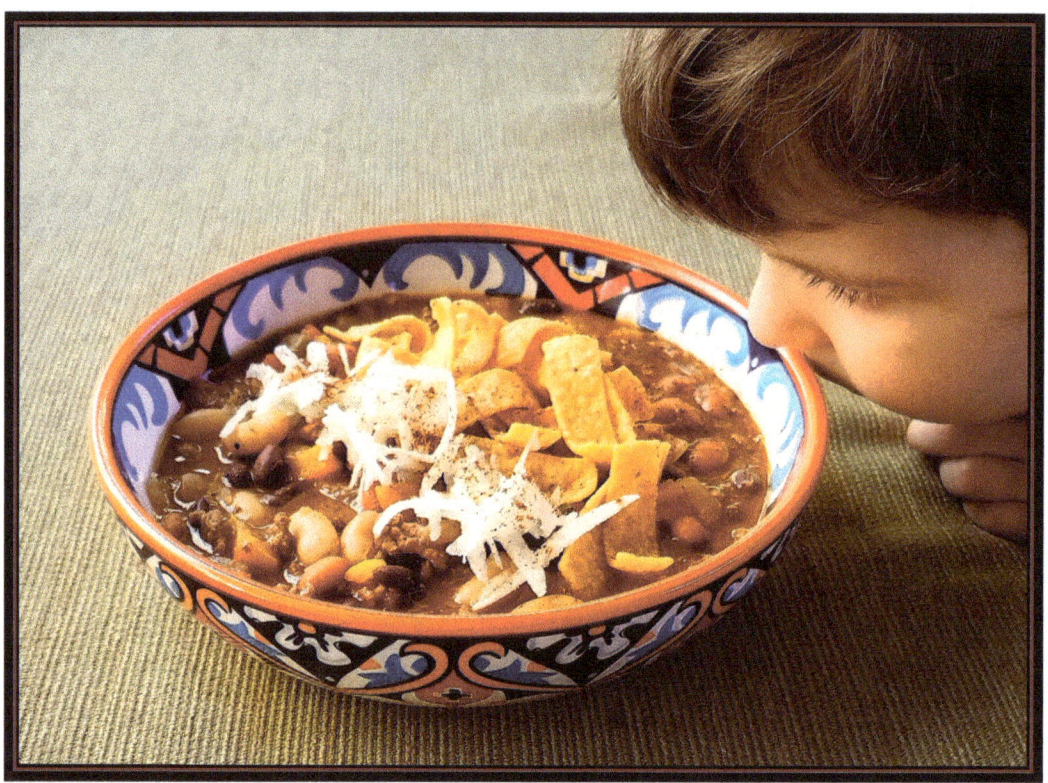

2 tablespoons olive oil
1 pound ground beef sirloin
2 cups onion, coarsely chopped
1 tablespoon minced garlic
3 large bell peppers (preferably 3 different colors), cored and coarsely chopped
3 (15.5-ounce) cans of sturdy beans (preferably 3 different colors), drained and rinsed
14.5-ounce can low-sodium chicken broth
12 ounces dark beer (any variety of a brown ale or stout, or even an amber type)
14.5-ounce can diced tomatoes, with juice
8 ounces roasted and chopped green chile, with juice

2 tablespoons cornmeal
1 tablespoon chili powder
1 tablespoon hot sauce
1½ teaspoons salt
1 teaspoon black pepper
1 teaspoon cumin
1 teaspoon dry oregano
       (2-3 tablespoons fresh, minced)
½ teaspoon cayenne pepper

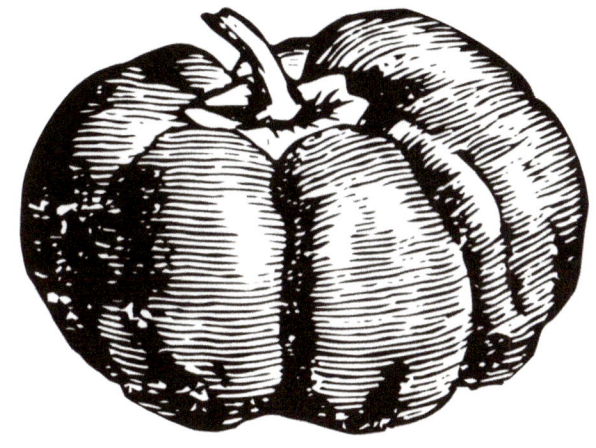

OPTIONAL GARNISH:

Fritos
Shredded jicama
Chili powder
Any of the **CHARMING CHILI GARNISHES** would be great.

COAT a 6-quart saucepan with cooking spray. Sauté the oil, beef, onion, and garlic over rather high heat until the pink is gone from the meat. Add the peppers and sauté another 5 minutes. Add the remaining ingredients and bring to a boil. Cover and cook on a rather low heat (a rolling simmer) 30 minutes; stir a few times. Cook another 30 minutes, uncovered, on medium heat (a gentle boil). Stir a few times, especially at the bottom of the pot. Season, if desired. Garnish, as desired. Cover and chill leftovers. Serves 6-8.

Omit the meat and change the broth to vegetable or even water. Add a large chopped up green bell pepper and another can of beans. How about chickpeas or black-eyed peas?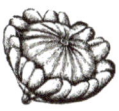

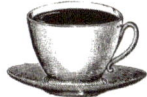 *This keeps exceptionally well for a few days, but it also freezes well. Double the batch, cook it in a 12-quart saucepan, portion it out, and you'll have some hearty dinners planned. OR—plan to cook it awhile longer (anywhere from 30-45 minutes, uncovered, depending on your heat) to make it thick enough to top some hot dogs.*

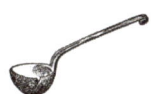

Bodacious Brisket Soup

Once in a while, I go nuts and buy a giant brisket, throw a spicy rub on it, and bake it for a few hours. My recipe makes a gravy, so I usually serve mashed potatoes with it. Usually I serve some sort of green vegetable with it, like peas or green beans. Then everybody tears into it, but you still end up with a ton of it leftover. One day, I figured I would make a soup with the typical brisket accompaniments just to do something different with my leftover slab of meat—so here it is.

Now, if you don't happen to have a brisket hanging around, you can use other items such as BBQ beef or pork, roast beef, or pulled pork. You might even find a few varieties of prepared brisket in your market. Your choice of meat product will dictate the seasoning in the soup; obviously, a BBQ-type of meat will make your soup a bit sweeter, and a plain roast beef might require extra seasoning. You can play it by ear.

2 tablespoons salted butter
1 tablespoon minced garlic
1½ teaspoons salt
1 teaspoon black pepper
1 teaspoon dry thyme
    (2-3 tablespoons fresh, minced)
1 cup carrot, peeled and coarsely chopped
1 cup celery, coarsely chopped
1 cup onion, coarsely chopped
1 quart low-sodium beef broth
1½ cups water
2 tablespoons lemon juice
2 bay leaves
1½ pounds russet potatoes; peeled, then cut into ½" chunks
1½ pounds leftover, cooked, seasoned brisket; cut into roughly ½" chunks
1 cup frozen peas

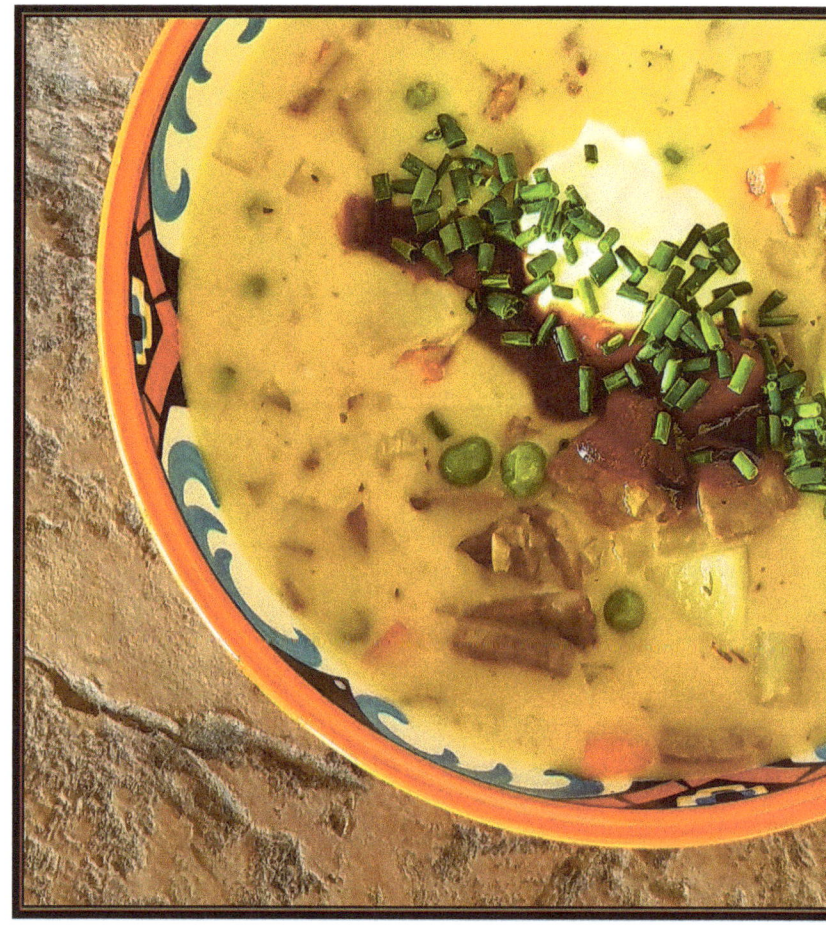

1 cup heavy cream
½ cup dry white wine, such as Chardonnay
6 tablespoons all-purpose flour

OPTIONAL GARNISH:

Sour cream or crème fraîche
Minced chives
BBQ sauce
Bacon bits
Chili sauce
Shredded cheese, any variety

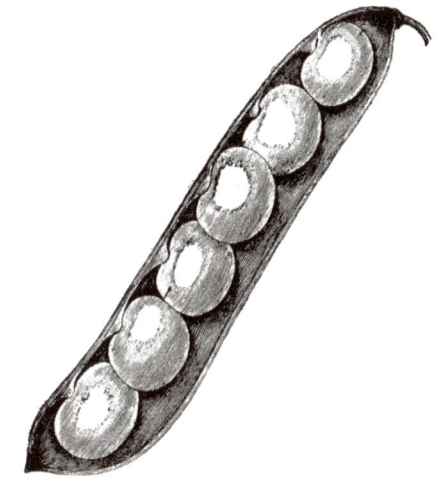

COAT a 6-quart saucepan with cooking spray. Melt the butter over rather high heat and sauté the garlic, salt, pepper, thyme, carrot, celery, and onion 5 minutes. Add the broth, water, lemon juice, bay leaves, potatoes, and brisket and bring to a boil. Cook, uncovered, on a medium rolling simmer, 15 minutes. Stir a couple of times. Add the peas and raise heat a notch; cook another 15 minutes.

WHISK the remaining ingredients well in a 4-cup glass measuring cup. Add a cup of hot soup to this and mix in. Add all to the pot and cook another few minutes on a rolling simmer until it thickens. Stir a few times. Remove bay leaves. Season, if desired. Garnish, as desired. Cover and chill leftovers; don't freeze. Serves 6-8.

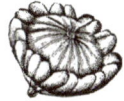 Change the broth to water or vegetable broth. For an effortless vegetarian version, I would increase my potatoes to 2 pounds, and increase the carrot, celery, onion, and peas to 2 cups each.

As I said above, your meat might be spicy enough. My brisket recipe is fairly spicy, so I usually don't need to adjust the seasoning much. I've made it with a prepared "seasoned" brisket and I've made this with BBQ pork; both varieties of meat completely changed the character of the soup. And, of course, it certainly lends itself to the addition of green chile or salsa.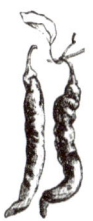

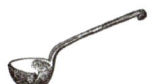

Pasta e Fagioli

Here's an extra hearty version of an Italian classic, made with—you guessed it—pasta and beans. You'll be glad to make a big batch of this soup because it freezes quite well! But it is also easy to cut the recipe in half, and it will keep in your refrigerator for a few days.

2 tablespoons olive oil
2 tablespoons minced garlic
1 pound ground beef sirloin
1 cup carrot, peeled and cut into ¼" slices
1 cup celery, cut into ¼" slices
1 cup onion, coarsely chopped
2 (14.5-ounce) cans diced tomatoes, with juice
2 quarts low-sodium beef broth
2 (15.5-ounce) cans cannellini beans, drained and rinsed
2 (14-ounce) jars prepared pizza sauce
½ cup prepared pesto sauce, any variety
1 teaspoon salt
1 teaspoon black pepper
1 teaspoon dry basil (2-3 tablespoons fresh, minced)
1 teaspoon dry oregano (2-3 tablespoons fresh, minced)
1 teaspoon hot sauce
1 cup orzo
1 cup frozen peas

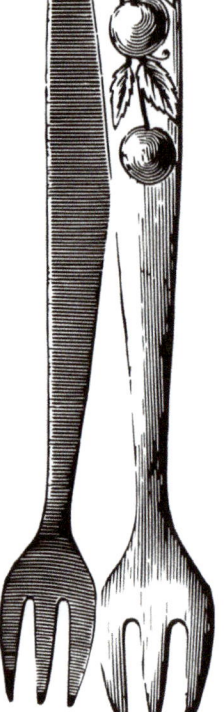

OPTIONAL GARNISH:

Shredded fresh Parmesan and/or Romano cheese
Chopped tomatoes
Minced fresh herbs; such as basil, sage, or oregano

COAT an 8-quart saucepan with cooking spray. Sauté the oil, garlic, beef, carrot, celery, and onion over rather high heat until the pink is gone. Add the tomatoes, broth, beans, pizza and pesto sauces, salt, pepper, basil, oregano, and hot sauce and bring to a boil. Cover and simmer on lowest heat 45 minutes. Stir a few times. Add orzo and peas. Raise heat and cook on medium heat, uncovered, 20-25 minutes or so, until the orzo is cooked to your liking. Maintain a good rolling simmer; stir every 5 minutes, especially at the bottom of the pot. Season, if desired. Garnish, as desired. Cover and chill leftovers. Serves 8-10.

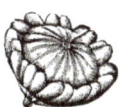 Change the broth to vegetable and omit the beef. Thinly slice a pound of cremini mushrooms instead.

Green chile (8 ounces roasted and chopped, with juice, will be up to the challenge) is surprisingly good in this classic Italian soup, or you could simply increase the amount of hot sauce. A sprinkling of crushed red pepper flakes wouldn't hurt.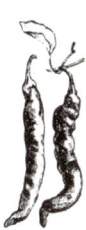

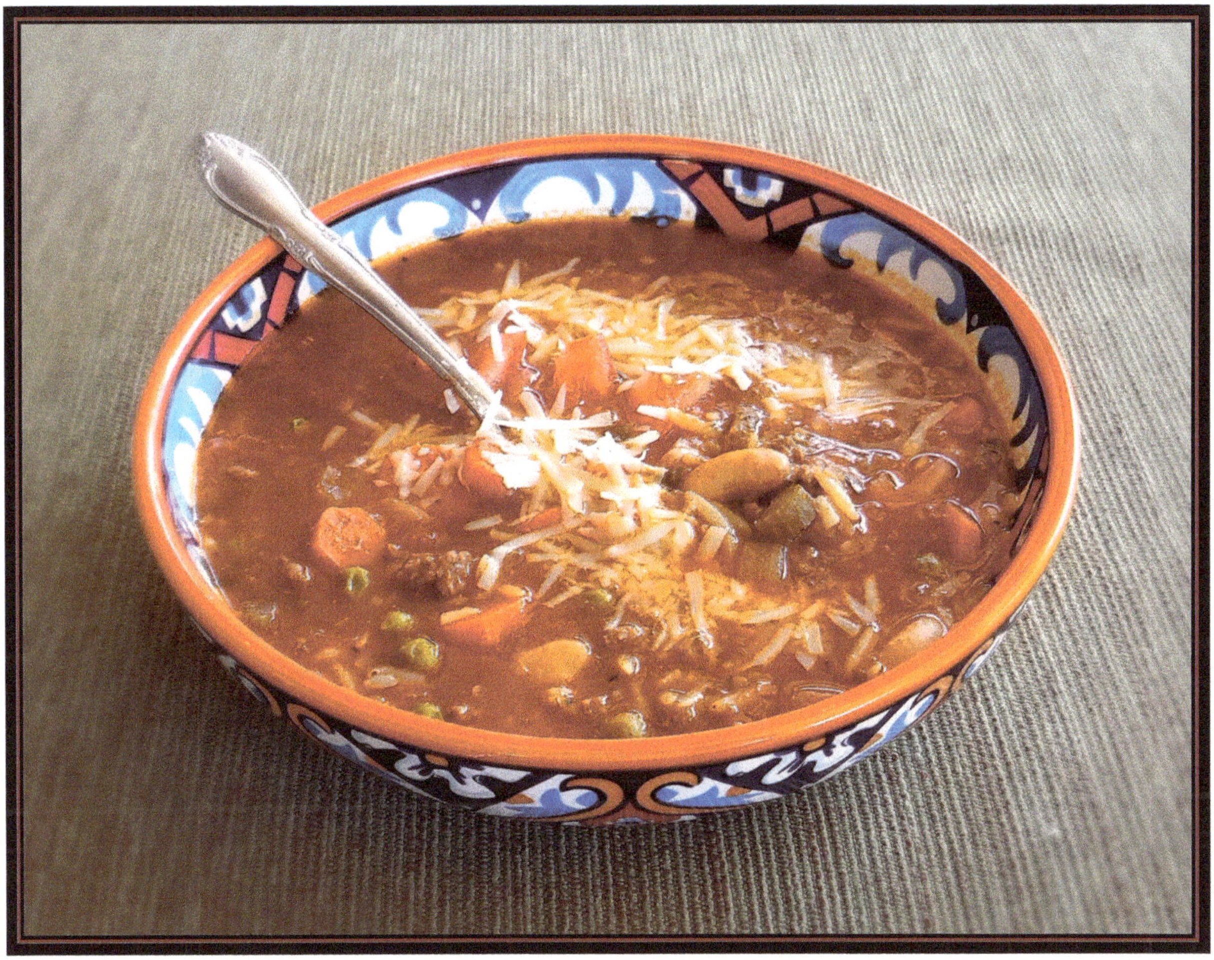

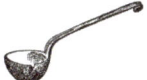

Chapter One: Beef   23

Cheeseburger Soup

I once went out to one of the trendy restaurants in Albuquerque's oh-so-chic neighborhood called Nob Hill (which is definitely a defined and charming area, though I'm always surprised how far its borders extend according to local businesses hoping to cash in on the cachet of being called "Nob Hill"), and reluctantly decided to order a cup of "Cheeseburger Soup" since nothing else sounded that fantastic. It ended up being a delicious choice; so much so, that I figured I'd have to invent my own. One of my recipe testers suggested that ground turkey is a tasty and healthier variation here.

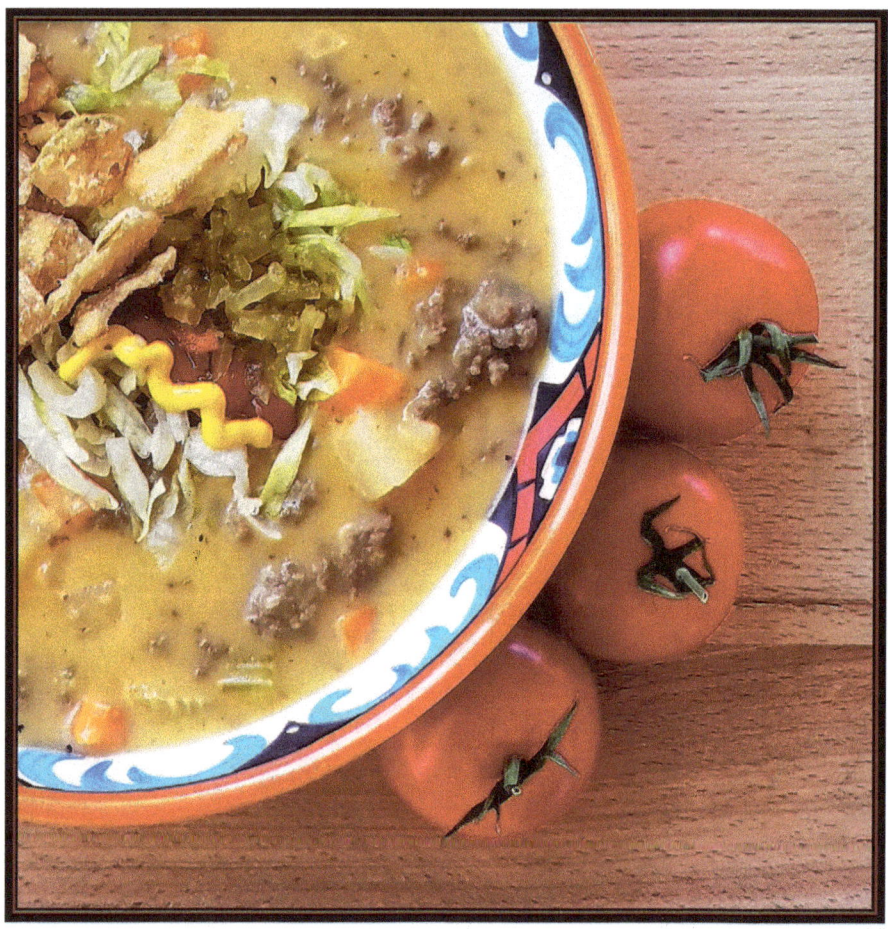

2-2¼ pounds ground chuck
1 teaspoon onion powder
1 teaspoon garlic powder
1½ teaspoons salt, divided

¼ cup salted butter
1 cup carrot, peeled and coarsely chopped
1 cup celery, coarsely chopped
1 cup onion, coarsely chopped
1 tablespoon minced garlic
1 teaspoon black pepper
1 pound potatoes, cut into ½" chunks (peeled or not; it depends on the variety you use)
2 quarts low-sodium chicken broth
2 teaspoons liquid smoke
1 pound Velveeta, shredded (or use a sharp Cheddar; Velveeta melts very well, however)
2/3 cup all-purpose flour

OPTIONAL GARNISH:

Garnish with pretty much anything you might put on a hamburger! I know it sounds a little strange, but that is what the restaurant served, and it worked. In the photo, I have ketchup, mustard, relish; lettuce and crispy fried onions in a can (such as French's). Diced tomatoes and/or avocado would be nice, as would bacon bits.

COAT a 6-quart saucepan with cooking spray. Fry the meat, onion and garlic powders, and 1 teaspoon salt over very high heat, breaking it up as you cook, until the pink is gone; stir frequently. Drain and set aside. Don't bother washing out the pot.

COAT the pot with more cooking spray. Melt the butter over very high heat. Add the carrot, celery, onion, garlic, pepper, and the remaining ½ teaspoon salt and sauté over moderately high heat for 5 minutes. Add the potatoes, broth, and liquid smoke and bring to a boil. Cook on medium (a rolling simmer), uncovered, 20 minutes. Stir a few times. Add the meat and cook another 3 minutes. Toss the cheese and flour in a large bowl with your hands. Mix into the soup and cook another 3-4 minutes, uncovered, over medium heat. Stir to melt. Season, if desired. Garnish, as desired. Cover and chill leftovers; don't freeze. Serves 8-10.

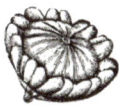
Since the whole point of this soup is "burger," I would use your favorite ground meat substitute. However, you could also chop up 2 pounds of cremini mushrooms instead; they'll give the illusion of meat. Use a vegetable broth as a substitute, not water.

This soup is definitely conducive to the addition of spice! Green chile or salsa would be fine (a cup or so), or your favorite chili sauces to taste, such as Sriracha.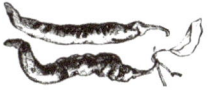

Chapter One: Beef   25

Dragon Fire Chili

This chili is designed to be served simply in a bowl with your favorite carb accompaniment. However, if you throw a bunch of Fritos into a spacious bowl first, top with chili, and then add garnishes such as shredded cheese, scallions, tomatoes, and onions, you'll end up with a luscious Frito Pie. Or, you could cook this for an extra 30-60 minutes over very low heat, until it thickens quite a bit. Then it'll be perfect to top some hot dogs or baked potatoes. Be sure to stir it frequently!

2-2¼ pounds ground chuck
¼ cup minced garlic
3-4 cups onion, coarsely chopped
2 tablespoons cornmeal
2 tablespoons chili powder
1 tablespoon hot sauce
2 bay leaves
2 teaspoons cumin
1 teaspoon salt
1 teaspoon black pepper
1 teaspoon dry oregano
      (2-3 tablespoons fresh, minced)
8 ounces roasted and chopped green chile, with juice
2 (14.5-ounce) cans diced tomatoes, with juice
2 (15.5-ounce) cans pinto beans, drained and rinsed
24 ounces dark or amber beer, room temperature

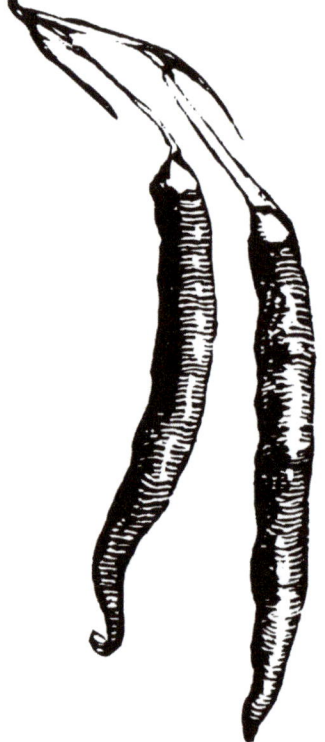

OPTIONAL GARNISH:

Crispy tortilla strips
A dollop of sour cream
A sprinkling of chili powder
Any of the **NICE NEW MEXICAN & MEXICAN GARNISHES** will work!
And, of course, any of the **CHARMING CHILI GARNISHES** would be delicious.

COAT a 6-quart saucepan with cooking spray. Sauté the beef, garlic, and onion until the pink is mostly gone, over very high heat, breaking up the meat and stirring frequently. Add the remaining ingredients and mix well. Bring to a boil. Set heat to medium/low and cook 2 hours, uncovered. Stir a few times, especially near the end of cooking. Keep at a gentle, bubbling simmer; adjust heat as needed. Discard bay leaves. Season, if desired. Garnish, as desired. Cover and chill leftovers. Serves 6-8.

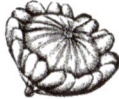 Use your favorite ground beef substitute, or a 2-pound combination of desired coarsely chopped vegetables (carrot, celery, summer squash, more beans, more onion…).

Substitute ground turkey and/or pork; veal and/or chicken.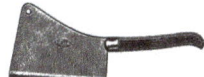

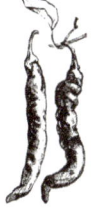 Too spicy? You could omit the hot sauce or the chili powder or the green chile; or simply cut them all in half for a milder chili. Not spicy enough? Beard the dragon and increase according to your tastes; some people have a high tolerance, especially those of us who live in New Mexico.

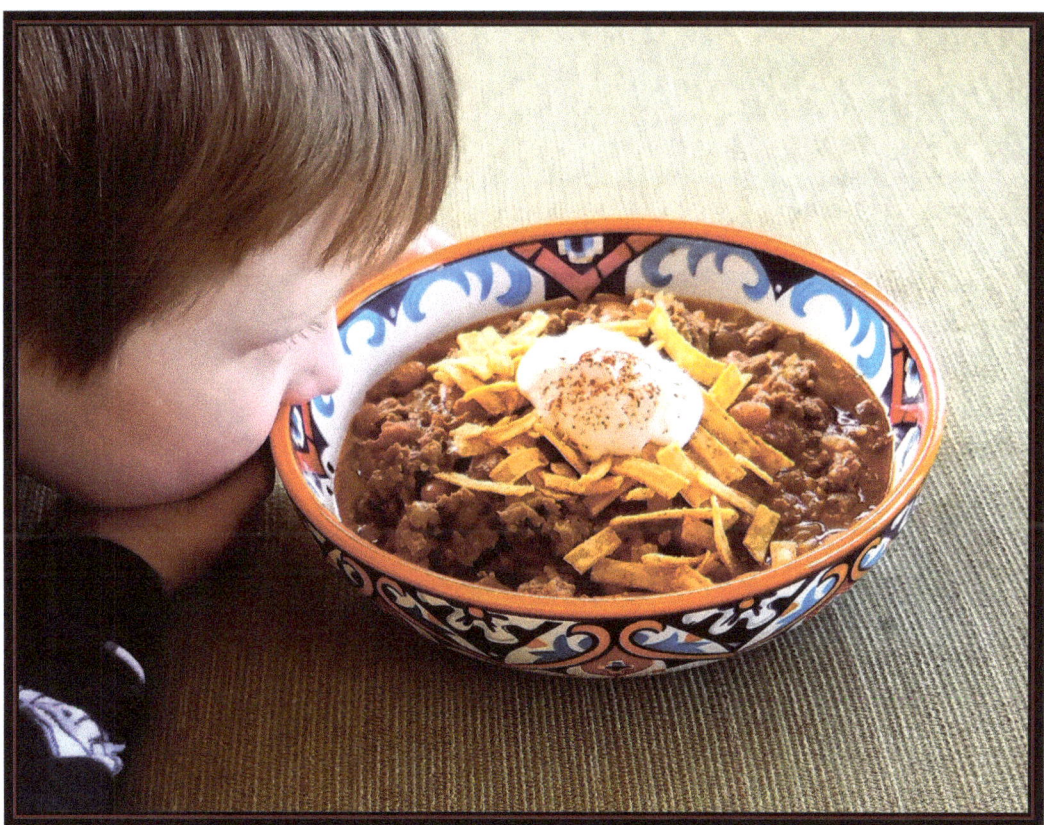

Chapter One: Beef   27

Coconut Beef Stew

Feel free to use parsnips or carrots in this mellow, yellow stew.

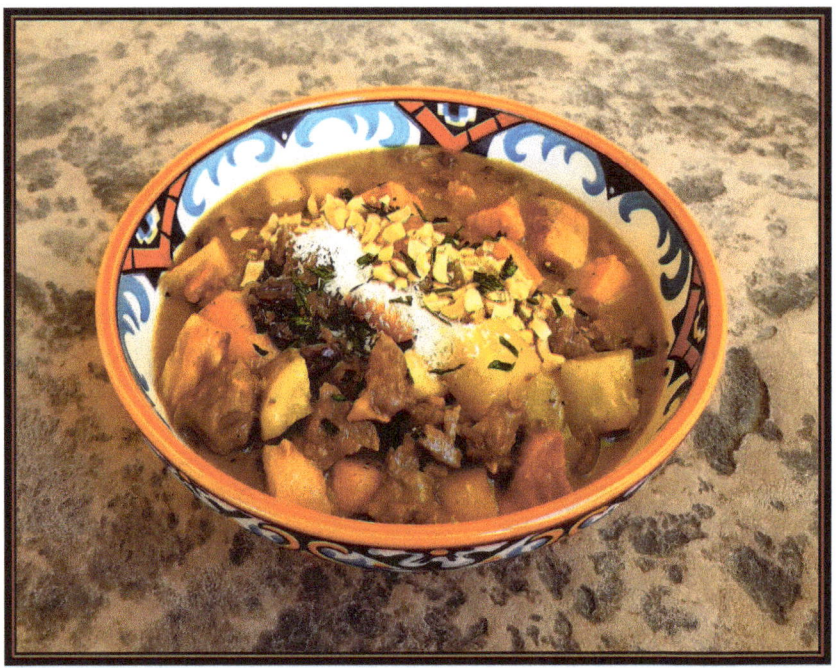

2 tablespoons salted butter
1½ teaspoons salt, divided
1 teaspoon black pepper, divided
1 tablespoon hot Madras curry powder
2 cups onion, coarsely chopped
2½ pounds beef stew meat, cut into 1" chunks
1 tablespoon packed golden brown sugar
½ cup raisins
14.5-ounce can low-sodium beef broth
1 pound parsnips, peeled and cut into 1" chunks
1 pound sweet potatoes, peeled and cut into 1" chunks
2 tablespoons peanut oil
1 teaspoon smoked paprika
13.66-ounce can unsweetened coconut milk
2 tablespoons all-purpose flour
8 ounces zucchini; partially peel, cut off stems, then cut in quarters lengthwise, and cut into 1" chunks

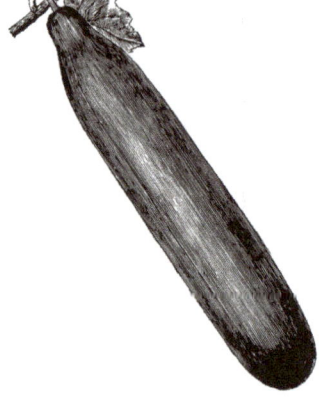

OPTIONAL GARNISH:

Nuts, such as peanuts or cashews, finely chopped
Raisins
Unsweetened coconut flakes
Minced fresh parsley or chives
Crème fraîche

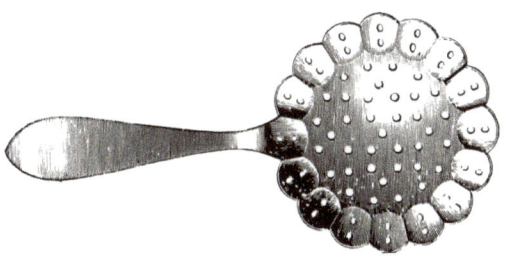

COAT a 6-quart saucepan with cooking spray. Melt the butter over moderately high heat, then sauté ½ teaspoon salt, ½ teaspoon pepper, curry, onion, and meat until the pink is mostly gone, 6-8 minutes. Add the brown sugar, raisins, and broth. Bring to a boil, then cook on the lowest heat 1 hour, covered. Stir twice.

MEANWHILE, preheat oven to 425°. Coat an 11" by 7" baking dish with cooking spray. Place the parsnips and sweet potato in the prepared pan. Drizzle the peanut oil over all, then sprinkle with paprika and remaining salt and pepper. Stir to combine. Roast 45 minutes; stir once, halfway through roasting. Let stand in the pan (you can prepare these vegetables in advance, if desired; cover and refrigerate up to 24 hours before use).

IN a 4-cup glass measuring cup, whisk together the coconut milk and flour. Add this to the pot along with the zucchini. Bring to a boil again, then cook over a medium heat (a gentle boil), uncovered, 15 minutes. Add the roasted vegetables and cook another 10-15 minutes, until vegetables are tender. Stir a few times. Season, if desired. Garnish, as desired. Cover and chill leftovers; don't freeze. Serves 6-8.

Substitute vegetable broth. To make it easy, I would simply increase the required vegetables: 3-4 cups onion, 1½ pounds each of the parsnips and sweet potatoes, and 1 pound zucchini. You'd want to roast the vegetables for a whole hour in a 13" by 9" dish. If you did this, you'd start by roasting the vegetables, then follow the first paragraph's instructions regarding the initial sauté and addition of the brown sugar, raisins, and broth. Omit cooking on the lowest heat for one hour. Then skip to the final paragraph's instructions.

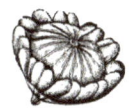

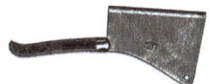 Chicken broth and meat (a combination of boneless, skinless breasts and thighs, or just one or the other) would make a good substitute.

You could definitely spice this up; for a sweet-hot version, you could add some more Asian-influenced items such as mango chutney or tamarind sauce, be bold and add chili paste with garlic, or increase the curry to 2 tablespoons.

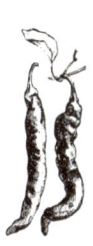

Oodle Noodle Soup

I was nearing the end of choosing recipes to include or invent for this cookbook, so I asked Bob for soup suggestions. He mentioned a vintage Campbell's soup called beef noodle. He apparently used to love this, but my own memory of this soup was not so favorable. I remembered it being tomato-based, with a few meager and minuscule chunks of beef and some broken pieces of a linguine-type of pasta. Some research about this rather obsolete soup yielded a few basic ingredients, though I have seen it lately at my supermarket, so I guess it is not as obsolete as I thought it was. Anyway, I fudged around with the idea and decided to go BIG with the beef and noodles.

Bob said this is the BEST soup I have ever made, but he is often rather hyperbolic when it comes to food.

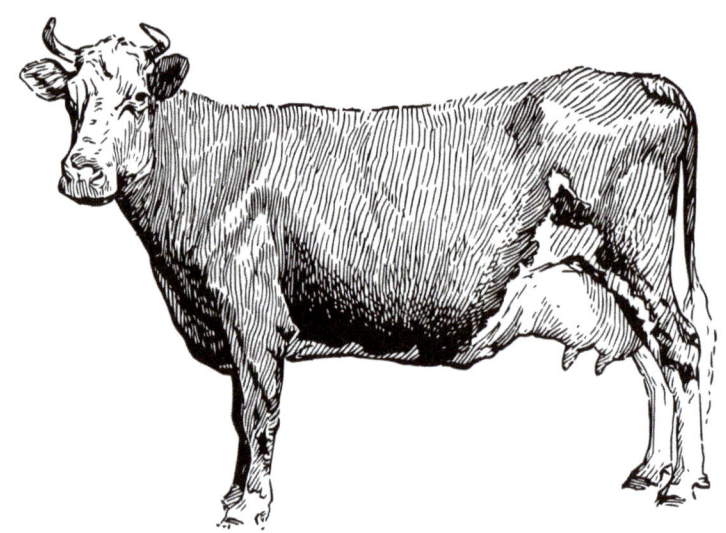

1 tablespoon vegetable oil
1 pound ground beef sirloin
1½ teaspoons garlic powder
1½ teaspoons onion powder
1 teaspoon black pepper
1 teaspoon garlic salt
1 teaspoon onion salt
¾ cup water
2 tablespoons Worcestershire sauce
6-ounce can tomato paste
2 quarts low-sodium beef broth
8 ounces extra wide egg noodles
    (or other medium-sized pasta)

OPTIONAL GARNISH:

6-ounce can fried onions (such as French's)
1-2 cups of thinly sliced scallions

COAT a 6-quart saucepan with cooking spray. Sauté the oil, beef, and the 5 seasonings over rather high heat, breaking up the meat until the pink is gone. Whisk the water, Worcestershire sauce, and tomato paste well in a 2-cup glass measuring cup. Add this mixture and the broth to the pot and bring to a boil. Add the noodles and boil again. Cook, uncovered, on a medium/high heat (a gentle boil) about 20 minutes or so. Stir a few times, until the noodles are done to your liking. Season, if desired. Garnish, as desired. Cover and chill leftovers. Serves 6-8.

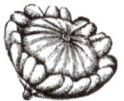 You would definitely want to use a vegetable broth instead of the beef broth. One pound of any ground meat substitute would be fine, but the best vegetarian substitute would be a pound of coarsely chopped cremini mushrooms.

I don't know, I guess you could add my typical spice recommendations to this, but I never do. Even Bob doesn't, and that's saying something. It's so tomato-y and noodle-y, onion-y and garlic-y, you probably just won't want to.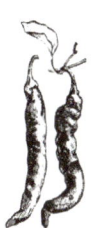

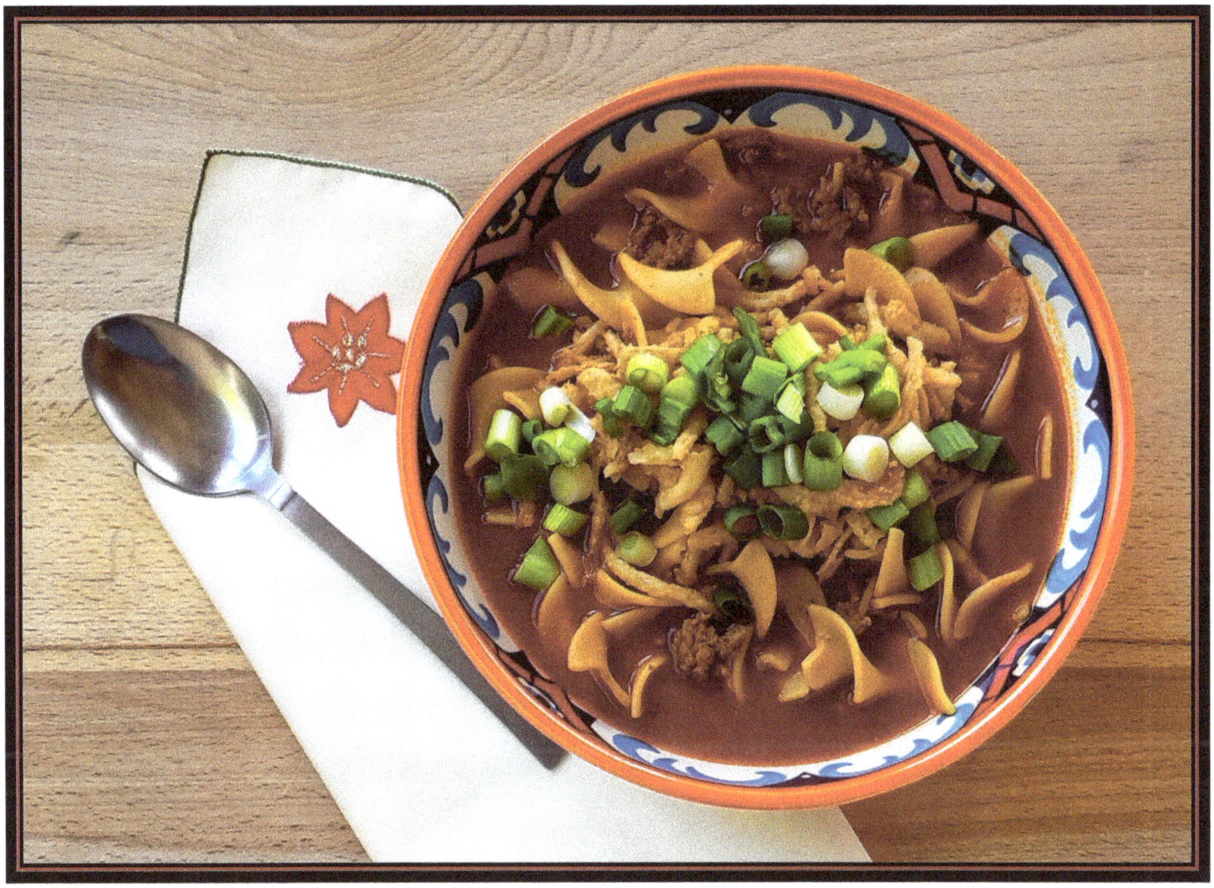

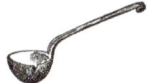

Chapter One: Beef

CHAPTER TWO
CHICKEN

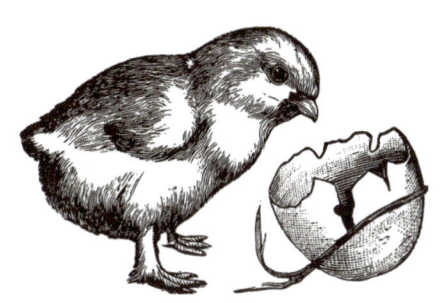

Rev It Up Posole

Awesome Avgolemono

Troy's Terrific Thai Turkey Soup

Robert the Bruce's Cock-a-Leekie Soup

Walter's Bitchin' Buffalo Soup

Elegantly Sufficient Egg Drop Soup

Nothing Wrong with Mulligatawny

Casbah-Rockin' Chicken Stew

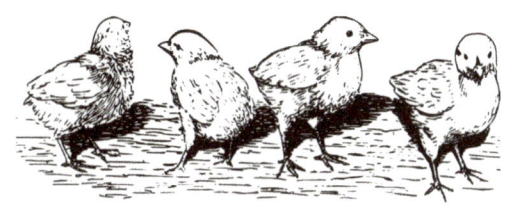

Mmm... So Spicy Miso Soup

Turkey Black Bean Soup

Callista's Amazing Avocado Chicken Soup

Ten-Alarm Butternut Chicken Chili

Sopa de los Burqueños

Stracciatella Bella

BONUS: "Rey's Savory Quarter-Portion"

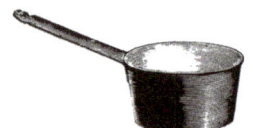 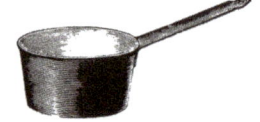

Chapter Two—Chicken
(TURKEY & OTHER ASSORTED POULTRY)

Of course, turkey can always substitute for chicken in all of this chapter's recipes. Cornish game hens, duck, goose, pigeon, pheasant, and squab are not popular around my house, but you can always experiment with different birds and see what you might like to use.

I'm afraid I don't have any interesting chicken stories. I do have a few roadrunners living around my neighborhood, however. They are the state bird of New Mexico, and if you observe them closely, you'll be able to see their rather obvious, though far-removed, kinship with dinosaurs. Roadrunners are kind of like petite velociraptors.

I would never recommend substituting roadrunner for chicken. Although I said one should never say never, way back in the stocks/broths section, I really mean it here. NEVER substitute a roadrunner for a chicken.

Rev It Up Posole

Ground chicken or turkey will also work well in this posole. Since there's a V8 in this, it will help you get your motor going.

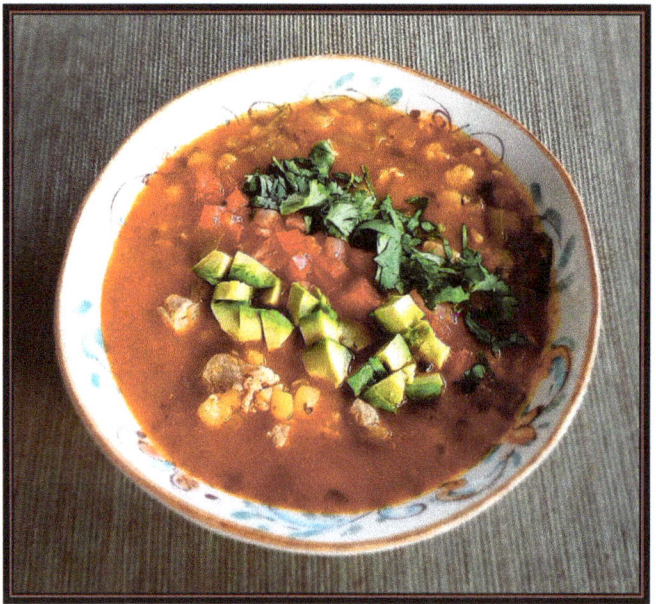

1 tablespoon vegetable oil
2 cups onion, coarsely chopped
1 tablespoon minced garlic
1-1¼ pounds boneless, skinless chicken thighs, cut into ¾" chunks
1 quart low-sodium chicken broth
11.5-ounce can V8 (12 ounces is also fine, or 1½ cups)
8 ounces roasted and chopped green chile, with juice
2 (15.5-ounce) cans yellow hominy, drained and rinsed
     (if you like, or 3 cups cooked hominy;
      white hominy is also fine)
1 teaspoon dry oregano (2-3 tablespoons fresh, minced)
1 teaspoon lime juice
½ teaspoon salt
½ teaspoon black pepper
½ cup fresh cilantro, minced (optional)

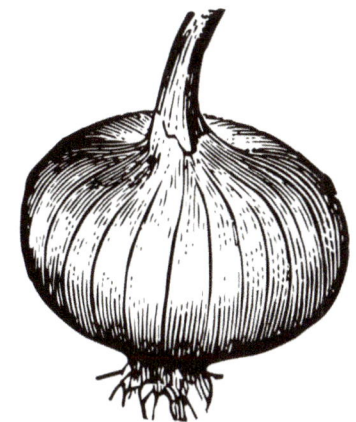

OPTIONAL GARNISH:

Diced avocado
Chopped fresh cilantro
Fresh diced tomatoes
Or try any of the other **NICE NEW MEXICAN & MEXICAN GARNISHES.**

COAT a 4-quart saucepan with cooking spray. Sauté the oil, onion, garlic, and chicken over very high heat until most of the pink is gone. Add the remaining ingredients and bring to a boil. Reduce heat to low and maintain a rolling simmer. Cook, uncovered, 45 minutes; stir a few times. Season, if desired. Garnish, as desired. Cover and chill leftovers. Serves 4-6.

Change your broth and substitute two (15.5-ounce) cans of pinto beans, drained and rinsed. Or try any other bean you like; a combination of black beans and cannellini beans would be great.

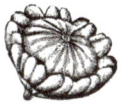

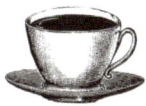

If you have trouble getting V8, just substitute the same amount of tomato juice or sauce with an additional ½ teaspoon of both celery salt and onion salt. Conversely, you could also substitute a pureed 14.5-ounce can of tomatoes. If you would like to use fresh tomatoes, chop about a pound or so into rather small chunks; you would still need to add the additional seasonings listed above for either of these options.

Awesome Avgolemono

This soup was how I introduced my husband to Greek food. Our usual restaurant serves a relatively thin version of this classic soup mainly as an appetizer. I decided to develop a heartier dish, which is substantial enough to serve alone for dinner. Bob still hasn't acquired a taste for hummus or many other Greek specialties, however. Check out the anecdotal information for a quickie recipe, if you don't want to mess around with preparing a whole bird.

8 cups water
2½ teaspoons coarse sea salt
1½ teaspoons whole peppercorns, black or mixed
A whole chicken, approximately 4½-5 pounds

USE a 4-cup glass measuring cup for the entire recipe and don't bother to wash it out. Combine the water, salt, and peppercorns in a 6-quart saucepan. Remove any giblets from the chicken and add to the pot. Rinse off chicken and add to the pot. Bring to a boil then simmer on low, covered, for 30 minutes. Turn chicken over and cook on low, covered, another 30 minutes. Strain into a very large bowl. Set the chicken aside to cool in the colander. Rinse out the saucepan and pour 8 cups broth back into the pot. When the chicken is cool enough to handle, remove all the meat and shred it into bite-size pieces. Discard all skin, bones, and giblets. Set aside 4 cups of chicken; save any extra broth or meat for other recipes.

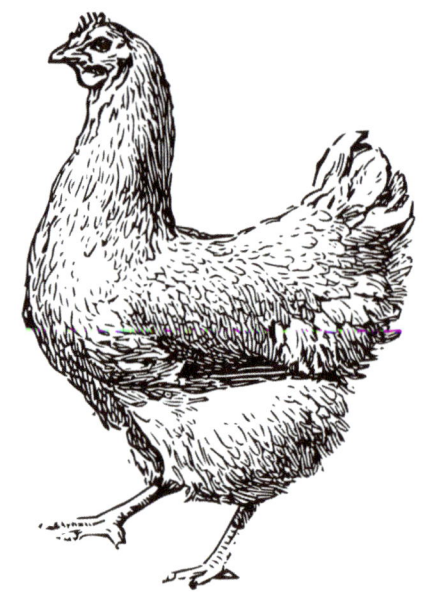

1 cup onion, coarsely chopped
1 cup carrot, peeled and thinly sliced
2/3 cup long-grain rice (or orzo)
2/3 cup lemon juice, room temperature
4 large eggs, room temperature
1 teaspoon salt
1 teaspoon black pepper

OPTIONAL GARNISH:

Minced fresh parsley
Finely shredded carrot
Chopped hard-boiled eggs

BRING the 8 cups broth to a boil in a 6-quart saucepan, then add the onion, carrot, and rice. Boil again, then cook on medium, uncovered, 20 minutes. Stir a few times. After it has cooked 18 minutes, whisk the lemon juice and eggs together in the 4-cup glass measuring cup. SLOWLY whisk 1 cup of the hot broth into the egg mixture. Then SLOWLY whisk the egg mixture into the pot, using a back and forth and side to side motion. Add the reserved 4 cups of chicken and the salt and pepper. Cook another 3-4 minutes on medium/low, uncovered, until everything is tender; stir a few times. Season, if desired. Garnish, as desired. Cover and chill leftovers; reheat slowly. Serves 6-8.

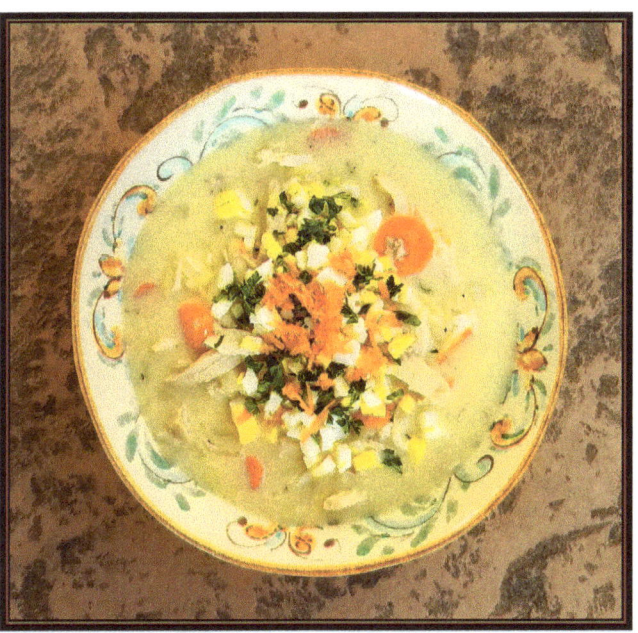

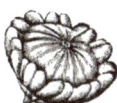

Change to a vegetable broth and omit the chicken. The easiest option would be to double the onion, carrot, and rice quantities, but you might also consider using a pound of your favorite vegetables to substitute for the chicken, cut or sliced thinly, as necessary.

Yes, well, perhaps we all love spice, but the lemon flavor is so prominent here, you'd probably regret adding any spice.

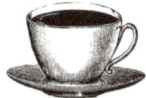

For a speedy soup, omit the initial whole chicken preparation and simply prepare in a 6-quart saucepan. Substitute 2 quarts of low-sodium chicken broth and use 1 pound cooked chicken, diced or shredded.

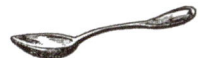

Chapter Two: Chicken

Troy's Terrific Thai Turkey Soup

My son-in-law was a chef in a former life, so we often chat about recipes. I don't know what brought the subject up, but somehow he suggested that your basic curry powder and red chile were a natural pairing. This was a revelation.

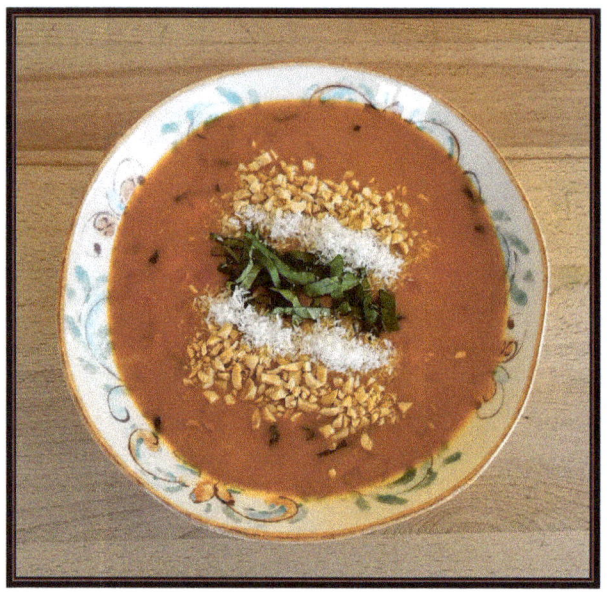

¼ cup salted butter
4 teaspoons hot Madras curry powder
1 tablespoon packed golden brown sugar
1 tablespoon chili powder
1 teaspoon ground coriander
1 teaspoon white pepper
1 cup carrot, peeled and coarsely chopped
1 cup onion, coarsely chopped
1 cup red bell pepper, cored and coarsely chopped
4-ounce jar red curry paste (such as Thai Kitchen)
2 tablespoons fish sauce
1 tablespoon lime juice
2 quarts low-sodium chicken broth (or use Turkey Frame Broth, on page xxvi)
1 pound cooked turkey, coarsely chopped
1 cup short grain rice
2 (13.66-ounce) cans unsweetened coconut milk
1 cup loosely packed fresh basil leaves, cut into thin slices

OPTIONAL GARNISH:

Chopped salted peanuts
Unsweetened coconut
Chopped fresh basil or cilantro

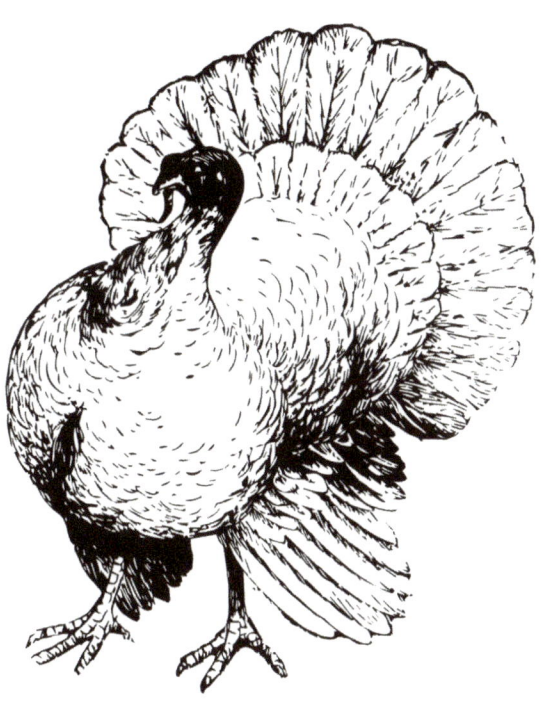

MELT the butter over very high heat in a 6-quart saucepan. Add the curry, brown sugar, chili powder, coriander, pepper, carrot, onion, and bell pepper and sauté 5 minutes. Add the curry paste, fish sauce, and lime juice and mix in well. Add the broth and bring to a boil. Add the turkey, rice, and coconut milk and bring to a boil again. Cook on a medium heat (a rolling simmer), uncovered, 30 minutes. Stir frequently; scrape up any brown bits that accumulated at the bottom of the pot. Add the basil and mix in; cook another minute or so. Season, if desired. Garnish, as desired. Cover and chill leftovers. Serves 6-8.

Change your broth to vegetable or water, and instead of the turkey, slice up half a pound of mushrooms and half a pound of peeled zucchini.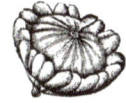

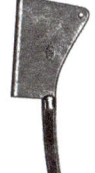 Forget the turkey and substitute a pound of raw, peeled, medium shrimp. You would add the shrimp about three or four minutes before you are done cooking.

This is already pleasantly spicy, so I'm not sure you would want to add spice, but you might consider using a jar of green curry paste instead of the red for variety.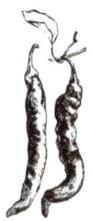

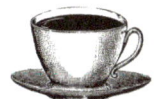 *This is a great recipe to use after Thanksgiving, if you have made a 20-pound bird and if you leave some flesh on your carcass. After you make the Turkey Frame Broth (see page xxvi), you'll probably be able to strip a pound of turkey off the frame to make this soup. However, I usually substitute chicken for both the meat and the broth; I always try to avoid cooking whole turkeys whenever possible.*

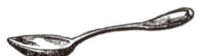

Chapter Two: Chicken   39

Robert the Bruce's Cock-a-Leekie Soup

This is a traditional Scottish soup and quite substantial. I have named it for the famous King of Scotland, Robert I (a.k.a. Robert the Bruce, 1274-1329). He was quite an amazing fellow, and apparently my husband was named for him. Bob never liked the name Bruce; I don't really know why, considering King Robert's history. This king actually chose the unicorn to be his country's national animal. That's pretty fantastic.

Would Robert the Bruce have eaten cock-a-leekie soup? Probably not; the dish made its first appearance around the 16th century. Would he have liked to have eaten it? Probably; it's a hearty dish that would have kept his troops toasty (and regular...) on many of those cold Scottish marches. Of course, the soup requires chicken and leeks; but it also has an unexpected ingredient—prunes. You might think they are an odd addition, but please don't omit them! If you would like to make an easier, quicker version, use a 6-quart pot, 10 cups of low-sodium chicken broth, and a pound of chopped, cooked chicken; skip all of the preliminary chicken cooking.

10 cups water
1 tablespoon salt
A whole chicken, approximately
    5 pounds, rinsed;
    remove giblets

PLACE water and salt in an 8-quart saucepan. Add the chicken and giblets. Bring to a boil, then cook, covered, on medium/low heat for 30 minutes. Turn chicken over and cook another 30 minutes on medium/low heat, covered. Drain into a very large bowl; when cooler, measure out 10 cups (reserve any extra broth for other recipes). Set chicken in another bowl. When chicken is cool enough to handle; remove skin, and shred into bite-size chunks—you should end up with 4-5 cups worth of meat. Set aside. Discard all skin, bones, and giblets. Rinse out the pot and reuse it.

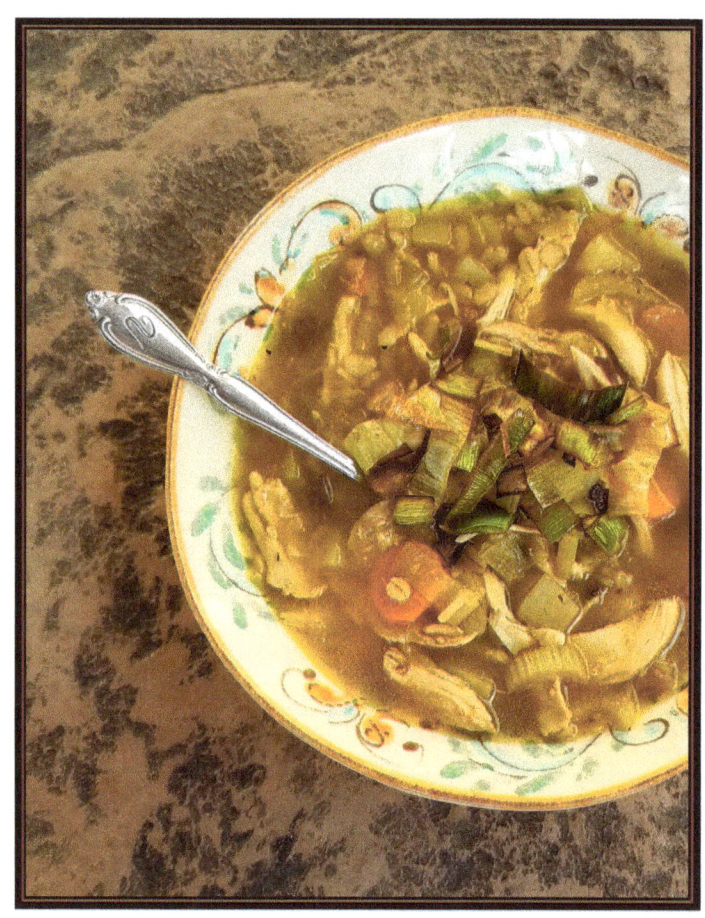

¼ cup salted butter
2 teaspoons salt
1 teaspoon sugar
1 teaspoon black pepper
1 teaspoon dry thyme (2-3 tablespoons fresh, minced)
1 cup carrot, peeled and thinly sliced
1 cup celery, thinly sliced
5 cups leeks, cleaned well and cut into ½" slices (use the white and light green parts)
10 cups prepared broth (add a little water, if necessary)
8 ounces potato, cut into ½" cubes (peeled or not; any type of potato is fine)
4 ounces prunes, coarsely chopped
½ cup quick barley

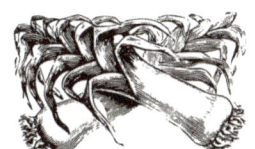

Optional Garnish:

Various minced fresh herbs, such as thyme or marjoram
Chop up some additional prunes and sprinkle on top.
Fry up some extra sliced leeks in some brown butter.

MELT butter, salt, sugar, pepper, and thyme in the 8-quart saucepan over moderately high heat. Add the carrot, celery, and leeks and sauté 8-10 minutes; stirring frequently, until the leeks brown just slightly. Add the broth, potato, prunes, and barley; bring to a boil. Cook, uncovered, on a gentle rolling simmer 30 minutes. Stir a few times. Add the reserved chicken and continue to cook, uncovered, 8-10 minutes, until everything is tender. Season, if desired. Garnish, as desired. Cover and refrigerate leftovers; don't freeze. Serves 8-10.

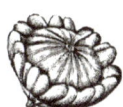

Switch out the broth for vegetable and simply increase all of the already-required vegetables; thus, 2 cups each of carrot and celery, 6 cups of leeks, and a whole pound of potatoes. I wouldn't bother to increase the prunes, however.

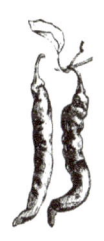

You could add spice, but this soup has a distinctive flavor already; you might not want to detract from it.

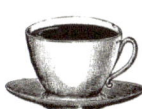

This was invented because of Narnia. In The Silver Chair, *we see our brave mighty girl, Jill Pole, being petted and cooed over by a rather hideous Queen Giantess. Later, she is treated to what C. S. Lewis calls a dinner, though it was apparently closer to tea time. This ample meal consisted of "hot roast turkey, and a steamed pudding, and roast chestnuts, and as much fruit as you could eat." That sure does sound like a dinner to me, maybe one you would serve on a holiday like Thanksgiving. The first course (before the giant turkey dinner) was a cock-a-leekie soup.*

Walter's Bitchin' Buffalo Soup

My other son-in-law is addicted to Buffalo chicken wings, so I invented a soup just for him. This isn't as messy as wings, but it still packs a punch. You can certainly cut the amount of hot sauce in half, if you like it milder. Frank's Hot Sauce is the traditional brand to use in Buffalo-style dishes, but you are welcome to use your favorite kind instead.

¼ cup salted butter
2 cups red onion, coarsely chopped
2 cups celery, thinly sliced diagonally
½ cup all-purpose flour, divided
¼ cup cornmeal
¾ teaspoon salt, divided
¾ teaspoon black pepper, divided
1 teaspoon cayenne pepper, divided
1-1¼ pounds boneless, skinless chicken breasts,
    cut into ¾" chunks
6 cups low-sodium chicken broth
½ teaspoon garlic powder
½ teaspoon smoked paprika
¼ cup hot sauce
½ cup water

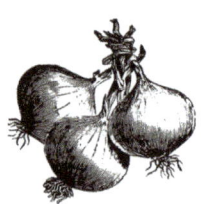
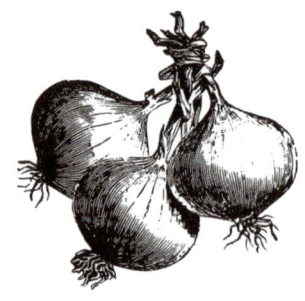

OPTIONAL GARNISH:

Generous dollops of the Gorgonzola cheese mixture listed below (other options for this creamy garnish would be dollops of sour cream or crème fraîche, or you could even use prepared Ranch salad dressing)
A cup of celery, thinly sliced diagonally
Additional hot sauce

FOR THE GORGONZOLA CHEESE:

8 ounces light sour cream
2 tablespoons heavy cream
¼ teaspoon salt
¼ teaspoon black pepper
6 ounces Gorgonzola cheese, crumbled

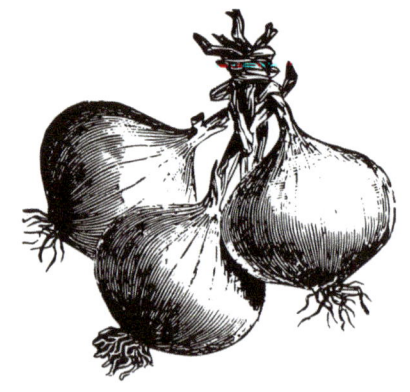

LIBERALLY coat a 6-quart saucepan with cooking spray. Melt the butter over rather high heat. Add the onion and celery and sauté 5 minutes. Whisk ¼ cup flour, cornmeal, ¼ teaspoon salt, ¼ teaspoon pepper, and ½ teaspoon cayenne pepper in a medium bowl. Add the chicken to the flour mixture and toss to coat well. Add all to the pot and sauté over moderately high heat another 5 minutes. Stir often. Add the broth, garlic powder, paprika, hot sauce, and the remaining salt, pepper, and cayenne. Bring to a boil, then cook on low, covered, 20 minutes. Stir twice, scraping up any browned bits.

MEANWHILE, combine the sour cream, cream, salt, and pepper in a medium bowl. Add the Gorgonzola and mix in well. Let it stand at room temperature.

WHISK the water and the remaining ¼ cup flour well. Add to the pot, whisking, and raise heat a notch or two. Cook, uncovered, about 3 minutes, until the soup thickens. Season, if desired. Garnish, as desired. Cover and chill leftovers. Cover and chill the Gorgonzola cheese separately. Serves 4-6.

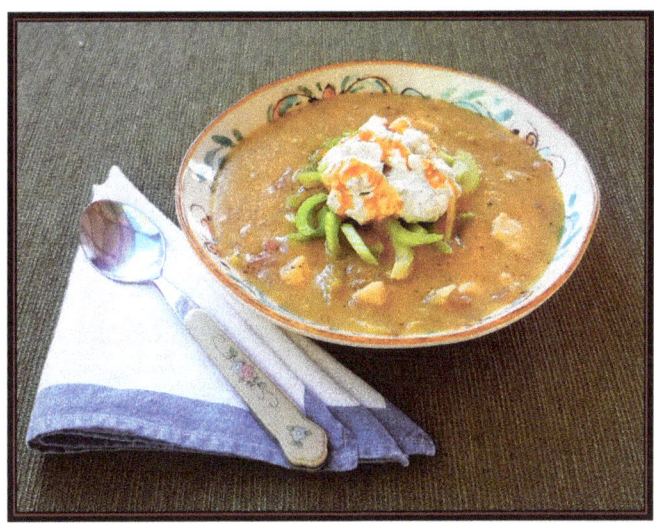

Change your broth to vegetable and use a pound of peeled potatoes, either regular or sweet, cut into ¾" chunks. You can coat these in the flour mixture as described above.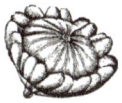

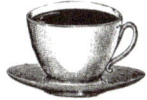 *You can definitely use stronger Bleu cheese varieties here, if you like, or skip it and just use sour cream. That combination of hot sauce, celery, chicken, and stinky cheese can't be beat, however. Leftover Gorgonzola cheese garnish would be nice on a baked potato, scrambled eggs, or mixed in with some cooked pasta.*

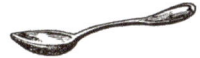

Chapter Two: Chicken   43

Elegantly Sufficient Egg Drop Soup

Who says egg drop soup is only for tiny cups to start your meal? The ubiquitous appetizer can certainly be hit or miss at your local Chinese restaurant. I decided to make it a truly filling soup, packed with vegetables and chicken. Now it's dinner! If there is a soul-pleasing chicken-y soup, this is it.

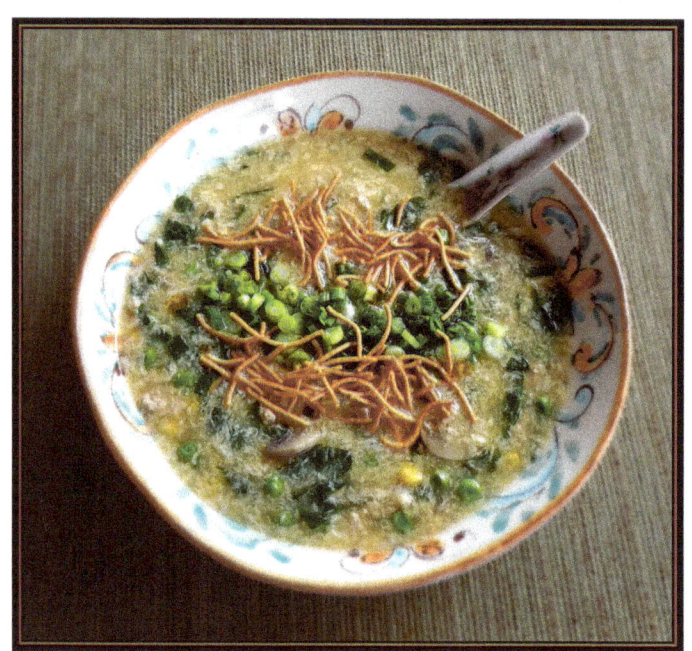

2 tablespoons toasted sesame oil
1 pound ground chicken
1 cup frozen corn
1 cup frozen peas
1 teaspoon salt
1 teaspoon white pepper
1 tablespoon minced garlic
1 tablespoon crushed ginger
5-6 ounces fresh baby spinach,
    chopped coarsely
4 ounces fresh mushrooms,
    thinly sliced
2 quarts low-sodium chicken broth
½ cup water
6 tablespoons cornstarch
2 tablespoons soy sauce
2 tablespoons aji-mirin
    (sweet cooking rice wine)
4 large eggs

OPTIONAL GARNISH:

Thinly sliced scallions and/or radishes
Crispy rice sticks or chow mein noodles
A drizzle of toasted sesame oil
A few fresh bean sprouts

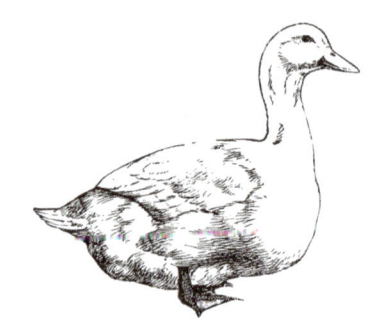

COAT a 6-quart saucepan with cooking spray. Heat the oil over rather high heat; add the chicken and sauté until all the pink is gone, breaking up the meat. Add the corn, peas, salt, pepper, garlic, ginger, spinach, mushrooms, and broth; bring to a boil. Cook on a rolling simmer, uncovered, 3 minutes. Stir a few times.

whisk the water, cornstarch, soy, and aji-mirin in a 4-cup glass measuring cup. Add to the soup and boil until it thickens; about 2 minutes. Whisk the eggs in the 4-cup glass measuring cup well. Reduce heat to low and add eggs in a slow, steady stream using the whisk to mix gently. Mix left to right; back to front. The eggs should become thready. Season, if desired. Garnish, as desired. Cover and chill leftovers. Serves 6-8.

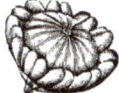
Change your broth to vegetable. You could simply omit the ground chicken and use another quarter pound of mushrooms and another half a cup each of the corn and peas, but a ground meat substitute would also work out well.

Ground pork would be an excellent substitute.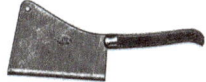

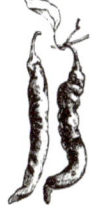
Need some spice? Of course, you can go with the green chile route (4-8 ounces, roasted and chopped, with juice), but why not add a few tablespoons of Sriracha? Or chili paste with garlic? Or make it easy by setting these condiments on the table.

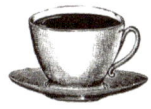
This was the last recipe to receive an official name, and it's sort of a mouthful. I finally settled on a phrase from my late mother, which she would use whenever she was fed up with us girls asking for more food. She would declare in a rather regal tone, "I think you've had an elegant sufficiency," and that would be the end of that. I've just started using the phrase around my grandchildren to keep up with the tradition. I'm sure they will be happy to hear it often, haha…

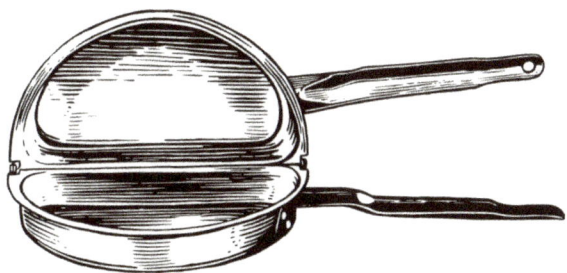

Chapter Two: Chicken   45

Nothing Wrong with Mulligatawny

I had heard of "Mulligatawny" as an exotic soup when I was a teenager in the 1970s, but it never really penetrated my consciousness until the 1990s when I saw the now-famous "Soup Nazi" episode of the television series *Seinfeld*. The character of Newman was positively giddy when he received his order. Will this soup make you giddy? Perhaps, and there would be nothing wrong with that. Be sure to use a Granny Smith apple; you need the tartness to stand up to the other flavors.

¼ cup salted butter
1 teaspoon minced garlic
1 tablespoon garam masala
1 tablespoon hot Madras curry powder
½ cup carrot, peeled and finely chopped
½ cup celery, finely chopped
½ cup onion, finely chopped
14.5-ounce can low-sodium chicken broth
14.5-ounce can petite diced tomatoes, with juice
¾ teaspoon salt
½ teaspoon black pepper
½ teaspoon dry thyme (1-2 tablespoons fresh, minced)
½ teaspoon turmeric
¼ teaspoon cayenne pepper
½ cup red lentils
4 ounces cooked chicken, diced
8 ounces Granny Smith apple; peeled, cored, and chopped coarsely
13.66-ounce can unsweetened coconut milk

OPTIONAL GARNISH:

Chopped fresh cilantro
Finely chopped cashews
Finely chopped slivered almonds
Unsweetened coconut

COAT a 4-quart saucepan with cooking spray. Melt the butter over medium heat. Add the garlic, garam masala, curry, carrot, celery, and onion and sauté over a low heat 8-10 minutes, stirring frequently (don't worry about any browning on the bottom of the pot).

Add the broth, tomatoes, the 5 seasonings, lentils, chicken, and apple and bring to a boil. Cook, covered, on lowest heat for 30 minutes. Stir a few times, scraping up any browned bits. Add the coconut milk and raise heat to medium/high. Cook on a gentle boil, uncovered, 4-5 minutes, until the vegetables and lentils are very tender. Season, if desired. Garnish, as desired. Cover and chill leftovers. Serves 3-4.

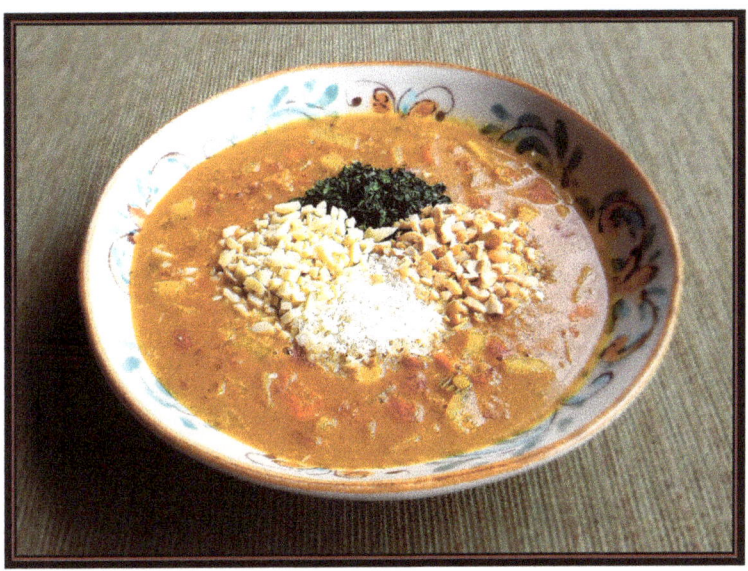

You'd need a broth substitution, of course, and simply omit the chicken and substitute a chopped summer squash (peeled, if it seems bitter).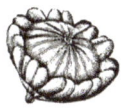

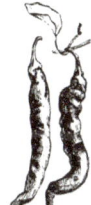 This soup is nicely spicy as is. Be sure to cut back on the various seasonings if you are sensitive to spice.

Mulligatawny is an English soup with Indian origins dating back to the late 1700s; it basically means "pepper water." Sometimes it is served with rice mixed into it, but I prefer the red lentils. Ordinary lentils should work as well, but the red ones are more delicate. Cook up a small pot of rice, if you would like to serve a scoop with your soup.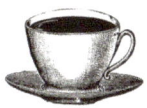

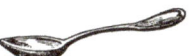

Chapter Two: Chicken   47

Casbah-Rockin' Chicken Stew

I've pushed the spice limits in this stew, to the point where it is one of the few recipes that Bob doesn't like. Plus, it has chickpeas (garbanzo beans) in it, which he mostly dislikes, except when they are in something like a three-bean salad. I love them, especially in hummus, or anywhere I can get them. This has a medieval influence about it, since I've mixed raisins with the chicken; it also has a sort of North African taste. So, I make it in a small batch, since I'm usually the only one who eats it. Chloë likes it quite a lot; perhaps you will, too!

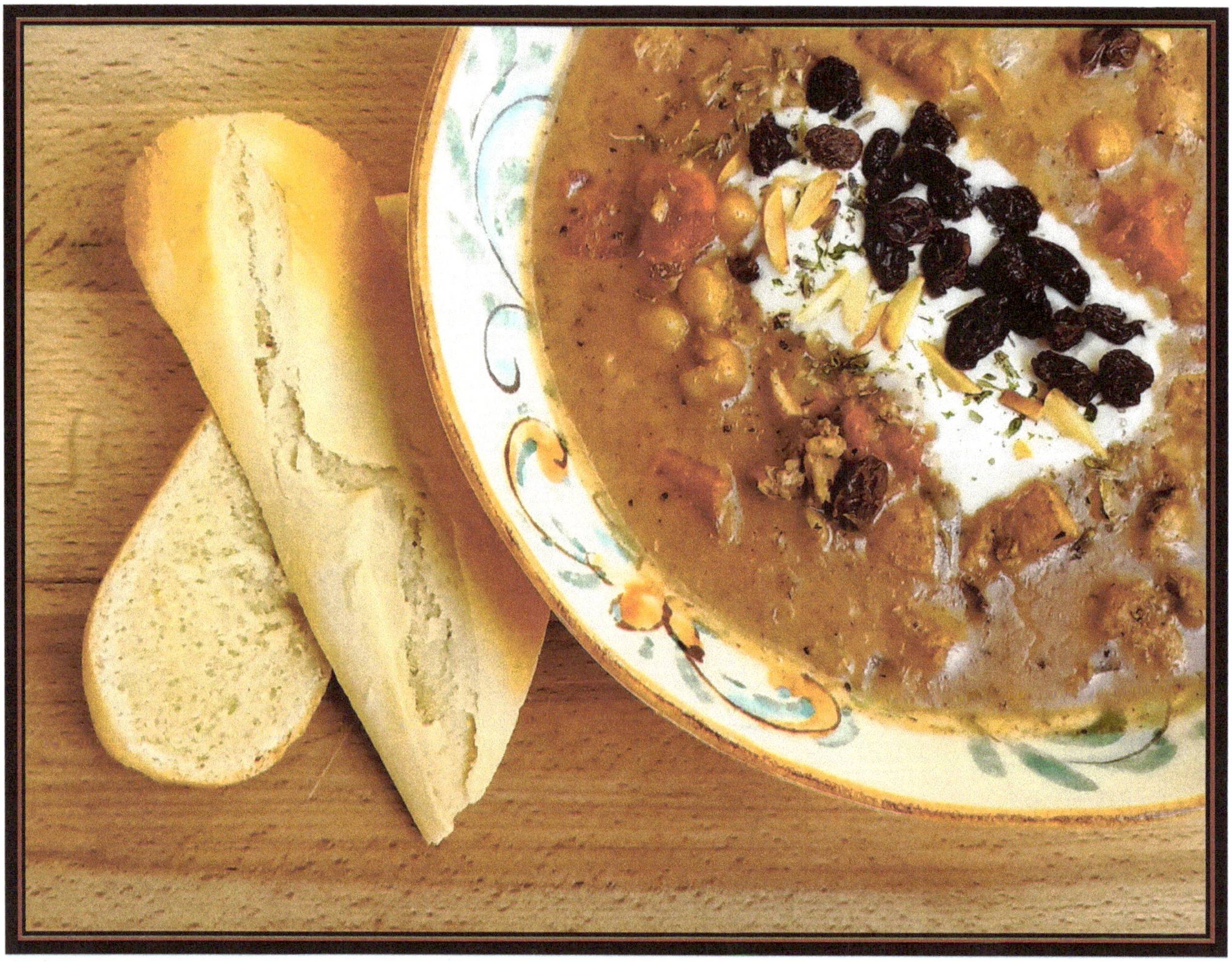

¼ cup salted butter
½ teaspoon dry thyme (1-2 tablespoons fresh, minced)
½ teaspoon dry basil (1-2 tablespoons fresh, minced)
½ teaspoon dry oregano (1-2 tablespoons fresh, minced)
1 teaspoon cinnamon
1 teaspoon ground cloves
1 teaspoon salt
1 teaspoon black pepper
1 teaspoon cumin
1 cup onion, coarsely chopped
1-1¼ pounds boneless, skinless chicken breasts, cut into ¾" bits
14.5-ounce can diced tomatoes, drained
15.5-ounce can chickpeas, drained
2 ounces raisins
2 ounces slivered almonds, lightly toasted
14.5-ounce can low-sodium chicken broth
½ cup heavy cream
2 tablespoons all-purpose flour

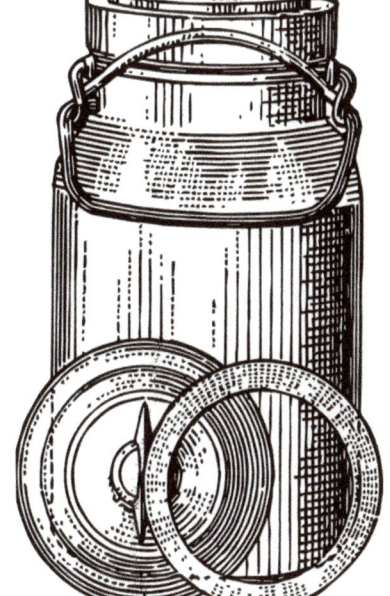

OPTIONAL GARNISH:

Crème fraîche
Lightly toasted slivered almonds
Raisins
A sprinkling of Easy Herbes de Provence (see page xxix), or any of the other herbs or spices mentioned in the recipe

COAT a 4-quart saucepan with cooking spray. Melt the butter and the 8 seasonings over rather high heat. Add the onion and chicken and sauté over rather high heat until most of the pink is gone, 5-7 minutes. Add the tomatoes, chickpeas, raisins, almonds, and broth and mix in. Bring to a boil then cook, covered, 20 minutes on low heat. Stir twice. Whisk the cream and flour in a 1-cup glass measuring cup; add a little of the hot broth to this, then add all back to the pot. Raise heat to medium; cook, uncovered, 4-5 minutes. Stir a few times. Season, if desired. Garnish, as desired. Cover and chill leftovers. Serves 3-4.

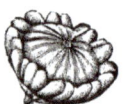 Use vegetable broth and two cans each of the tomatoes and chickpeas.

Hmm, spicy ideas... Nope!

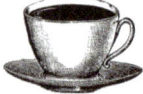 *This was invented as a Narnian recipe, which I originally called "Prince Rilian's Pigeon Pie." The stew lends itself to a puff pastry topping baked in individual bowls; hence, I felt I could get away with calling it a "pie." This was the scene in the book:*

> In a Dark Castle in C. S. Lewis's THE SILVER CHAIR, the characters of Jill, Scrubb, and Puddleglum encounter a mysterious, yet annoyingly charming nonetheless, Knight. He treats them to a feast of "pigeon pie, cold ham, salad, and cakes." He is obviously spellbound and tells his guests that he will "turn into the likeness of a great serpent, hungry, fierce, and deadly" unless he is strongly bound to a magical Silver Chair. The companions have been searching for a true sign as to their Prince's whereabouts. Fortunately for them, this Knight provides the correct sign and is indeed Prince Rilian, who is now released from his ten-year-long imprisonment.

I do wish they would hurry up and make this into a movie; I'd love to see the battle between our Narnian heroes and the Lady of the Green Kirtle, the witch who had held Prince Rilian captive. Now, if you want to be authentic to the book, you'd need to kill a few pigeons; pluck out their feathers, and otherwise dress them for inclusion in the stew. How many pigeons? I'm not sure, perhaps six would be sufficient. You can see why I'm calling for chicken, instead.

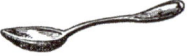

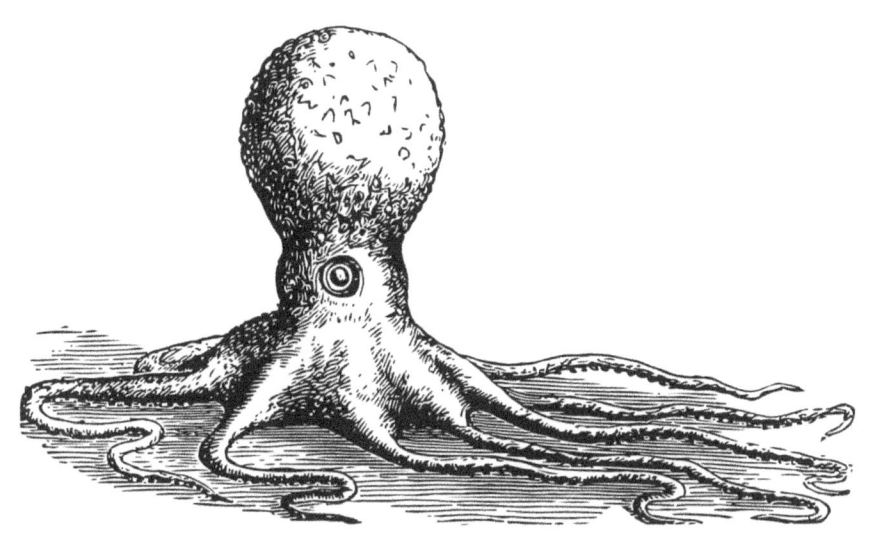
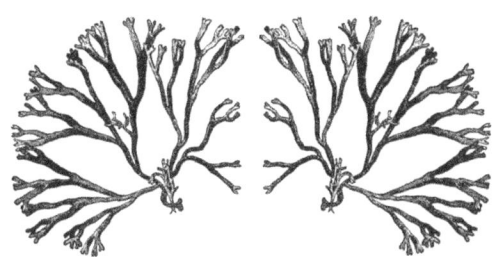
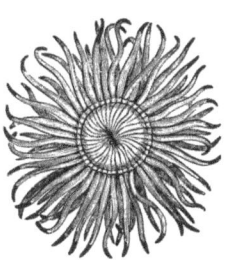

Mmm... So Spicy Miso Soup

(A.K.A. "Poe Pho")

This is the perfect place to try some exotic mushroom varieties such as enoki or brown clamshell; just leave them whole, and cut the stems down to an inch or two. As for the noodles, a flour-based type is preferred. Any sort of thin udon or even something like angel hair will work well.

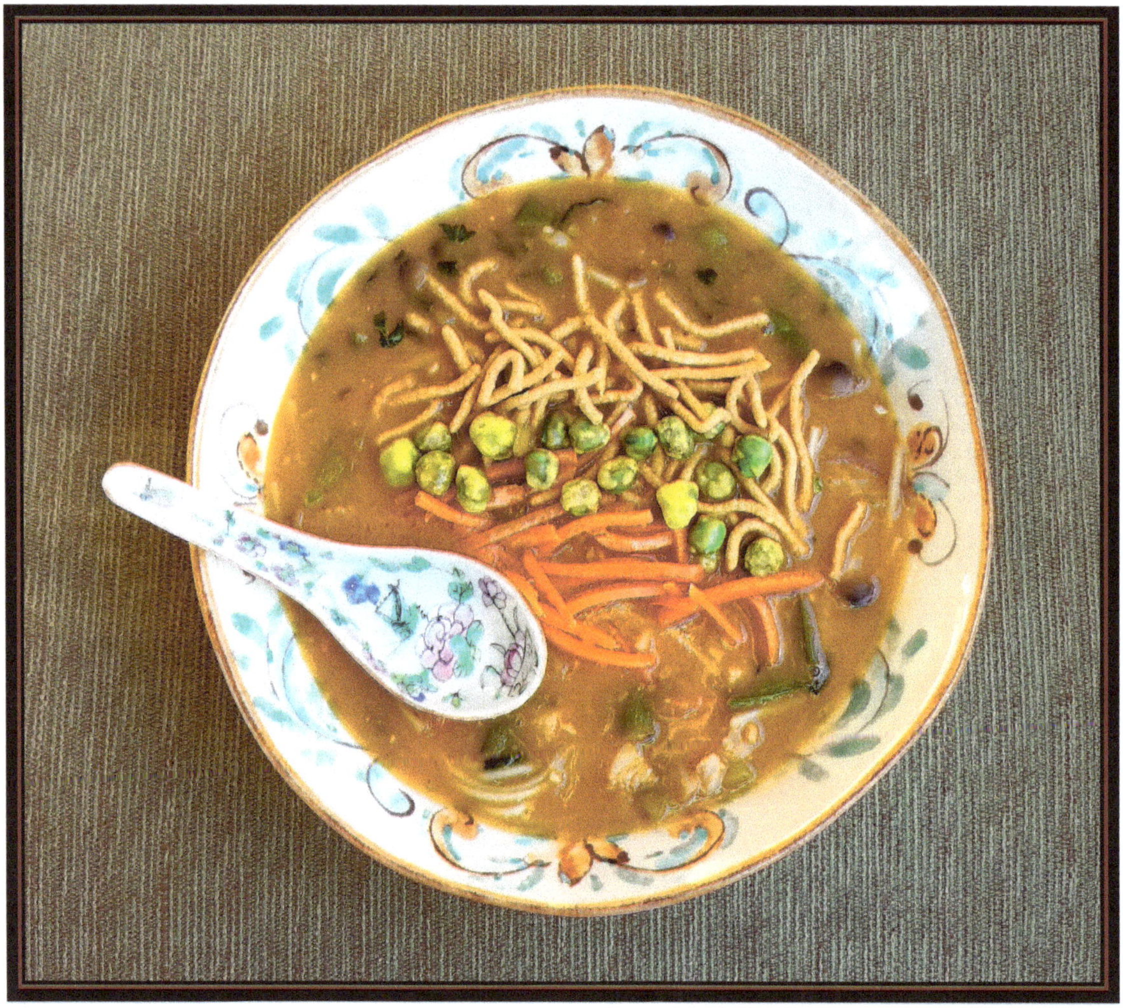

1 quart low-sodium chicken broth
1 cup water
¼ cup white miso (yellow is also fine; use red if you want to start off with
    a stronger and saltier flavor)
2 tablespoons soy sauce
1 tablespoon crushed ginger
1 tablespoon minced garlic
1 tablespoon Sriracha sauce (or more if you love it!)
1 tablespoon toasted sesame oil
1 cup cabbage, finely chopped
½ cup scallions, thinly sliced
½ cup carrot; peeled and shredded
    or cut into matchstick size
4 ounces mushrooms, thinly sliced
4 ounces snow pea pods; snip off stems,
    then cut vertically into thin slices
        (or just use 4 ounces frozen peas)
4 ounces cooked chicken, coarsely chopped
4 ounces very thin flour-type noodles or udon
½ cup loosely packed fresh basil,
    coarsely chopped

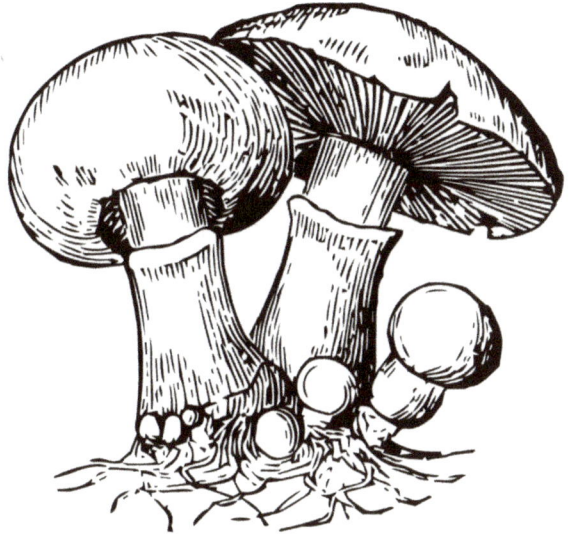

OPTIONAL GARNISH:

Shredded carrot and/or shredded cabbage
Wasabi peas
A drizzle of toasted sesame oil
Crunchy chow mein noodles or crispy rice sticks

COMBINE the broth, water, miso, soy sauce, ginger, garlic, Sriracha, and sesame oil in a 4-quart saucepan. Whisk well and bring to a boil. Cook on medium heat 5 minutes, uncovered. Add the cabbage, scallions, carrot, mushrooms, snow peas, and chicken and continue to cook on medium heat for 5 minutes, uncovered. Stir a few times. Break the noodles into halves or thirds and add to the pot. Raise heat and cook, uncovered, 5-10 minutes, until the noodles are done according to the package directions. Stir a few times. Mix in the basil and cook another minute. Season, if desired. Garnish, as desired. Cover and chill leftovers. Serves 3-4.

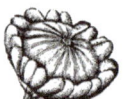 You could just use water instead of the chicken broth; omit the chicken and substitute a quarter pound of firm tofu, cut into ½" cubes.

Simply increase the Sriracha, or add your favorite Asian-influenced sauce.

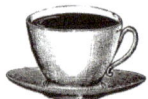 *I used this recipe in my* Star Wars *Internet writing. Here is the story, which takes place in* Star Wars: The Last Jedi:

> Perhaps before leading the rebels away from the Battle of Crait, Captain Poe Dameron found some time to make up a bit of soup. Or maybe he had already packed a thermos. If he prepared this soup on Crait, at least he wouldn't have any problems locating some salt. Finding a chicken might be problematic; would it be worthwhile to hunt for a vulptex? Hard to tell if those crystalline creatures would be appetizing, but you never know.

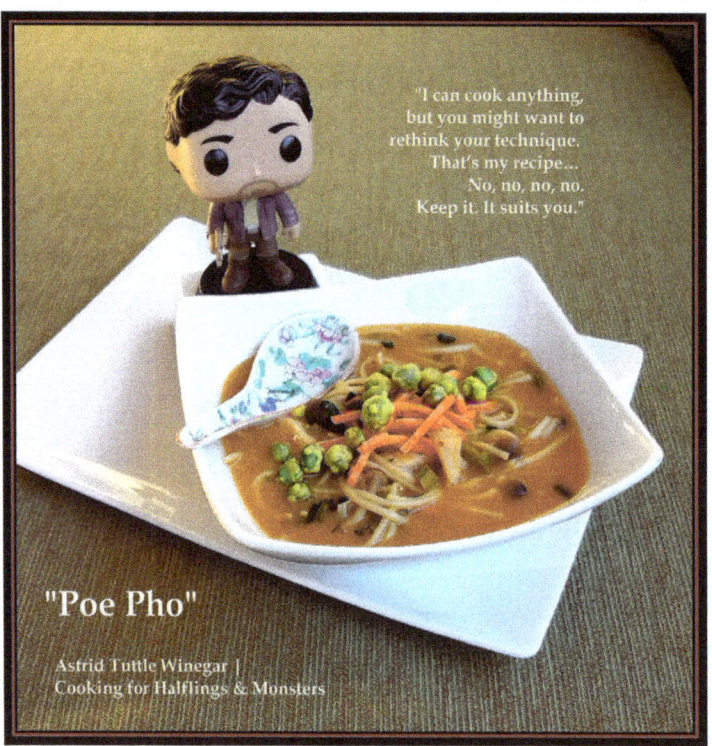

"Poe Pho"
Astrid Tuttle Winegar | Cooking for Halflings & Monsters

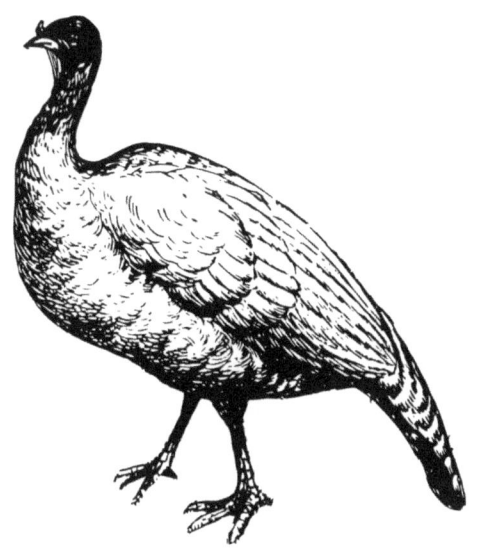
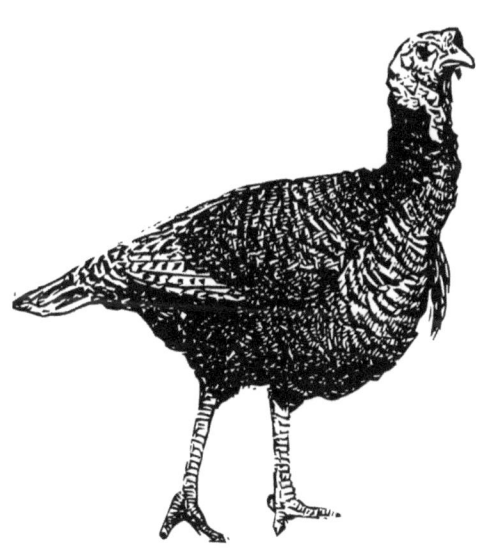

Turkey Black Bean Soup

Here's a great recipe to make after Thanksgiving, when you're looking for another way to use up some cooked turkey. Chicken will substitute perfectly.

2 tablespoons salted butter
1 tablespoon minced garlic
2 ounces precooked bacon, cut into ¼" slices
1½ cups carrot, peeled and thinly sliced
1 pound cooked turkey, cut into ½" cubes
2 (15.5-ounce) cans black beans,
    drained and rinsed
8 ounces roasted and chopped green chile,
    with juice
2 (14.5-ounce) cans low-sodium chicken broth
¼ cup cornmeal
¾ teaspoon salt
¾ teaspoon black pepper
¾ teaspoon dry thyme
    (1-2 tablespoons fresh, minced)
¾ teaspoon dry oregano
    (1-2 tablespoons fresh, minced)
¾ teaspoon chili powder
¾ teaspoon onion salt
1 cup heavy cream
6 ounces finely shredded Fiesta blend cheese

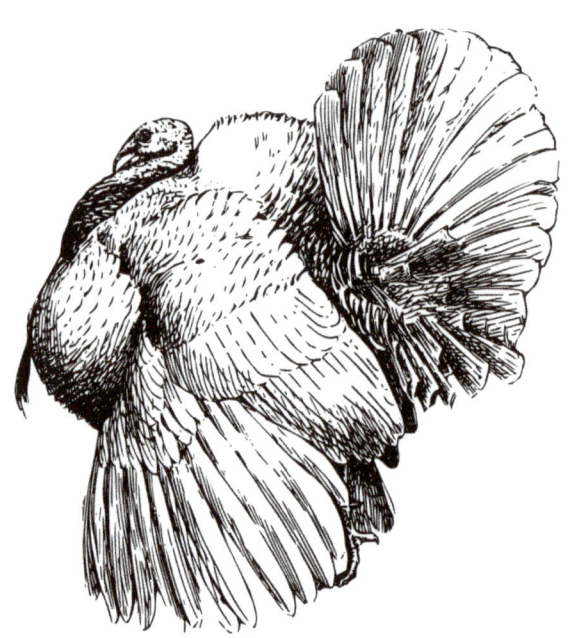

OPTIONAL GARNISH:

Crumbled Mexican cheese, such as queso Panela
Sour cream
A few spicy chips, such as Takis
Try any of the **NICE NEW MEXICAN & MEXICAN GARNISHES** you wish to use.

COAT a 6-quart saucepan with cooking spray. Melt the butter over moderately high heat. Add the garlic, bacon, and carrot, and sauté 5 minutes; stirring often. Add the turkey, beans, chile, broth, cornmeal, and the 6 seasonings. Bring to a boil. Cover and cook on lowest setting 20 minutes. Stir a few times. Add the cream and the cheese and raise heat to medium. Cook, uncovered, 5 minutes, until the soup is thicker, the cheese has melted, and the carrots are tender. Stir a few times. Season, if desired. Garnish, as desired. Cover and chill leftovers. Serves 4-6.

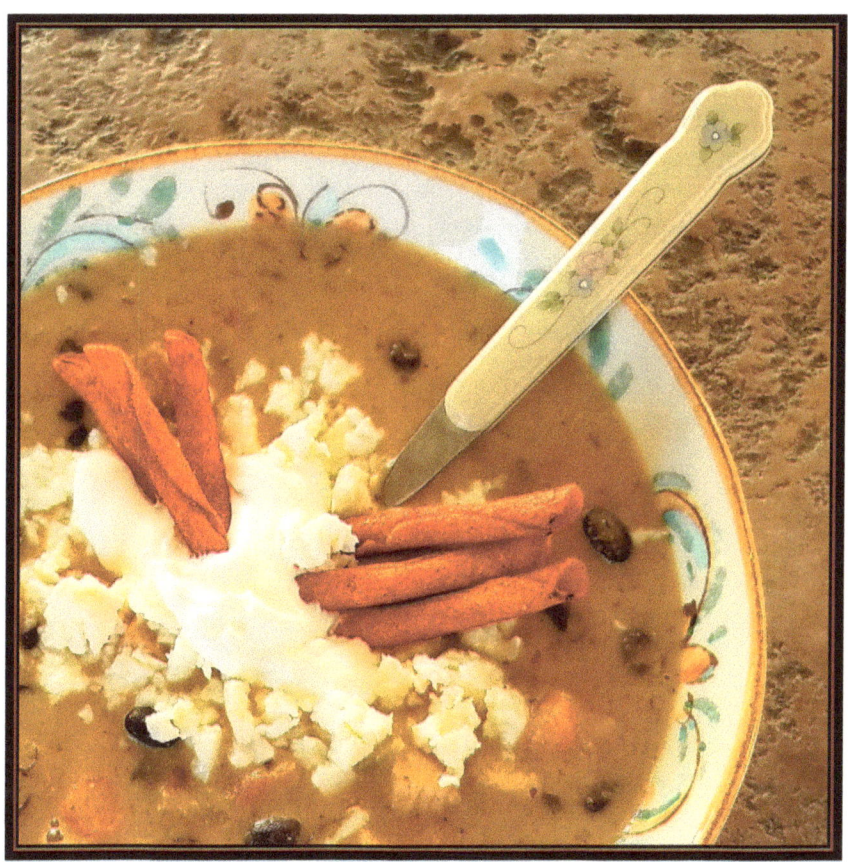

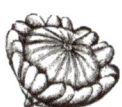 Change your broth to vegetable and substitute 1 pound (or 4 cups) of your preferred vegetables, cut into small chunks or sliced thinly. Just about any vegetable combination will work here: potatoes, celery, squash, peas, corn, onion, etc.

Change your broth to beef and use a pound of cooked ground beef or pork. Change your broth to clam juice or a seafood broth and add a pound of small raw shrimp (peeled, tails off) right near the end of cooking.

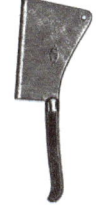

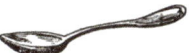

Chapter Two: Chicken   57

Callista's Amazing Avocado Chicken Soup

My daughter Callista was telling me about this soup she had whipped up on a whim. I told her it sounded amazing, but she hadn't written any of it down; she sort of remembered what she did, so I had to coax some memories out of her. This might not be exactly what she created, but she gave it a thumbs up. You wouldn't think that avocados would function well in a soup, and you might be concerned that they will turn brown after you store them for awhile. However, they last quite well in this soup—surprise!

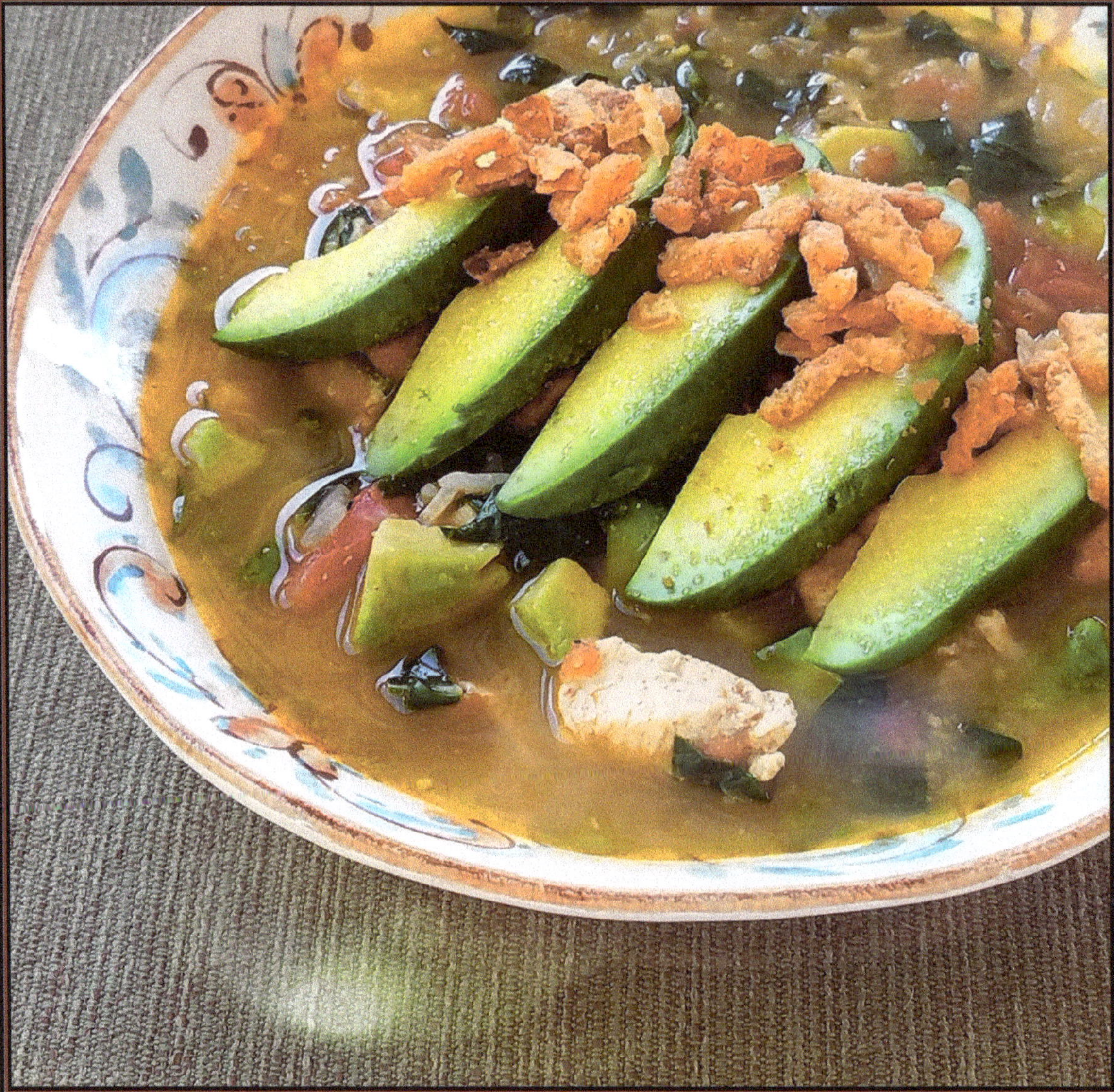

2 tablespoons salted butter
1 tablespoon minced garlic
1 teaspoon salt
1 teaspoon black pepper
1 teaspoon smoked paprika
1 teaspoon cumin
1 cup onion, coarsely chopped
1-1¼ pounds boneless, skinless chicken breasts, cut into ¾" chunks
1 quart low-sodium chicken broth
2 cups water
4 ounces roasted and chopped green chile, with juice
10-ounce can diced tomatoes with green chiles, with juice (such as Ro*Tel)
½ cup long grain rice
5-6 ounces fresh baby spinach, coarsely chopped
¾-1 pound avocados; peel, pit, and cut into ½" chunks (ripe, but not mushy)

OPTIONAL GARNISH:

Additional sliced or diced avocados
A sprinkling of pink Himalayan salt on the avocados (or coarse sea or kosher salt)
Crispy red peppers in a can (such as French's)
Crème fraîche
Many of the **NICE NEW MEXICAN & MEXICAN GARNISHES** will work well here, though preferably the lighter varieties.

COAT a 6-quart saucepan with cooking spray. Melt the butter over rather high heat. Sauté the garlic, salt, pepper, paprika, cumin, onion, and chicken until the pink is gone, 5-7 minutes. Add the broth, water, chile, and diced tomatoes with green chiles and bring to a boil. Add the rice and bring to a boil again, then cook on a rolling medium simmer 20 minutes, uncovered. Stir a few times. Add the spinach and cook another 1-2 minutes. Stir the avocados in gently and cook just for a few seconds. Season, if desired. Garnish, as desired. Cover and chill leftovers. Serves 4-6.

Substitute one pound of chopped summer squash varieties, such as yellow or zucchini, and substitute vegetable broth for the chicken broth.

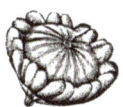

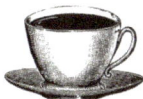

I've never frozen this soup, so I can't tell you how avocados will freeze. It never lasts that long; it's such a comforting soup, sort of a New Mexican version of a chicken noodle soup. You'll feel your sinuses opening up when you eat this, and you'll be glad.

Chapter Two: Chicken   59

Ten-Alarm Butternut Chicken Chili

You've heard of a five-alarm fire, perhaps. This chili is ten-alarm because it has twice as much fire power, though it mellows out as a leftover. If you need to go back to five, omit either the green chiles or the jalapeños, or you can make it the day before you want to serve it, then cover and chill it.

2 tablespoons salted butter
1 teaspoon sugar
1½ teaspoons salt, divided
1½ teaspoons black pepper, divided
½ teaspoon chipotle powder
1½ pounds butternut squash cubes, cut into ¾" chunks (I sometimes buy this prepackaged for convenience if I can find it; the weight reflects the actual amount of cubed squash, so you'd need about a 2½-pound squash to obtain the required amount)
4 ounces fresh jalapeños; cut off stems and ends, then cut into ¼" slices
2 tablespoons olive oil
1 tablespoon minced garlic
1 cup red onion, coarsely chopped
1-1¼ pounds boneless, skinless chicken thighs, cut into ¾" chunks
14.5-ounce can low-sodium chicken broth
12 ounces beer; any variety will do
½ teaspoon dry thyme (1-2 tablespoons fresh, minced)
15.5-ounce can pinto beans, drained and rinsed
15.5-ounce can cannellini beans, drained and rinsed
4 ounces roasted and chopped green chile, with juice
3 tablespoons cornmeal
½ cup heavy cream

Optional Garnish:

Finely shredded Fiesta blend cheese
Crispy jalapeños in a can or a bag
Sour cream or crème fraîche
Chipotle or chili powder
Any of the **Nice New Mexican & Mexican Garnishes** will work nicely.
Any of the **Charming Chili Garnishes** would be lovely.

PREHEAT oven to 350°. Coat an 11" by 7" baking dish with cooking spray or grease lightly. Melt butter in a 6-quart saucepan, then mix in sugar, ½ teaspoon salt, ½ teaspoon pepper, and chipotle powder. Add squash and jalapeños and mix well. Pour into prepared dish. Roast 45 minutes, until the squash is fork tender. Stir a couple of times. Remove and let stand in the dish. Don't bother washing out the pot.

MEANWHILE, coat the pot with cooking spray. Sauté the oil, garlic, onion, and chicken over rather high heat until the pink is gone; stir frequently. Add broth, beer, thyme, remaining salt and pepper, beans, chile, and cornmeal. Bring to a boil, then cook on medium/high (a gentle boil), uncovered, 30 minutes. Stir often; scrape up any browned bits. Add cream and mix in. Add the roasted vegetables and combine. Cook another 5 to 10 minutes, until the squash is very tender. Season, if desired. Garnish, as desired. Cover and chill leftovers. Serves 4-6.

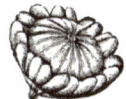 I would simply use two extra cans of beans, but a pound of other vegetables will also work well; whatever you like to throw in a chili.

Ground chicken will also work, as will ground beef, pork, or turkey.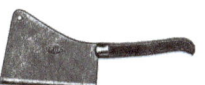

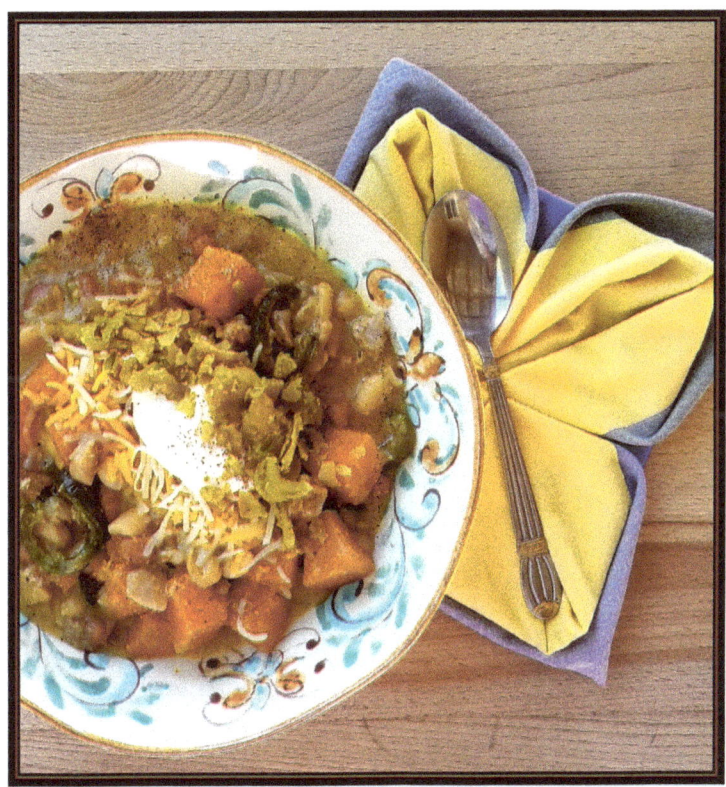

Sopa de los Burqueños

Your basic green chile chicken soup is ubiquitous in Albuquerque/New Mexican restaurants. It's even ubiquitous in non-New Mexican restaurants all around Albuquerque. And everyone claims their recipe is the best. Even award-winning. I've tried many, and I find that hard to believe for most of them. I've never entered mine in any contests, however, so I don't know if it would win or not. Restaurant versions can be too thick or too thin. They can have way too many vegetables in it. They sometimes don't seem to have any chicken at all in the bowl. Some resemble watered-down soup from a can.

Then there are other times when it can be sublime. So, I have attempted to create one of those sublime recipes. I've kept the variety of vegetables to a maximum of four—I don't waste time or space on bell peppers, potatoes, corn, or squash. The amount of chicken is generous. It is one of those ultimate comfort soup recipes. Check the anecdotal information at the end of the recipe for a quickie version.

Just use a 4-cup glass measuring cup for both wet and dry ingredients throughout the recipe, and don't bother to wash it out.

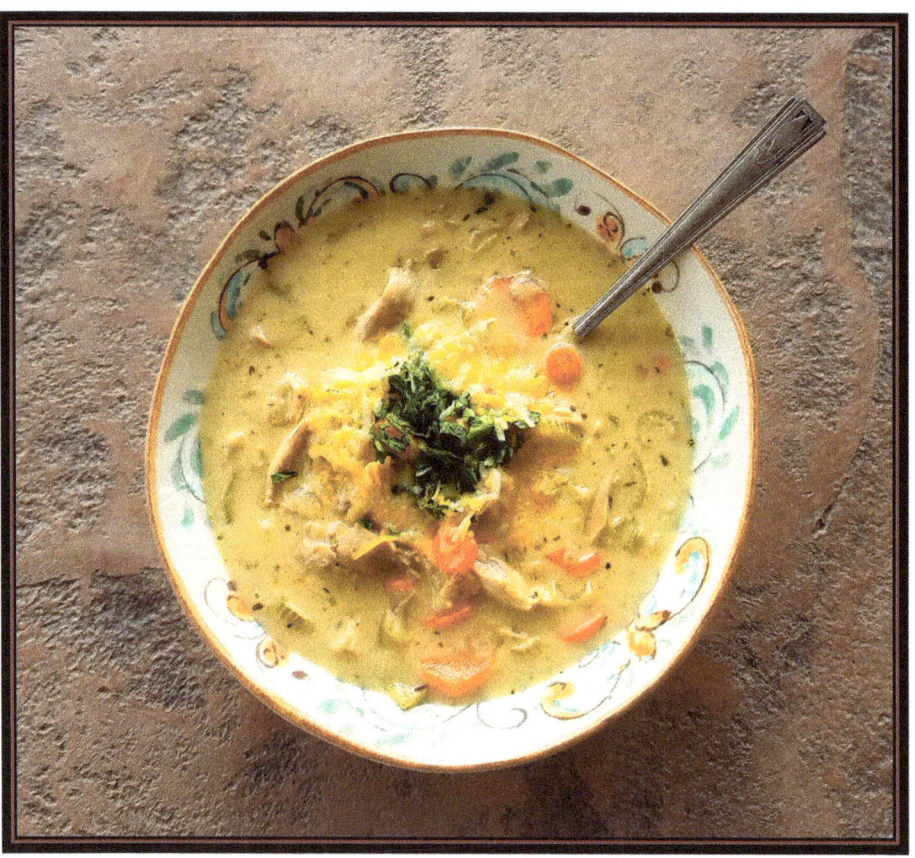

1 tablespoon salt
1 tablespoon whole peppercorns, black or mixed
8 cups water
A large unpeeled yellow onion, ¾ pound
A whole chicken, weighing 5-5½ pounds

COMBINE the salt, peppercorns, and water in an 8-quart saucepan. Wash the onion; cut into 6 wedges, and add to the pot. Rinse the chicken; cut off large neck fat and discard. Remove any giblets and add to the pot. Place the chicken in the pot and bring to a boil. Turn heat to lowest setting; cover and cook 45 minutes. Turn chicken over; cover and cook another 45 minutes on lowest setting. Place a large strainer over a very large bowl. Drain the chicken. Rinse out the pot and reuse it. When the chicken is cooler, remove all the meat and shred into 1-2" chunks and set aside; you should end up with 5 cups or so. Discard all onion, skin, bones, and giblets (will a lucky pet get some of those giblets?). You will need 8 cups of broth for the soup.

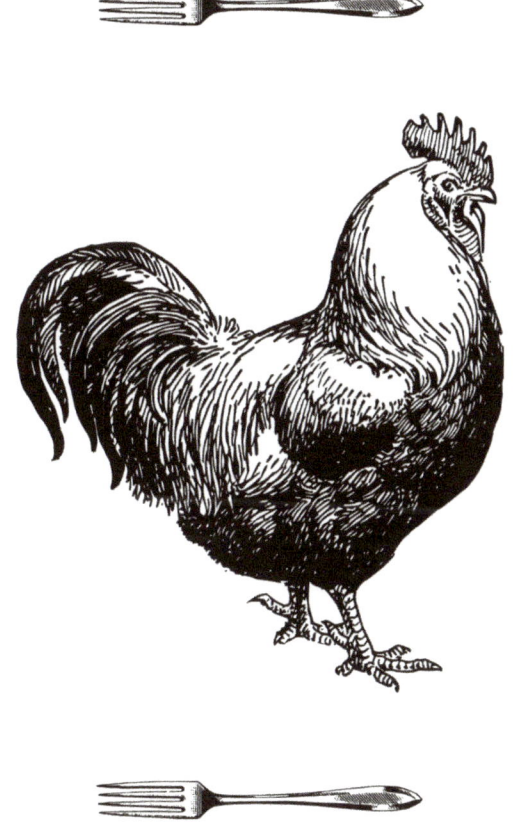

¼ cup salted butter
3 cups carrot, peeled and cut into ¼" slices
3 cups celery, cut into ¼" slices
3 cups onion, coarsely chopped
8 cups of prepared chicken stock (if you have leftover stock, reserve for another use)
12-13 ounces roasted and chopped green chile, with juice (1½ cups)
1 cup heavy cream
1 tablespoon dry oregano (2-3 tablespoons fresh, minced)
1 teaspoon salt
1 teaspoon black pepper
¾ cup water
¾ cup all-purpose flour

OPTIONAL GARNISH:

Chopped fresh cilantro
Finely shredded cheese, such as Cheddar or a Fiesta blend
Though any of the **NICE NEW MEXICAN & MEXICAN GARNISHES** will work out on this soup, you'll usually not see garnishes served much around Albuquerque. Yes, the soup is that good; why gild the lily?

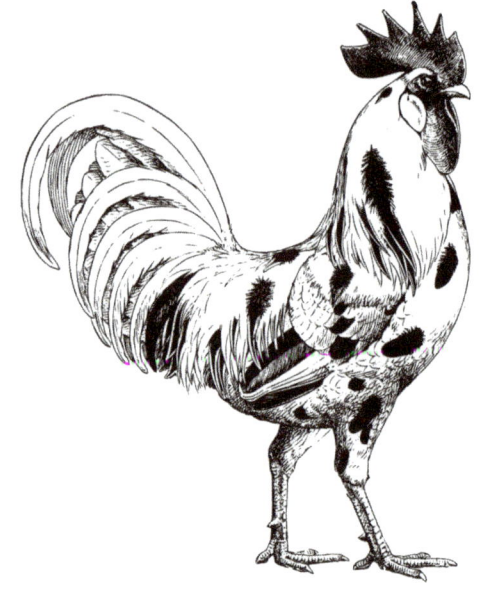

MELT the butter in the 8-quart saucepan over rather high heat. Add the carrot, celery, and onion and sauté 10 minutes. Add the stock and chile and bring to a boil. Reduce to a medium/high setting and cook 20 minutes, uncovered. Stir a few times. Add the reserved chicken and cook another 5 minutes. Add the cream and the 3 seasonings and raise the heat to get a boil going again. Combine the water and flour in the 4-cup glass measuring cup with a whisk. Add 1 cup of the hot soup to the flour mixture and whisk well. Mix this into the pot and cook at a gentle boil, 5-8 minutes, uncovered, until the soup is thicker and the vegetables are tender. Season, if desired. Garnish, as desired. Cover and chill leftovers. Serves 8-10. It keeps well for quite a few days and also freezes well.

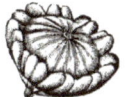 I know I was going on above about keeping the number of vegetables to a minimum, but if you switch to a vegetarian option, you would switch to a vegetable broth, of course, and coarsely chop about 5-6 cups of various vegetables, such as the ones mentioned above. Potatoes, bell peppers, peas, corn, beans, and squashes will all work out well; or perhaps you have some leftover items that need a new home. You could cut down on the total amount of carrot, celery, and onion, and replace them with your favorites for variety. Never cut down on the chile, however. Never. NEVER. (Yes, I'm aware of the irony inherent in my use of the word "never.")

For a quickie version, skip the entire section about cooking the whole bird and start with the butter/vegetable sauté. Use two quarts of low-sodium chicken broth and 1½ pounds of cooked chicken. Those grilled rotisserie chicken strips are perfect for this, coarsely chopped. Everything else remains the same.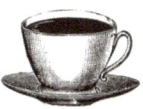

Burqueños are natives of Albuquerque, which includes our metropolitan area and extends to much of Central New Mexico. The term supposedly alludes to our particular accent, which none of us notice, of course. I moved here when I was six, so I do consider myself a Burqueña even though I was not born here. Quirky Albuquerque—where everybody eats a burrito for breakfast every single day if they can manage it (I can't manage this, though I certainly wish I could…), everybody has a Zia tattoo somewhere on his or her body (not on me; I have other tattoos), and everybody calls every single type of soft drink Coke (I am able to differentiate between various sodas). These stereotypical assumptions were spoofed in a funny online video called "Shit Burqueños Say," which is worth a watch, especially since it's only a couple of minutes long. Although I don't fulfill the Burqueña requirements listed above, I have encountered people who do. Sort of; hey, don't we all know people who endearingly embody local stereotypes?

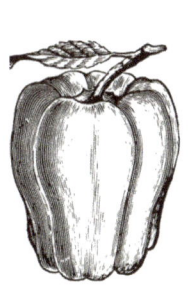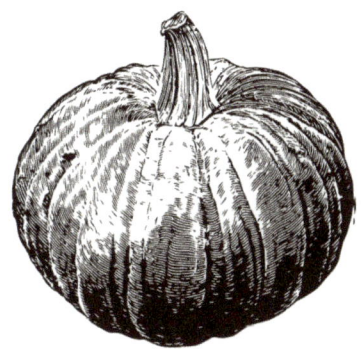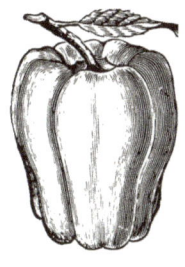

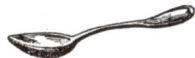

Chapter Two: Chicken   65

Stracciatella Bella

(A.K.A. "Hoth Broth")

This is the Italian version of egg drop soup; so savory, so comforting.

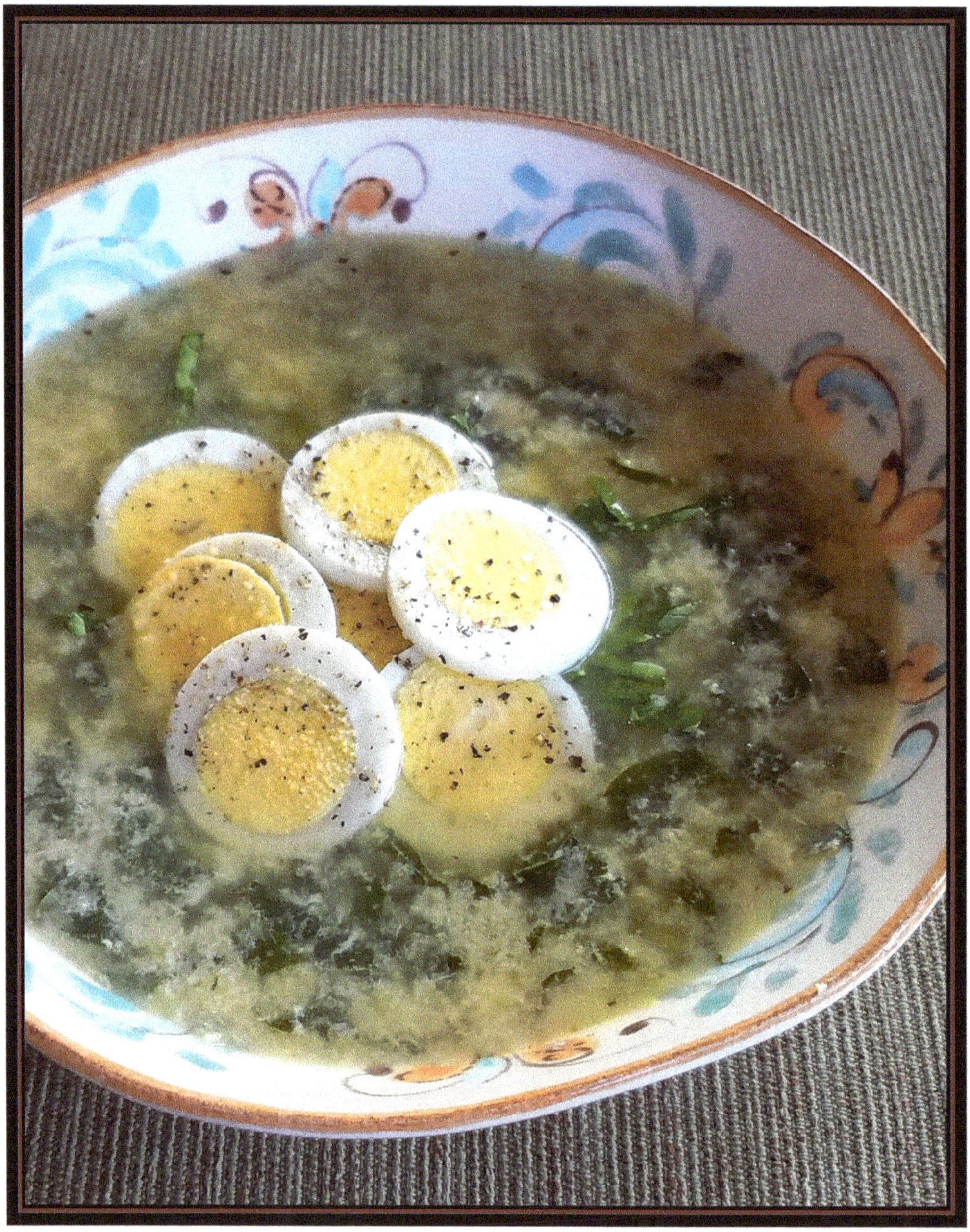

2 quarts low-sodium chicken broth
1 teaspoon salt
1 teaspoon black pepper
8 ounces cooked chicken, diced or shredded
5-6 ounces fresh baby spinach, cut into thin slices
1 cup packed fresh basil leaves, cut into thin slices
4 ounces fresh Parmesan and/or Romano cheese, finely shredded
4 large eggs

OPTIONAL GARNISH:

Sliced hard-boiled eggs with a sprinkling of coarse salt and/or freshly ground black pepper
Other minced fresh herbs, such as more basil
Finely shredded fresh Parmesan and/or Romano cheese

BRING broth to a boil in a 6-quart saucepan. Add the salt, pepper, chicken, spinach, basil, and cheese and bring to a boil again. Cook on medium (a gentle boil), uncovered, 10 minutes. Stir a few times. Whisk the eggs well in a 4-cup glass measuring cup. Turn heat to lowest setting. Slowly pour eggs into the pot and stir slowly back and forth and side to side with a fork or whisk to make thin threads; cook on low another minute. Season, if desired. Garnish, as desired. Cover and chill leftovers. Serves 6-8.

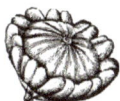 Change broth to vegetable and substitute half a pound of thinly sliced mushrooms for the chicken.

If spice brings you comfort, go ahead and add green chile (4 ounces) or throw in a teaspoon or so of crushed red pepper flakes.

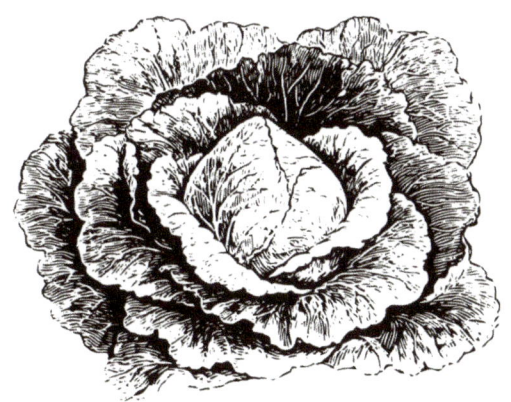

Chapter Two: Chicken   67

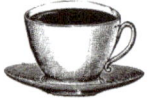 *This was a recipe I used for my* Star Wars *Internet writing, hence the "a.k.a." designation in the title. Life has a habit of surprising you, sometimes unpleasantly. Oddly enough, the timing for this particular post occurred during the month of January, 2017, right after we lost our Princess. And then her mother followed so soon, to add to the tragedy. Now, I'm not in the habit of writing elegies; I'm more of a bottle-everything-up-and-occasionally-weep-quietly-in-my-bedroom type of person. I definitely did some weeping during the awful year that called itself 2016. On New Year's Eve and Day of 2017, however, Bob and I wanted to do something cheerful, so we decided to watch the Austin Powers movie trilogy. It had been many years since we had seen them. And there was Carrie Fisher, in an uncredited role as a family therapist to Dr. Evil and his son Scott. She was a generous soul.*

Here is the post (which references a scene in Star Wars: The Empire Strikes Back*) with its accompanying photograph:*

> Well, it's January and pretty cold, maybe not Hoth cold, exactly, but cold. Perhaps you need a delicious chicken soup to warm you up. If only Han Solo had thought about packing a thermos filled with a nourishing soup like this, he wouldn't have had to cut open that tauntaun. Poor Luke Skywalker—injured and traumatized by a vicious wampa, then unceremoniously stuffed inside a stinky tauntaun just to stay alive. Luke was probably having nightmares about the wampa the whole time he was stuck in that unfortunate animal's guts. It's a safe bet that wampas are pretty foul-smelling, too.

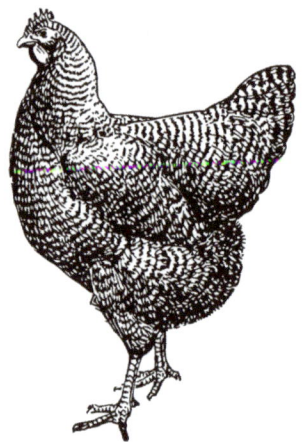 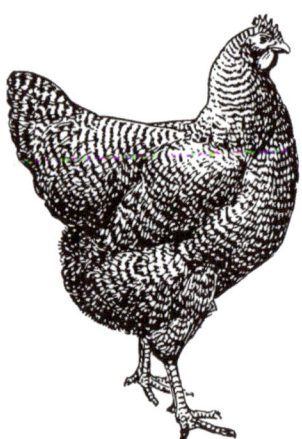

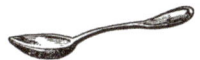

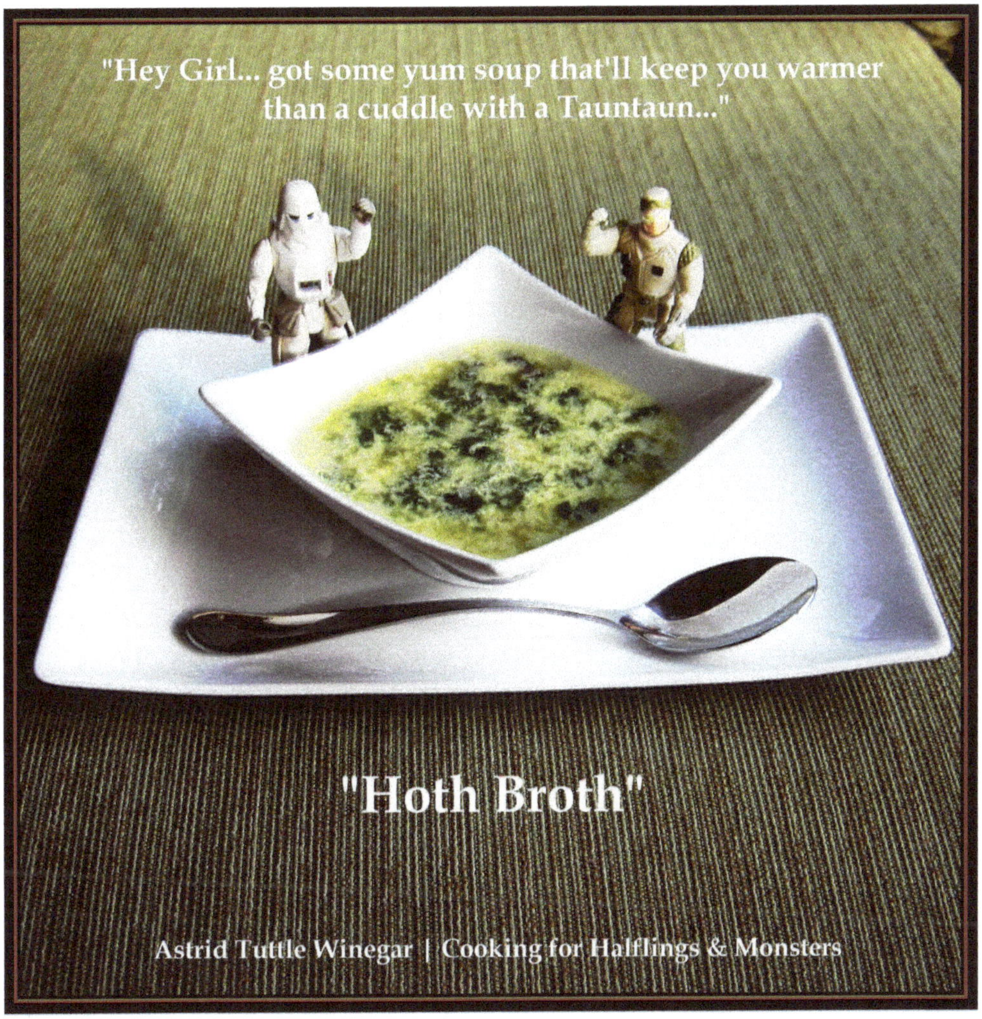

"Hey Girl... got some yum soup that'll keep you warmer than a cuddle with a Tauntaun..."

"Hoth Broth"

Astrid Tuttle Winegar | Cooking for Halflings & Monsters

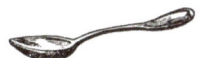

BONUS: "Rey's Savory Quarter-Portion"

(A.K.A. PUFFY SPINACH BREAD)

Even though I have a chapter on bread products, I'm including this item here after the "Hoth Broth" not only because it is a Star Wars recipe, but also because it uses a few spinach leaves. It's an odd little product, which I invented after *Star Wars: The Force Awakens* was released. Here is the story:

> Unfortunate Rey has to work all day in the blistering Jakku sun, gathering junk to trade with the rather vile Unkar Plutt. One day, her haul netted her a "quarter-portion," which she took home and hydrated for her supper. Her meal is merely nutritious, but not joyful. Now, if only Rey could see into the future—Jedi skills? A Millennium Falcon?? Kylo Ren???
> On second thought, maybe it's better not to know…

Now… I know you're thinking my photo doesn't look EXACTLY like the film's version. I'm also using a microwave, fresh spinach, and cooking spray. (Get over it!) However, this is a very edible, savory little bread product, unlike the "polystarch" product produced in the film, which was apparently extremely UN-edible. It is weirdly sponge-like in texture, but strangely tasty and easy to make. One of my recipe testers compared it to the Indian bread *idli*, which is a spongy, steamed bread. Try it when you have a few leaves of spinach around, such as when you make the previous recipe.

¼ cup fresh buttermilk
6 large fresh baby spinach leaves
¼ cup cake flour
1 tablespoon semolina flour
1 tablespoon dry Parmesan cheese
    (Parmesan and/or Romano is fine)
½ teaspoon baking powder
½ teaspoon dry oregano (1-2 tablespoons
    fresh, minced)
½ teaspoon garlic powder
¼ teaspoon salt
Butter or margarine

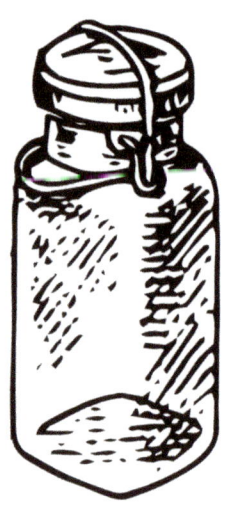

COAT a 12-ounce microwave-safe ceramic mug (preferably one that is rather open at the top) with cooking spray or grease lightly. Combine the buttermilk and spinach in a small food processor or blender and pulse until well combined. Add the remaining ingredients and process well. Pour into prepared mug. Microwave on HIGH 90 seconds. Let it stand in the microwave for 10 seconds. Invert onto a plate and serve while warm. Pull it apart and spread some butter or margarine over each bite. Leftovers? Probably not an issue, but you could cover and chill any leftover bits. Makes 1.

GOOD PAIRINGS:

- � Stracciatella Bella (a.k.a. "Hoth Broth")
- � Elegantly Sufficient Egg Drop Soup
- � It's a Nice Day for a Wedding Soup
- � Callista's Amazing Avocado Chicken Soup

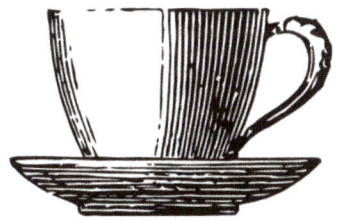

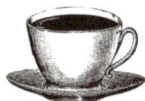 *Mug cakes and breads were sort of a rage for awhile. Mostly cakes now, I've been seeing all sorts of varieties at the grocery store. Beware of looking at the actual sugar content of those products! Yikes! Though I suppose we would all be surprised if we knew how much sugar was in all of our favorite sweets. I've paired this funky little carb with some of the soup recipes that utilize spinach, mainly so you can reserve a few leaves and whip this up for grins.*

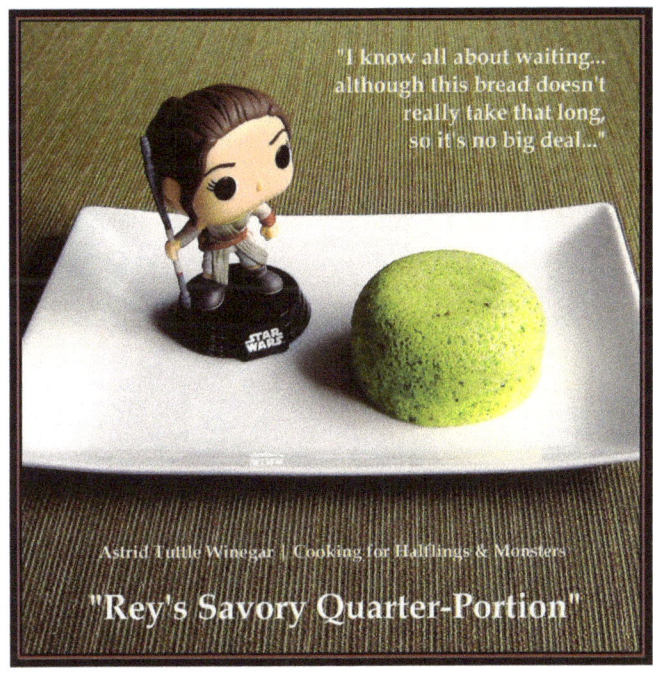

"I know all about waiting... although this bread doesn't really take that long, so it's no big deal..."

Astrid Tuttle Winegar | Cooking for Halflings & Monsters

"Rey's Savory Quarter-Portion"

Chapter Three

Pork & Seafood

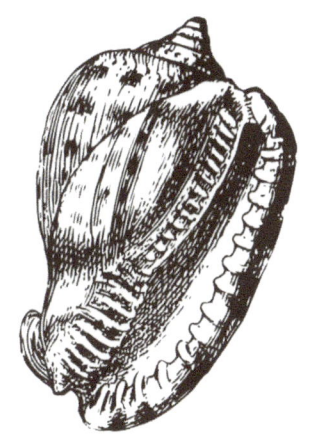

Donna's Christmas Eve Posole
Sassy Shrimp Posole
Notorious CSC
Carpe Caldillo
Esther's Manhattan Clam Chowder
Jumbo Gumbo
Butternut Risotto Soup
Asbjorn's New England Clam Chowder
Tecolote Chili
Funky Artichoke Bisque
Bob Hates Cauliflower Soup
Tater Ham Chowder
Chloë's Kale-apalooza

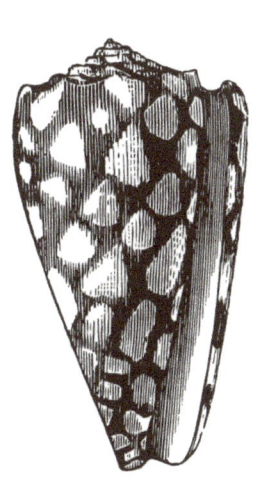

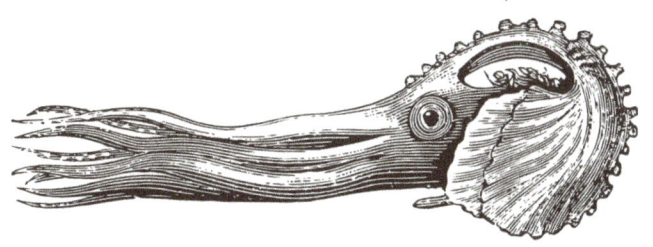

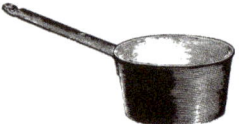 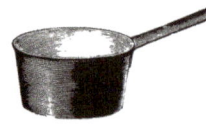

Chapter Three—Pork & Seafood

(ham, bacon, and sausage)

Though I have itemized various pork products, I have not differentiated between various seafood items. A few of the recipes in this chapter combine pork and seafood, so they fit together nicely. Bob is not the biggest fan of certain types of seafood, so I don't have a separate chapter for fish.

Donna's Christmas Eve Posole

My husband's cousin Donna supposedly didn't like posole of any kind. It turns out she just hadn't tasted the right posole. This was the first one she tried at our house around Christmas time back in the late 1980s and I'm proud to say she was converted. From then on, she always looked forward to having a bowl. For many years, I hosted the Winegar side of the family on Christmas Eve; she would come with her mother, who was an identical twin to my mother-in-law.

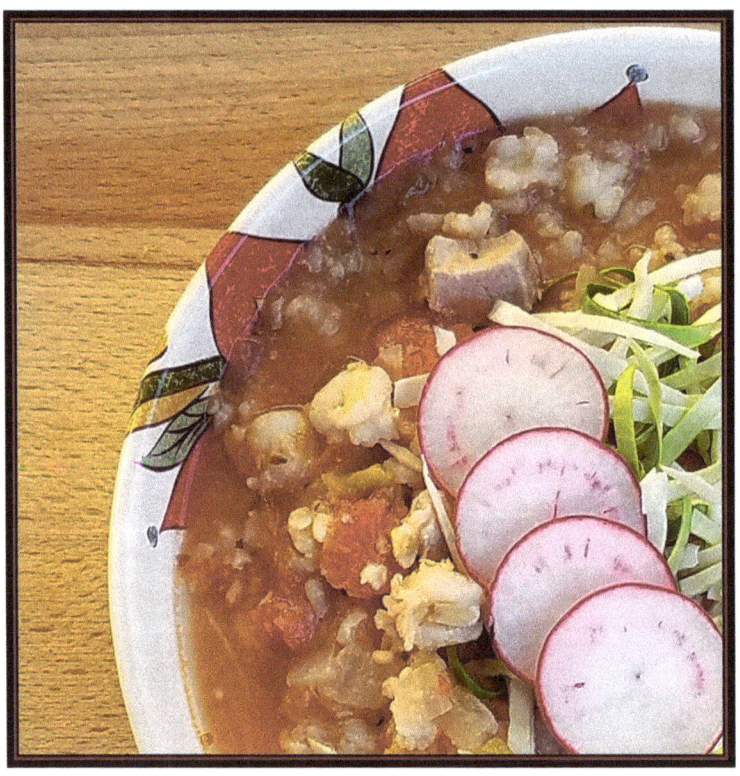

1 quart water
14.5-ounce can diced tomatoes, with juice
1 cup onion, coarsely chopped
2 (15.5-ounce) cans white hominy, drained and rinsed (if you like, or 3 cups cooked hominy; yellow hominy is also fine)
1 tablespoon minced garlic
1 teaspoon salt
½ teaspoon black pepper
½ teaspoon dry oregano (1-2 tablespoons fresh, minced)
½ teaspoon dry thyme (1-2 tablespoons fresh, minced)
1¼ pounds pork tenderloin or sirloin, cut into ¾" bits
8 ounces roasted and chopped green chile, with juice

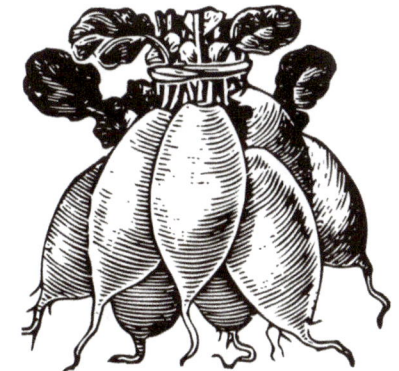

OPTIONAL GARNISH:

Shredded cabbage
Paper-thin radish slices
Just about any of your favorites from the NICE NEW MEXICAN & MEXICAN GARNISHES section will complement this posole.

COMBINE the water, tomatoes, onion, hominy, garlic, the 4 seasonings, and pork in a 4-quart saucepan. Bring to a boil, then simmer on lowest heat 1 hour, uncovered. Stir a few times. Add the green chile and continue to simmer on lowest heat for 30 minutes, covered. Season, if desired. Garnish, as desired. Cover and chill leftovers. Serves 4-6.

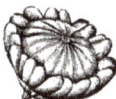 Replace the pork with a pound or so of coarsely chopped summer squashes; peel them or not. Or use an additional can of hominy and another cup of onion. Cook about 30 minutes less.

Chicken would be fine in this recipe, either white or dark meat.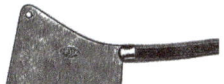

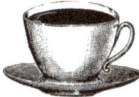 *I know cheap cuts of meat are all the rage in the culinary world, but please don't substitute extremely cheap cuts of pork; you'll end up trimming forever. This will freeze well, but why? It'll keep for a week or so and taste better with each day.*

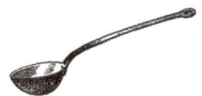

Chapter Three: Pork & Seafood

Sassy Shrimp Posole

Use raw, medium shrimp (36-40 per pound) for this ultra-light posole, and thaw as directed, if you are using frozen. Give them a rinse and a paper towel pat dry. If you use bigger shrimp, cut them in half. And if you use cooked shrimp, throw them in right at the end of cooking.

This posole is rather heavy on the cilantro. Do you hate cilantro? Apparently, quite a few people do; I guess it's one of those herbs you either love or hate. You can simply omit it, or you might want to substitute fresh parsley.

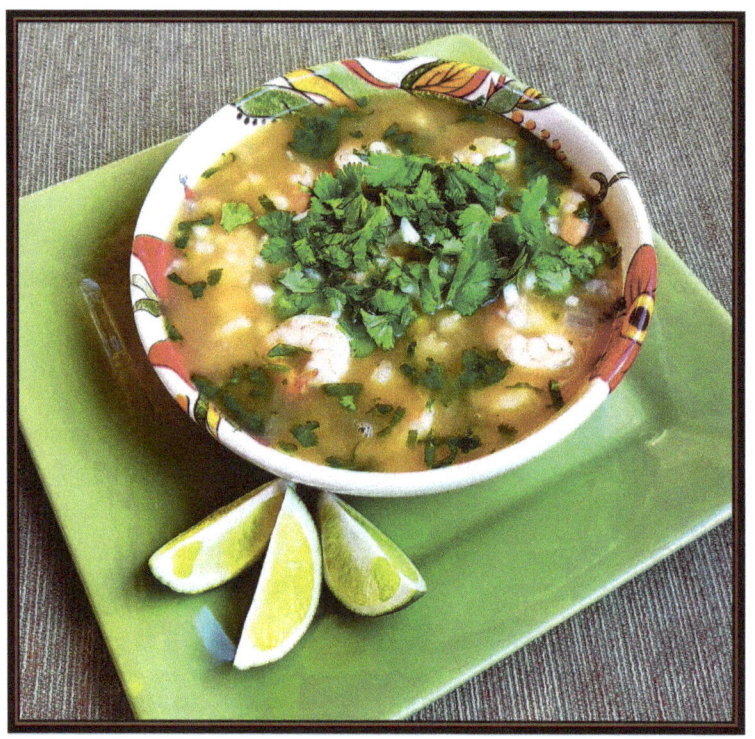

1 tablespoon vegetable oil
1 tablespoon minced garlic
1 cup onion, coarsely chopped
8 ounces roasted and chopped green chile, with juice
1 quart low-sodium chicken broth
1 cup water
2 (15.5-ounce) cans white hominy, drained and rinsed (if you like, or 3 cups cooked hominy; yellow hominy is also fine)
1 cup corn (fresh, frozen, or canned—drain first)

¾ cup fresh cilantro, finely chopped
½ teaspoon salt
½ teaspoon white pepper
1 pound raw medium shrimp,
      peeled and tails removed

OPTIONAL GARNISH:

Additional fresh chopped cilantro
Diced white onion
Lime wedges
Some of the **NICE NEW MEXICAN & MEXICAN GARNISHES** will work well with this posole, but especially the lighter vegetable ones.

HEAT the oil in a 6-quart saucepan on medium heat. Sauté the onion and garlic for 5 minutes. Add chile, broth, water, hominy, and corn and bring to a boil. Reduce heat to medium/high and cook 20 minutes, uncovered. Stir a couple times. Add remaining ingredients and, if necessary, raise heat to maintain a rolling simmer. Cook another 3-5 minutes, until your shrimp is just cooked through, but not overcooked. Season, if desired. Garnish, as desired. Cover and chill leftovers. Serves 4-6.

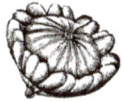 Use vegetable broth and substitute a pound of various summer squashes, chopped coarsely. You can peel them if you wish, or not, depending on their bitterness. Cook vegetables along with the corn and hominy.

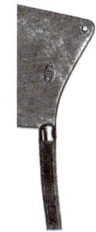

If you dislike seafood, try a pound of chicken, preferably breast meat. If cooked, add at the end. If raw, dice it up and sauté with the onion mixture.

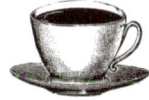 *Try using a combination of seafood, such as shrimp and bay scallops. Lobster, crab, or other fish will work well in this delicate broth.*

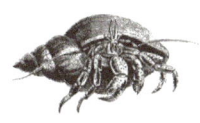 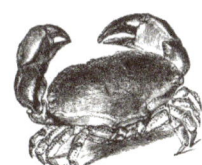 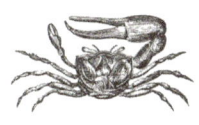

Chapter Three: Pork & Seafood   77

Notorious CSC

Otherwise known as Curry Shrimp Chowder (with a nod to my favorite Supreme Court justice), this recipe could definitely lend itself to a bisque treatment. Simply puree the soup before you add the shrimp, then place it back in your saucepan. Add the shrimp and heat for about a minute or so.

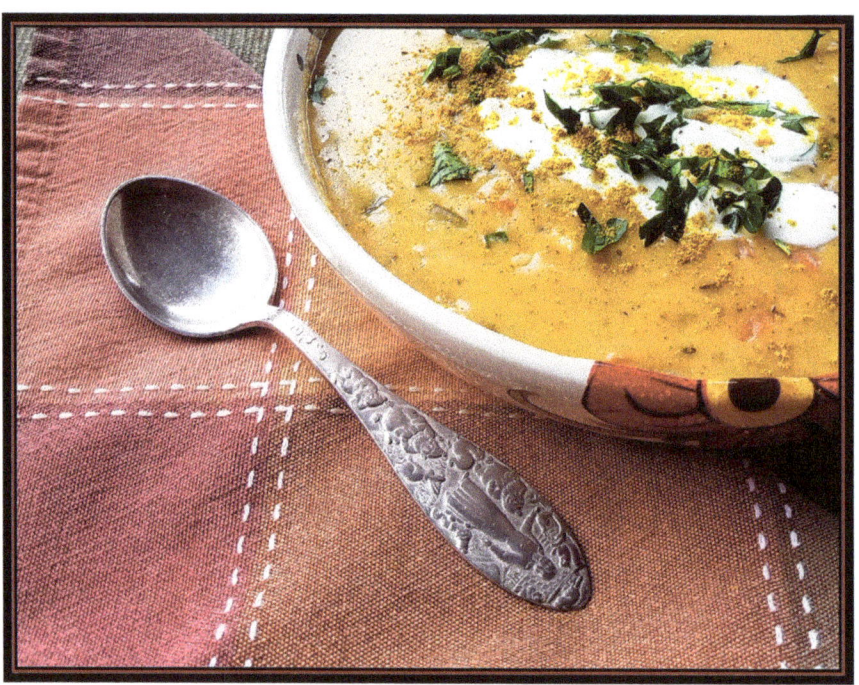

1 tablespoon salted butter
1 tablespoon olive oil
4 teaspoons hot Madras curry powder
1 teaspoon minced garlic
1 teaspoon salt
¾ teaspoon black pepper
¾ teaspoon dry thyme (1-2 tablespoons fresh, minced)
¾ teaspoon smoked paprika
¾ cup carrots, peeled and coarsely chopped
¾ cup celery, coarsely chopped
¾ cup shallots, coarsely chopped
1 quart low-sodium chicken broth

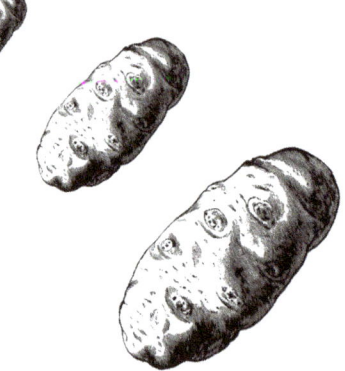

8 ounces potato, cut into ½" bits (peeled or not; it depends on the variety you use)
1 large bay leaf
½ cup heavy cream
¼ cup water
¼ cup cornstarch
8 ounces frozen tiny whole shrimp, cooked and peeled; thawed as directed (or you may use 4 [4-ounce] cans tiny shrimp, drained)

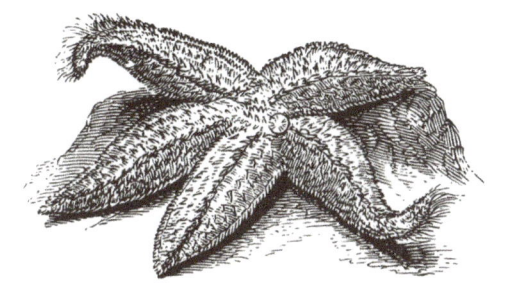

OPTIONAL GARNISH:

Crème fraîche
Minced fresh parsley or chives
An extra sprinkling of curry powder

COAT a 3-quart saucepan with cooking spray. Melt the butter and oil over medium heat. Add the curry, garlic, salt, pepper, thyme, paprika, carrot, celery, and shallots and sauté 8-10 minutes on a medium/low heat, stirring frequently. Add the broth, potato, and bay leaf and bring to a boil. Cook on lowest heat, covered, 20 minutes. Stir a few times; scrape up any browned bits. Add the cream and mix in. Whisk the water and cornstarch well in a 1-cup glass measuring cup. Raise heat to medium to start some bubbling, then whisk in the cornstarch mixture. Cook 2-3 minutes, uncovered, on a low simmer. Add shrimp and cook 1 minute. Remove bay leaf. Season, if desired. Garnish, as desired. Cover and chill leftovers; don't freeze. Serves 3-4.

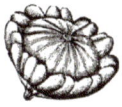 Replace the broth with vegetable broth and omit the shrimp. Substitute a cup or two of fresh or frozen corn and add with the potatoes.

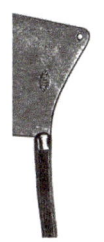 Omit the shrimp and substitute a half pound of other cooked meat, such as chicken or ham, cut into small bits; sausage or bacon would be good as well.

Well, of course, this could be delicious; how about half a cup of salsa or green chile? Yum. Or you could simply increase the amount of curry powder; try 2 tablespoons instead.

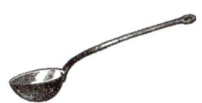

Carpe Caldillo

I used to teach Latin when I was a graduate student at the University of New Mexico. Now, that was quite a few years ago and much of my Latin has faded from my memory, but I figured I'd integrate it into this title. *Carpe*, of course, means "seize," and *caldillo* basically means "green chile stew prepared in a light broth with bits of meat." Simplify the concept and make this quick recipe, which will definitely make you want to "Seize the Green Chile Stew!" Pronounce it *car-pay-cal-dee-oh*. Any potato is fine, though I prefer to use something like thin-skinned gold potatoes here. You can use unpeeled red potatoes, or chopped fingerlings. I would peel russets, however.

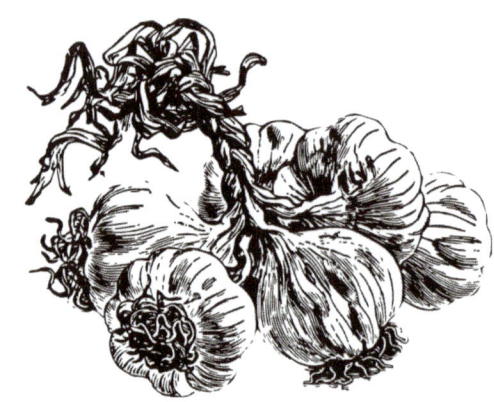

1 tablespoon vegetable oil
2 tablespoons fresh garlic, sliced paper thin
2 cups onion, coarsely chopped
1-1¼ pounds pork sirloin or tenderloin,
 cut into ¾" chunks
1 quart low-sodium chicken broth
1 pound potatoes, cut into ¾" chunks
 (peeled or not, it depends on
 the variety you choose)
14.5-ounce can petite diced tomatoes,
 with juice
8 ounces roasted and chopped green chile, with juice
1 teaspoon dry oregano (2-3 tablespoons fresh, minced)
¾ teaspoon salt
¾ teaspoon cumin
½ teaspoon black pepper

OPTIONAL GARNISH:

Table cream, sour cream, or crème fraîche
Sliced or diced avocado
Absolutely any of the **NICE NEW MEXICAN & MEXICAN GARNISHES** will be delicious in your bowl!

COAT a 6-quart saucepan with cooking spray. Sauté the oil, garlic, onion, and pork on rather high heat until the pink is mostly gone. Add the remaining ingredients and bring to a boil. Reduce heat to a low simmer; cover and cook 15 minutes. Stir occasionally. Raise heat to a rolling simmer and cook, uncovered, 15-20 minutes longer, until the potatoes are tender; stir a few times. Season, if desired. Garnish, as desired. Cover and chill leftovers; don't freeze. Serves 4-6.

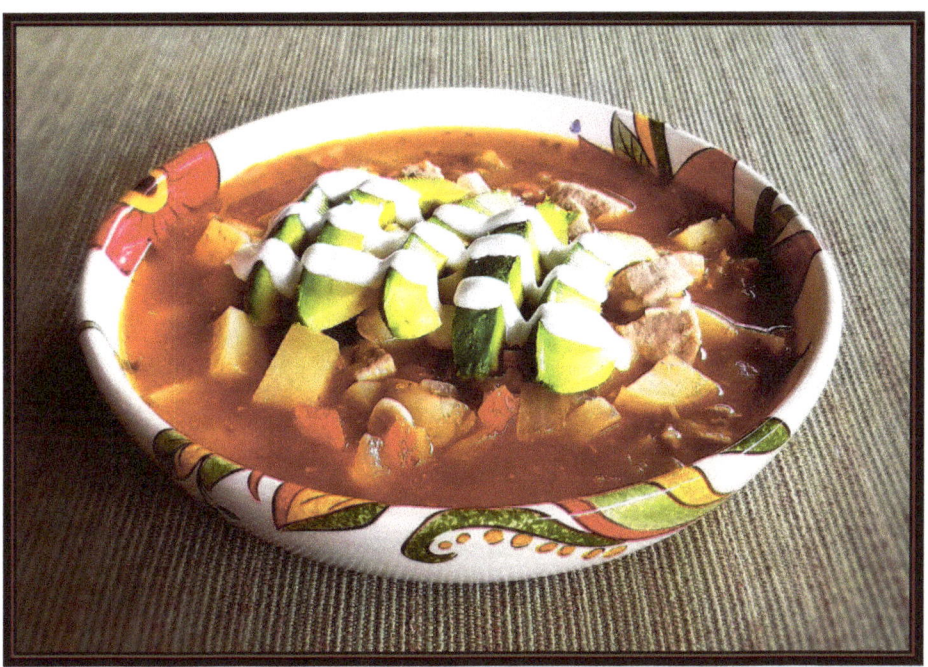

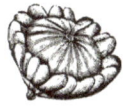 Substitute vegetable broth. Drain two (15.5-ounce) cans of pinto beans and add these with the tomatoes.

Traditionally, *caldillo* is often made with beef. You could substitute beef broth and cut up a pound of beef sirloin; everything else remains the same. You can even substitute a pound of any ground meat: beef or pork; chicken or turkey will also work well in this flexible stew.

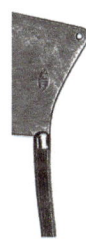

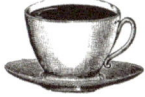 *Since everything should be cut into rather small chunks, this is a dish that can be completely ready in about an hour! It will taste like you've been slaving away for hours.*

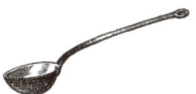

Chapter Three: Pork & Seafood

Esther's Manhattan Clam Chowder

This makes a fairly large amount of soup and is only hard to cut in half because of the small can of tomato sauce. So plan to make it when you know you're having a crowd of clam-lovers over, because you shouldn't freeze it (potatoes, you know). I came up with a chicken version to satisfy Bob, who won't eat clams. See the cleaver icon below for this delicious variation.

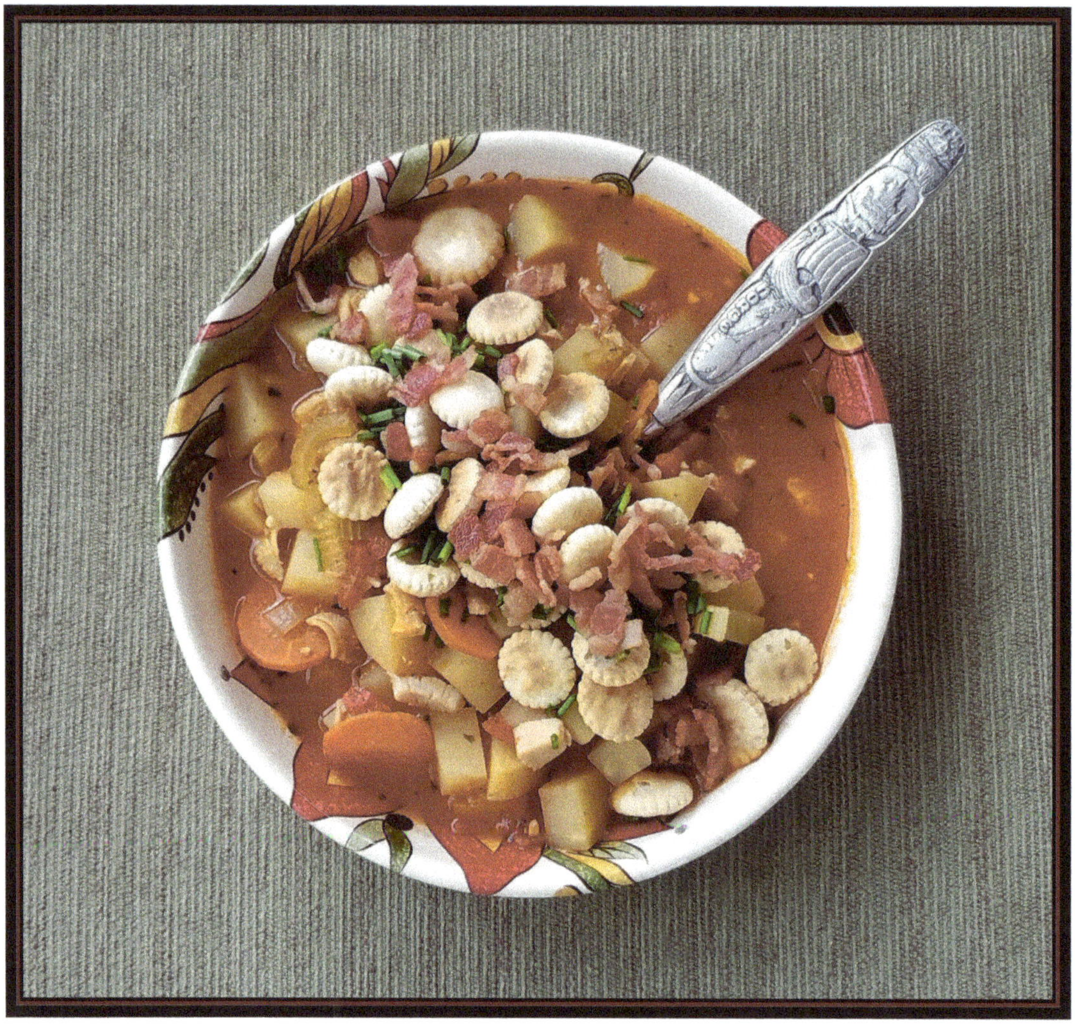

12 ounces premium raw bacon, cut into ¼" slices
1½ cups carrot, peeled and thinly sliced
1½ cups celery, thinly sliced
1½ cups onion, coarsely chopped
2 tablespoons minced garlic
2 pounds russet potatoes, peeled and cut into ½" bits
8-ounce can tomato sauce
28-ounce can petite diced tomatoes, with juice
3 cups clam juice, or other seafood broth
2 cups water
1 teaspoon Old Bay Seasoning
1 teaspoon dry thyme (2-3 tablespoons fresh, minced)
½ teaspoon black pepper
½ teaspoon salt
½ teaspoon hot sauce
4 (6½-ounce) cans chopped clams, with juice

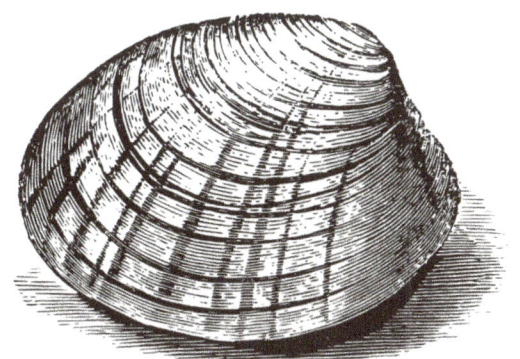

OPTIONAL GARNISH:

Oyster crackers or crumbled saltines
Finely chopped scallions or chives
Perhaps some more cooked, crispy, crumbled bacon

COAT a 6-quart saucepan with cooking spray. Fry bacon over fairly high heat for 6-8 minutes, stirring frequently, until it browns. Reserve 2 tablespoons fat; use a slotted spoon to remove bacon to paper towels. Discard remaining fat.

SPRAY pot again; add reserved bacon fat. Sauté the carrot, celery, onion, and garlic over rather high heat for 10 minutes. Stir frequently, scraping up the brown bits. Add the potatoes, tomato sauce, diced tomatoes, clam juice, water, Old Bay, thyme, pepper, salt, and hot sauce to the pot. Bring to a boil. Lower heat to medium/high and maintain a gentle boil 25 minutes, uncovered. Stir a couple of times. Add clams with their juice. Raise heat and cook another 5 minutes, until vegetables are tender. Mix in the reserved bacon. Season, if desired. Garnish, as desired. Cover and chill leftovers; don't freeze. Serves 8-10.

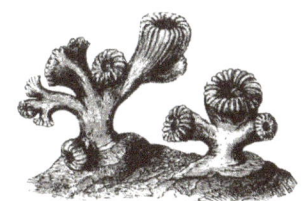

Omit the bacon preparation and substitute olive oil for the bacon fat. Change the clam juice to water or vegetable broth and substitute ¾ pound of diced summer squash. Or you could just increase the amount of carrot, celery, and onion to 2 cups each; this soup is actually not as meaty as you might assume.

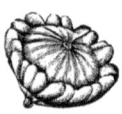

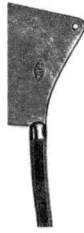

Two simple changes make this a soup that even my husband will eat. First change: omit the clam juice and replace it with 1 quart of low-sodium chicken broth. Second change: omit the canned clams and replace them with 8 ounces of diced cooked chicken.

You know the drill.

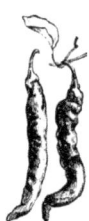

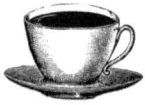

My mom (maiden name: Esther Ingebore Aslaksen—now there's a Norwegian name for you!) would whip up a big pot of clam chowder maybe three times a year, though I think she was the only one who really cared to eat it. My dad was picky about various foods, and of course, my sister and I were typical kids. She never gave me any recipes. Mom pined for a Manhattan chowder when she was quite elderly and living in a group home, so I finally decided to come up with my own version similar to what I remembered hers to be. I worked on this for awhile and this is about as close as it's going to get to my mom's mystery recipe. She was quite satisfied with it. Then she wanted me to make up a New England version, which I named for her father and have included later on in this chapter.

Now, if you decide not to use canned clams, you'll need 8 ounces of clam meat and 1½ cups of extra water. I would estimate you'd need about 4 dozen clams, poached in a couple cups of salted water. Wash them well, cook them until they open up, drain the liquid and reserve 1½ cups for the soup, then chop all the clam meat. I'm landlocked and not ashamed to use cans; plus, that's what my mom ALWAYS used and she was a native New Yorker!

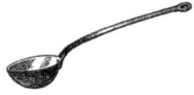

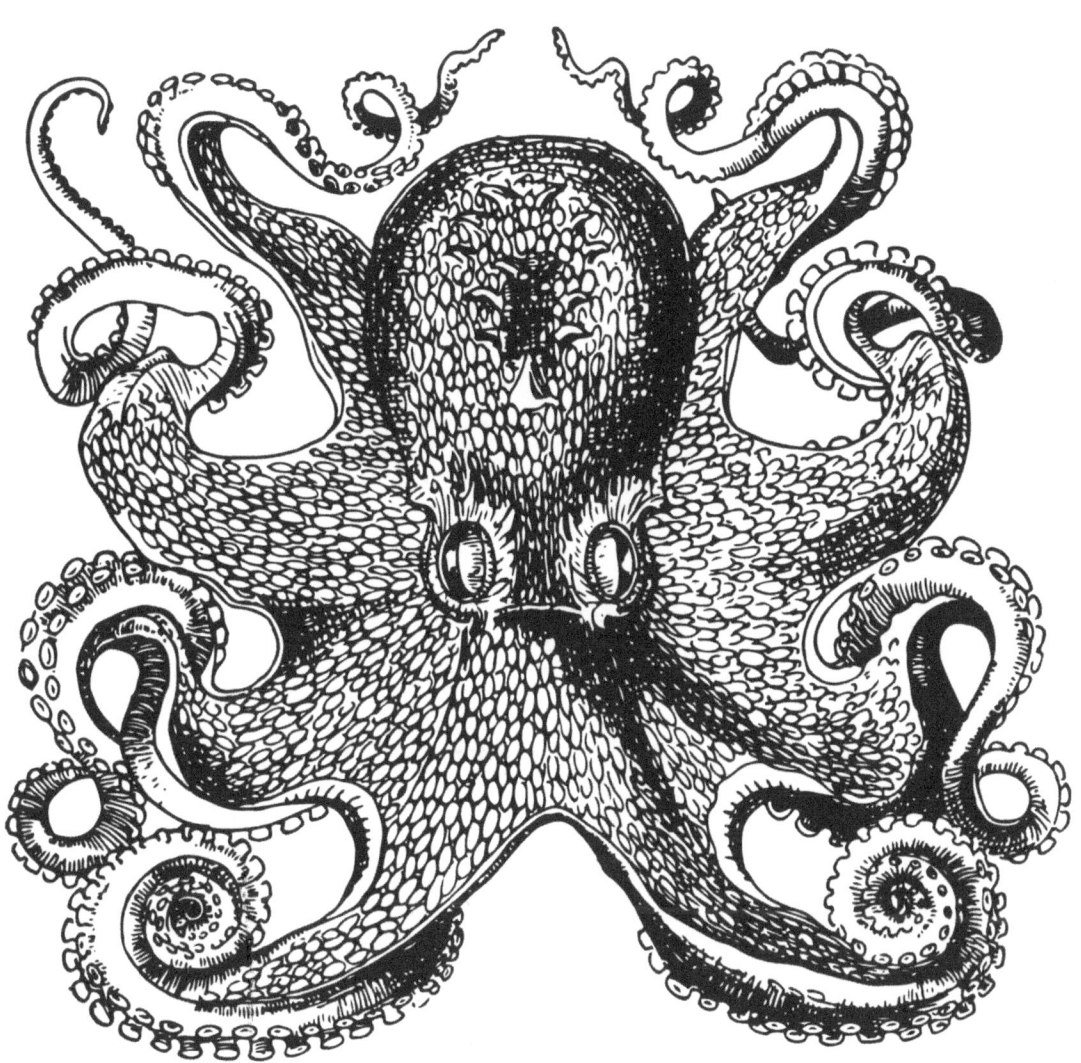

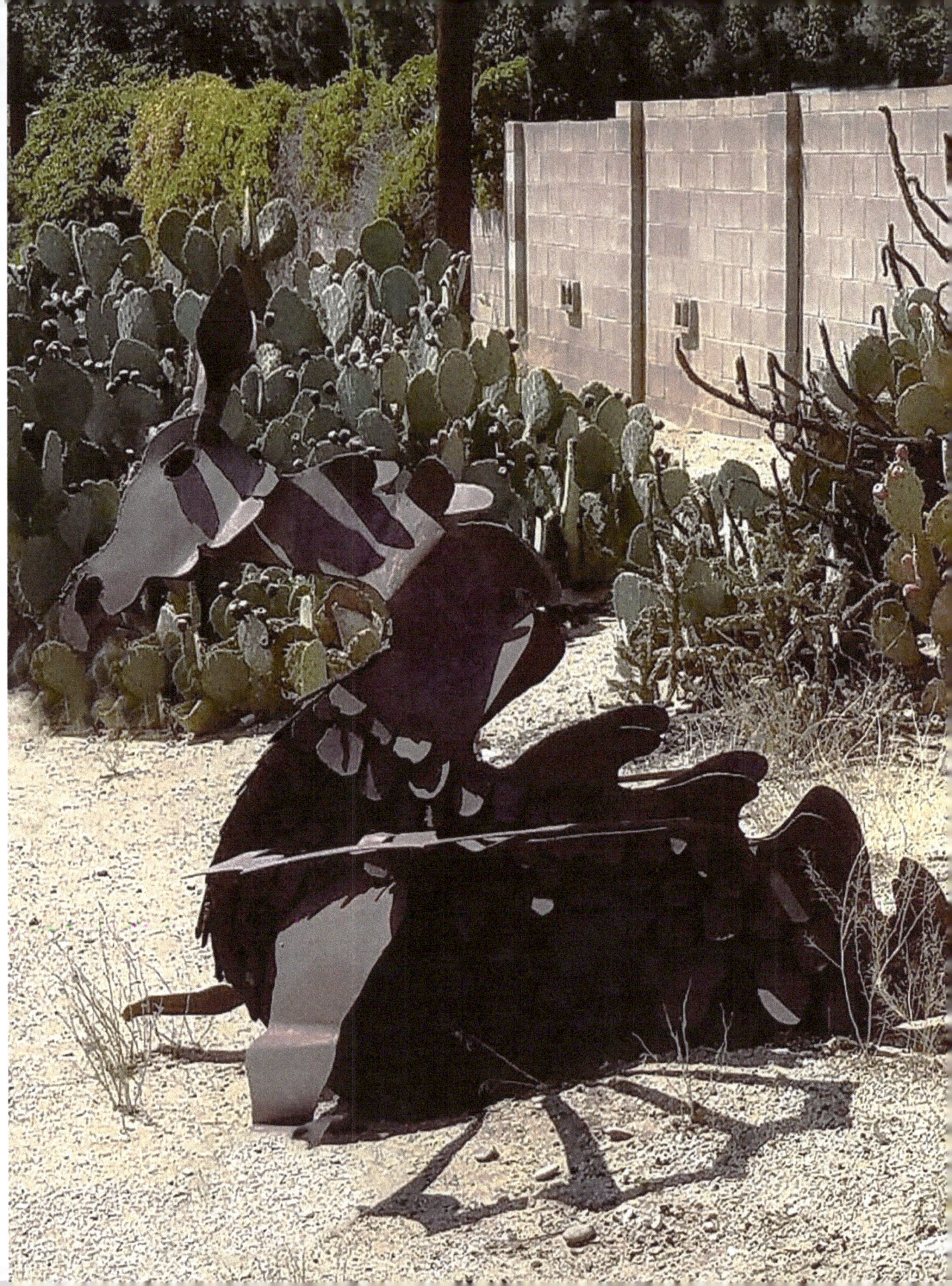

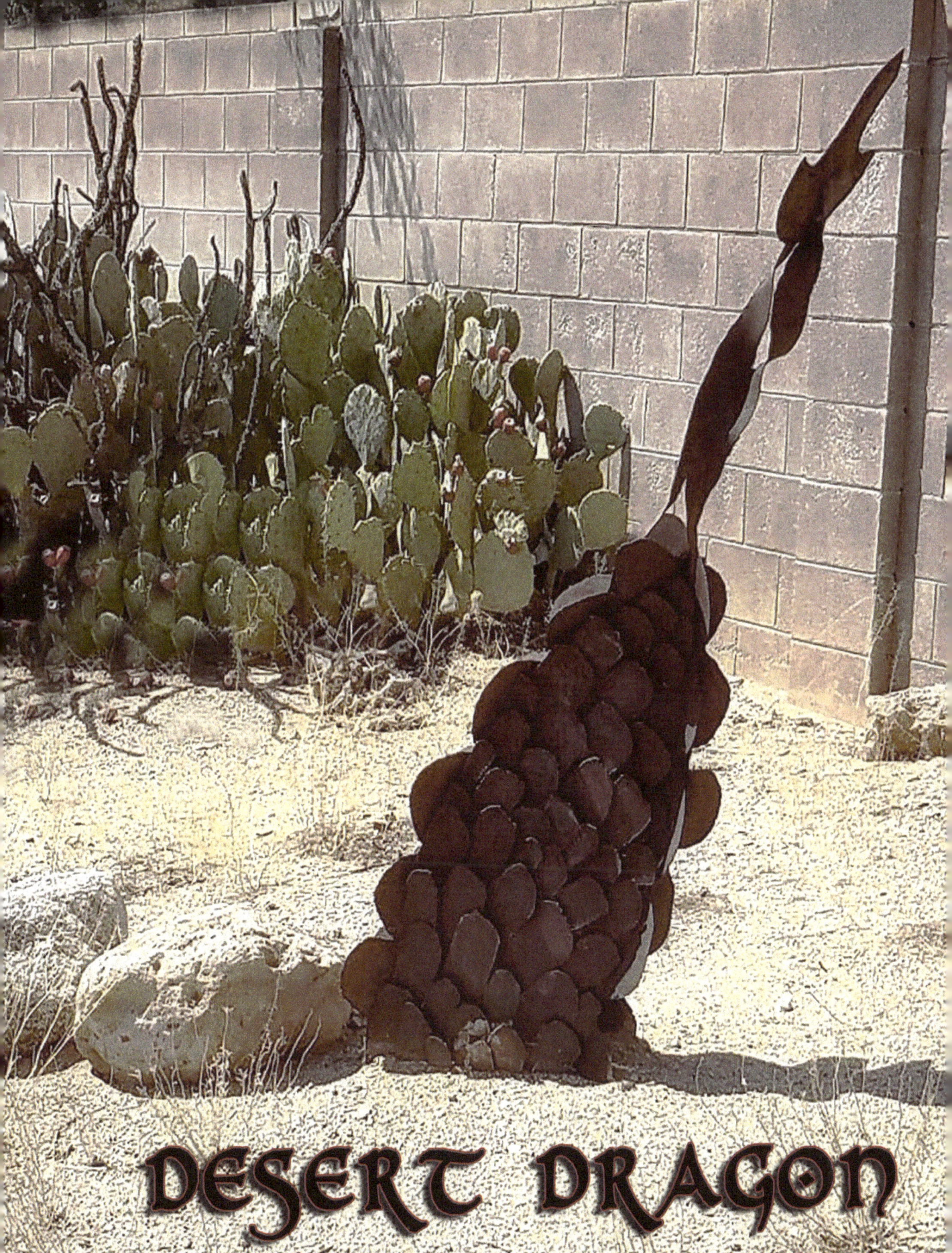

Jumbo Gumbo

Even though the word "gumbo" is apparently derived from a West African word for okra, it has evolved to encompass just about any New Orleans/Louisiana/Cajun stew/soup recipes that have emerged from the culinary cornucopia that represents the southern United States. Does this mean you must use okra in your gumbo? Are there absolute rules to follow when you make a gumbo? Gumbo is so controversial that people argue over whether it is a soup or a stew. Am I willing to enter the controversy surrounding this dish?

I'm not. So this is my version, which makes a fairly giant pot of soup and is a good excuse to invite some company over (though it does freeze well). Although the essential gumbo characteristics appear to be the following items listed below, in my opinion, the roux is the crucial component. That sets the stage for any sort of modification you would like to make. And you can certainly make modifications; gumbo is one of the most forgiving and flexible soups you can make. You can even start with a ready-made roux in a jar, but it's not hard to cook your own. Here are the must-haves for gumbo:

ONE: Start with a specially prepared roux, to which you add a traditional vegetable trinity; usually the *mirepoix* here consists of chopped yellow onion, celery, and green bell pepper. Will your gumbo suffer if you use red or white onion? Probably not too much, but using a different color for your bell pepper would definitely make a difference in the flavor. Not that that would be a horrible thing; it might turn out to be just fine.

Now, can you start your roux with just any type of fat? Opinions vary. I generally use vegetable oil. Some say you should start with butter, but these gumbo pundits appear to be in the minority. The venerable Leah Chase apparently used peanut oil. She gave Barack Obama a little slap on the hand when he started to put hot sauce on her gumbo without giving it a taste. Yes, you should always taste food first, before you presume to alter it (even if you are a former President of the United States).

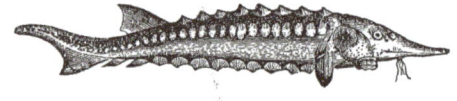

TWO: Get a generous amount of chopped okra in there (if you like it) and use at least two different varieties of meat products. Okra has a sort of inherent thickening quality.

THREE: White rice is essential, either in the soup or served as a scoop in the bowl, for the diner to mix in.

FOUR: Use some filé powder either near the end of cooking or as a garnish. Filé is made from dried and ground sassafras leaves. Whether you want to use this along with the okra is sort of a mystery, because filé powder is also supposedly a thickener (though

I've never noticed it behaving this way; maybe I haven't used enough of it to tell). I like to use it simply as a garnish sprinkled on top.

Well, as you might imagine if you've been reading this cookbook, okra is definitely not a vegetable that Bob likes, and it's one which doesn't thrill me either. I keep trying it, but I have a thing about fibrous vegetables. Okra has a rather unique texture which I've never been able to acquire a taste for; however, I found that a pound of frozen lima beans will work quite well here. Lima beans are also not one of Bob's favorites (sheesh!), but if they are mixed into something else, he doesn't mind them. If you like okra, you can definitely use the same amount of frozen chopped okra.

You can substitute crayfish (which are also known by many other names, such as crawdads, mountain lobsters, and my favorite—yabbies) for the shrimp, if you like! Treat their preparation as you would shrimp; meaning, thaw them as directed, peel them—you'll probably just utilize the tail meat in a dish such as this.

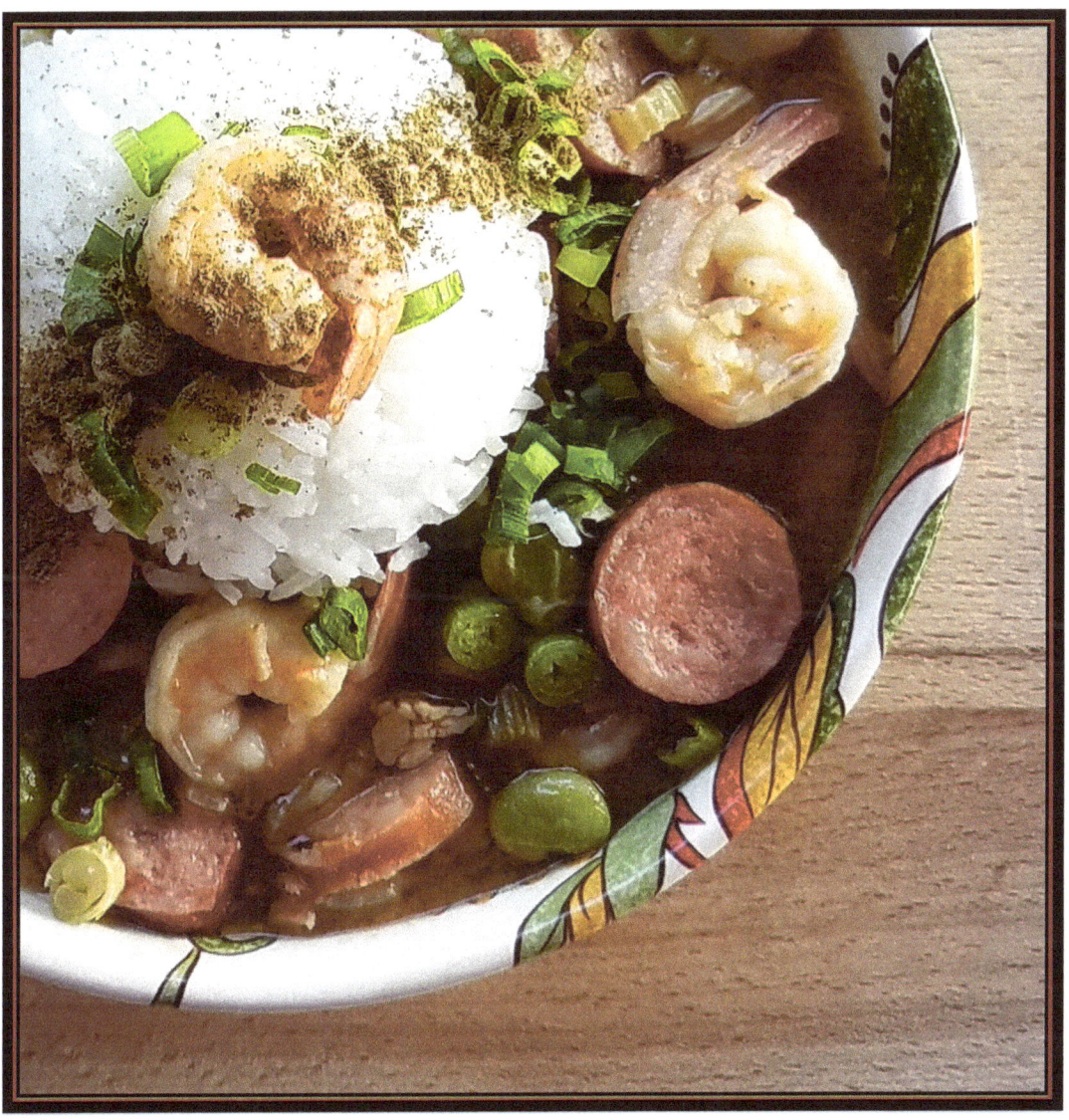

¾ cup vegetable oil, bacon grease, or peanut oil
1 cup all-purpose flour
1 tablespoon minced garlic
1½ cups yellow onion, coarsely chopped
1½ cups celery, coarsely chopped
1½ cups green bell pepper; cored,
    then coarsely chopped
2 quarts water
3 tablespoons Old Bay Seasoning
½ teaspoon coarse sea salt
½ teaspoon black pepper
½ teaspoon cayenne pepper
1 teaspoon hot sauce
½ cup white rice (long or short grain)
1 pound cooked chicken, diced or shredded
    into bite-size chunks
1 pound andouille sausage, cut into ¼" slices
    (any other smoked sausage will be fine)
1 pound frozen sliced okra (or lima beans)
1 pound raw shrimp (tail on or off; thaw according
    to package directions and give them a rinse;
    use medium or large shrimp)

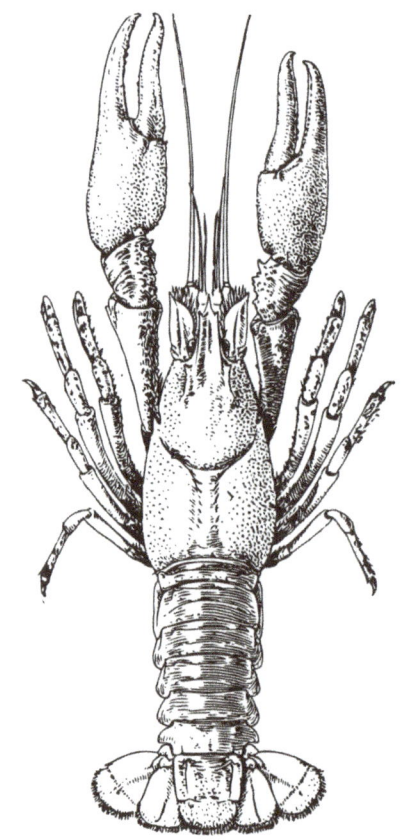

OPTIONAL GARNISH:

Extra cooked white rice (see anecdotal material for suggestions)
Thinly chopped scallions
Filé powder

HEAT oil over medium heat in an 8-quart saucepan. When it starts to bubble, whisk in the flour. Continue cooking, whisking frequently, over a rather low heat, about 10-15 minutes, until it turns to a shade of brown that resembles a light milk chocolate bar. Be patient with this step. If you end up with a bunch of black specks, you've burned it—discard it and start over.

    ADD garlic, onion, celery, and bell pepper to the pot and sauté for 5 minutes over moderate heat, stirring frequently. Add water, Old Bay, salt, pepper, cayenne, hot sauce, rice, chicken, sausage, and okra and bring to a boil. Cook on low, covered, 20 minutes. Stir a few times, especially at the bottom of the pot.

RAISE heat to medium/high to achieve a gentle boil, then cook 3 minutes, uncovered. Add shrimp and cook just until pink, 3-5 minutes, depending on the size of your shrimp. Season, if desired. Garnish, as desired. Cover and chill leftovers. Serves 8-10.

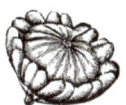

To replace the large amount of protein, you'd need a three-pound assortment of vegetables. Summer squashes, cauliflower, and beans would make nice substitutes. You can even use tomatoes, fresh or canned, though apparently they are a bit controversial.

Gumbo can be made with any sort of meat you can think of; just use three pounds worth of whatever you like.

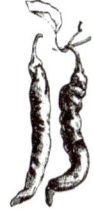

Extra heat can come from a spicier variety of sausage or additional hot sauce. Would red or green chile work? Yes, but you're probably tired of hearing about it by now.

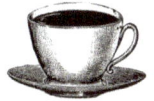

Let's say you can't stand okra or lima beans. You can either omit them completely, or substitute a pound of other frozen vegetables such as corn, peas, or green beans. Will that be authentic? Probably not, but the kitchen police are not going to come to your house anytime soon.

Although I have made this gumbo with some rice, it is nice to prepare extra. I would cook 2 cups of white rice in a 3-quart saucepan or a rice cooker and serve it on the side. Just use your basic rice recipe, or do this: combine 2 cups of rice and 1 quart water or low-sodium chicken broth in a 3-quart saucepan and bring to a boil. Stir once, cover, and set on the lowest heat. Cook 18 minutes, undisturbed. Turn off heat and let stand 15-20 minutes, covered and undisturbed. Stir it up when ready to serve.

Can you use jumbo shrimp when making this gumbo? If the oxymoronic qualities of this particular protein do not bother you, please feel free.

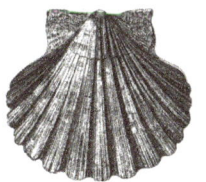 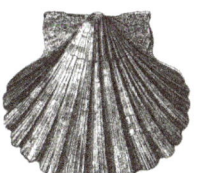 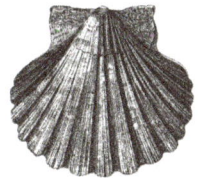

Chapter Three: Pork & Seafood

Butternut Risotto Soup

This is a lovely soup to make in the fall and winter seasons; it's quite hearty.

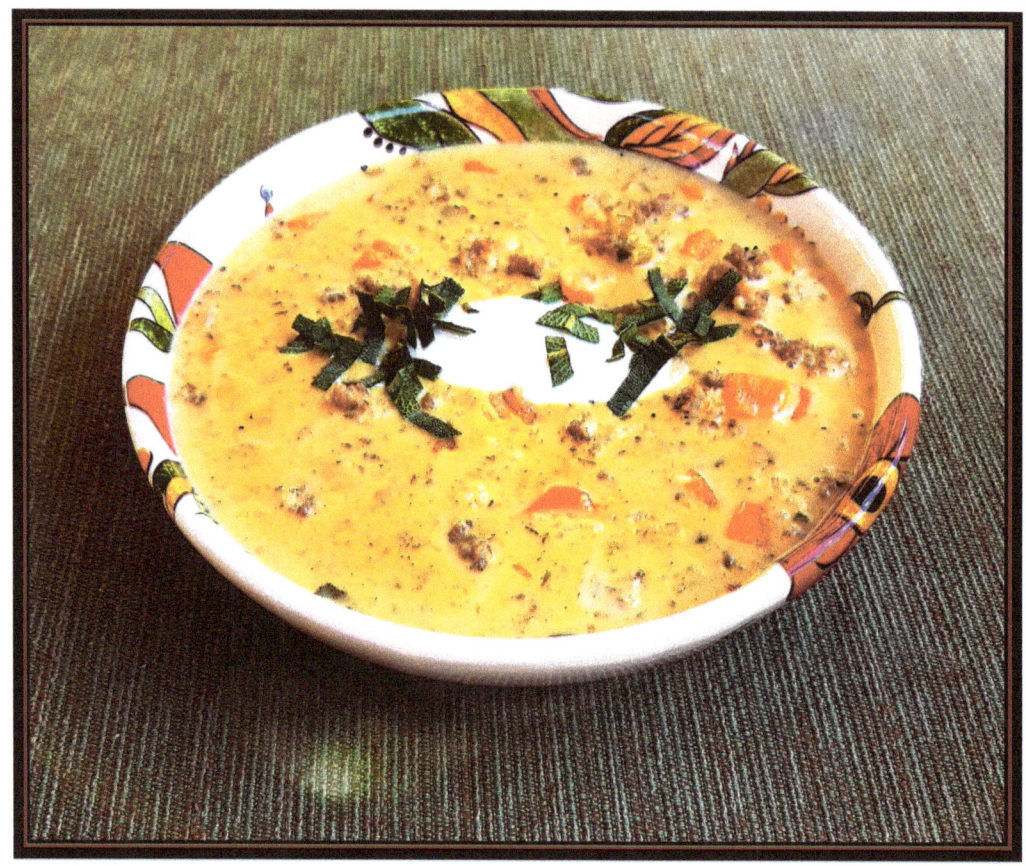

1 pound bulk sage sausage (any other flavors will be fine)
1 tablespoon salted butter
1 tablespoon olive oil
1 tablespoon minced garlic
1 teaspoon salt
1 teaspoon black pepper
1 teaspoon sage (2-3 tablespoons fresh, minced)
½ cup carrot, peeled and thinly sliced
½ cup celery, thinly sliced
½ cup onion, coarsely chopped

1 pound butternut squash, cut into ½" cubes
  (I usually just buy this already cut up
  in a package because I'm lazy)
½ cup dry white wine, such as Chardonnay
1 quart low-sodium chicken broth
½ cup Arborio rice
1½ cups heavy cream

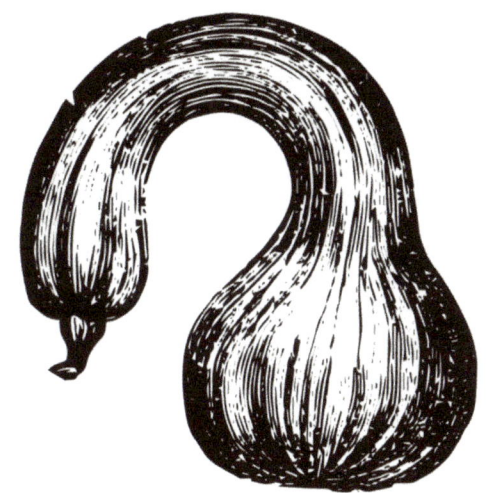

OPTIONAL GARNISH:

Crème fraîche or sour cream
Chopped fresh sage
Minced chives

COAT a 6-quart saucepan with cooking spray. Break up and fry the sausage over rather high heat until the pink is gone. Drain and set aside; reuse the pot. Spray the pot again. Sauté the butter, oil, garlic, salt, pepper, sage, carrot, celery, onion, and squash on a moderate heat 10 minutes, stirring often. Add the wine and bring to a boil. Boil 1 minute. Add the broth and rice and bring to another boil. Cook on a low simmer, covered, for 25 minutes. Stir a few times, scraping up any browned bits. Add the cream and the sausage. Raise heat to high/medium and cook 3-4 minutes, until everything is tender. Season, if desired. Garnish, as desired. Cover and chill leftovers. Serves 4-6.

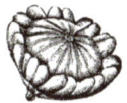 Change the broth to vegetable and use your favorite ground meat/sausage substitute. Or you could simply double the amount of squash, or use a pound of sliced mushrooms.

A pound of any ground meat or poultry will be fine, turkey, chicken, pork, or beef.

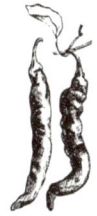 This soup is definitely a good candidate for the addition of green chile, but you might consider using a hot sausage instead of the sage variety. Or both, if you dare…

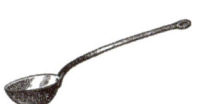

Chapter Three: Pork & Seafood   93

Asbjorn's New England Clam Chowder

This is named for my maternal grandfather. The oldest of 11, Asbjorn Kristian Aslaksen was born in 1892, in Moss, Norway. He left school after the sixth grade, but that didn't stop him from pursuing a lifetime of gainful employment. He worked at six years old, carrying baggage from ships; he apprenticed as a blacksmith, spent three years in the Falkland Islands as a whaler, then served in the Norwegian navy from 1915-1920. Asbjorn emigrated to Brooklyn, New York, in 1924; his only daughter Esther was born in 1928. He was a master machinist in the Brooklyn Navy Yard from 1938-1959 and worked on the Battleship Missouri. His busy career culminated in a stint as a naval inspector from 1959-1964. Then he retired to enjoy life, cooking, and fishing out on Long Island. In 1969, he and my grandmother followed us to Albuquerque, where he spent much of his time hunting for rocks with his senior group, polishing them, and making jewelry. The move to New Mexico with our milder weather probably extended his life by a few years—he died of emphysema in 1976, when I was almost 14.

My sister and I loved to visit Mama and Farsi (short for *Bestefar*, which is Norwegian for grandfather) at their apartment. It was filled with rock projects, tile projects, and paint-by-number sets. My strangest food memory of Farsi was his predilection for having a bowl of cottage cheese and pouring a tablespoon of soy sauce over it. I suppose I ate this when I was a child, but I really can't imagine eating this now. Maybe I should give it a shot sometime…

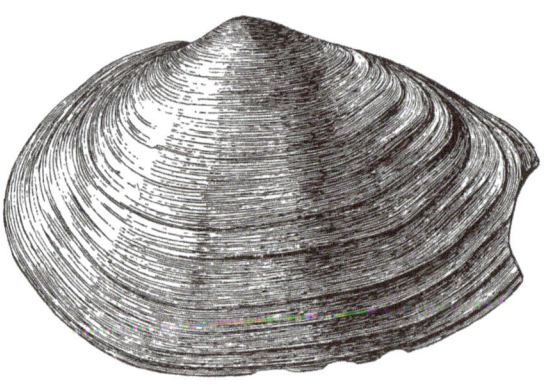

2 tablespoons salted butter
¾ cup carrot, peeled and cut into ¼" bits
¾ cup celery, cut into ¼" bits
¾ cup shallots, cut into ¼" bits
3 tablespoons all-purpose flour
2 cups clam juice, or other seafood broth
8 ounces russet potato, peeled and cut
    into ½" bits
½ cup heavy cream
½ teaspoon salt
½ teaspoon white pepper
½ teaspoon dry thyme (1-2 tablespoons fresh, minced)
2 (6½-ounce) cans chopped clams
4 ounces frozen tiny whole shrimp, cooked and peeled; thawed as directed
    (or you may use 2 [4-ounce] cans tiny shrimp, drained)
1 tablespoon lemon juice

OPTIONAL GARNISH:

Minced green herbs (such as parsley, chives, or dill)
Cooked and crumbled bacon
Oyster crackers, or crumbled saltines

COAT a 3-quart saucepan with cooking spray. Melt the butter over moderately high heat, then sauté the carrot, celery, and shallots 5 minutes. Mix in the flour. Add the clam juice and potato and bring to a boil. Cover and cook on lowest heat 20 minutes; stir a few times. Add the cream and the 3 seasonings. Raise heat to medium and cook 4-5 minutes, uncovered, stirring frequently, until the vegetables are tender. Drain the clams (and shrimp, if you are using a canned variety) and add clams and shrimp to the pot. Cook another couple of minutes or so. Turn off the heat and add the lemon juice. Season, if desired. Garnish, as desired. Cover and chill leftovers; don't freeze. Serves 3-4.

Omit the clam juice, clams, and shrimp. Substitute vegetable broth and a couple cups of desired vegetables, cut into small chunks, such as: another 8 ounces of potato, or something like a combination of frozen peas, corn, or lima beans. Add these variations with the potato and broth.

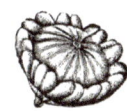

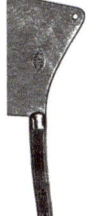

Change the clam juice to low-sodium chicken broth and add 8 ounces of diced, cooked chicken or turkey, or use ground, cooked sausage.

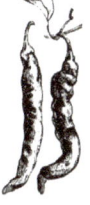

4 ounces of roasted and chopped green chile, with juice, would be lovely without being overpowering.

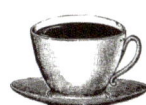

As I said previously in "Esther's Manhattan Clam Chowder," you can use fresh clams here. You'll only need about 2 dozen clams. Wash them well, then poach in a couple cups of salted water. Cook them until they open up and drain the liquid. You can use this broth in this recipe, though you might still need some additional clam juice. Chop the clams and add to the soup. You could also use other shrimp products (frozen, or ones you have cooked yourself), but they should be cut into rather small bits.

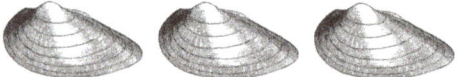

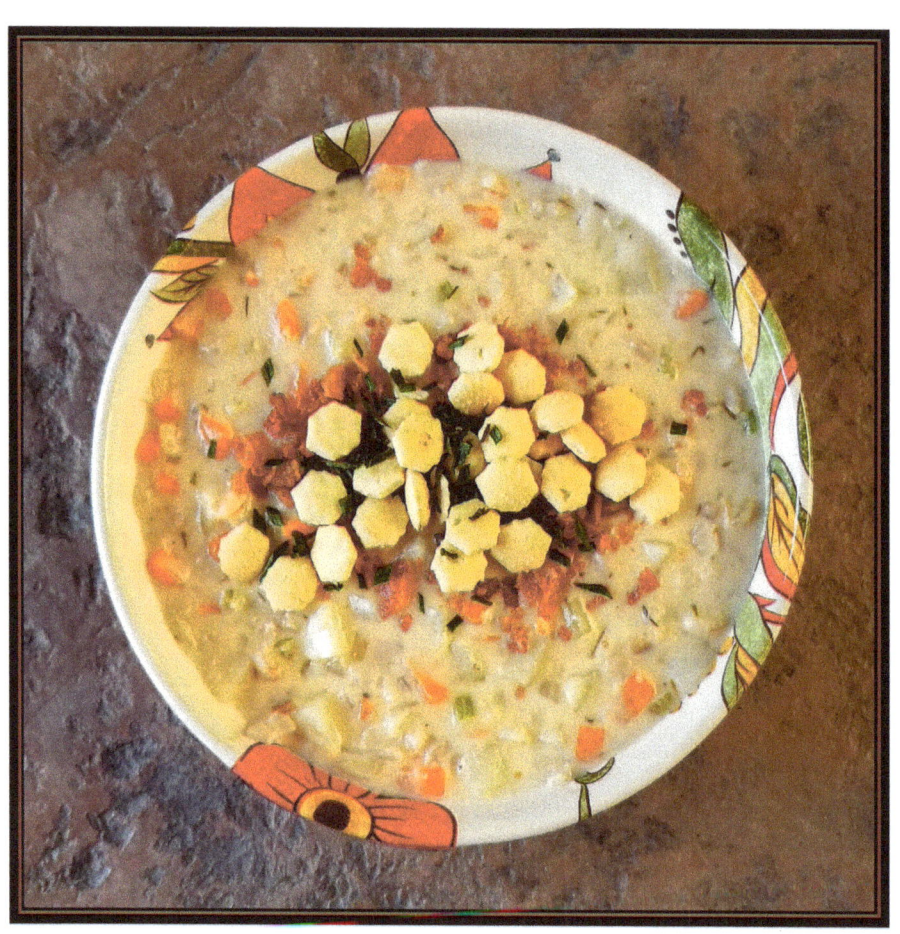

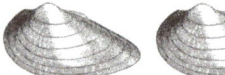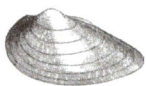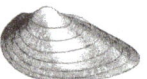

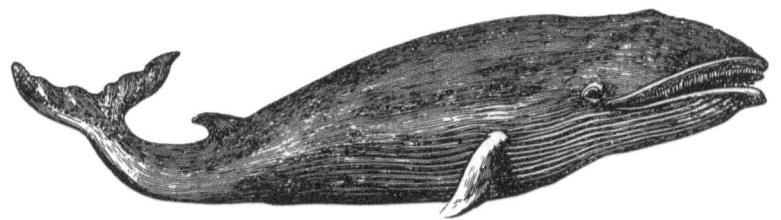

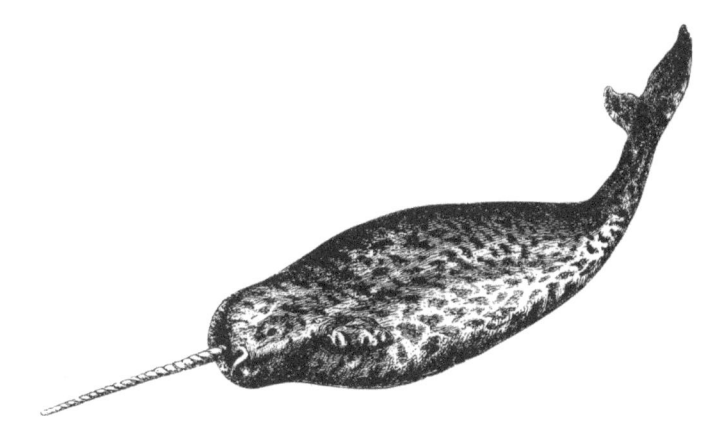

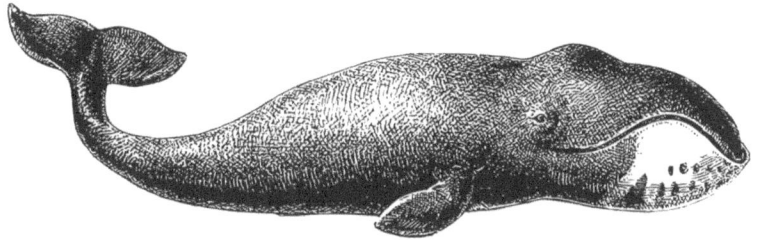

Tecolote Chili

This recipe was invented as a riff on a popular local restaurant's little starter bowl of chile beans. You might have seen this restaurant on the Food Network, since its architecture is rather unusual. The Owl Café started down in San Antonio, New Mexico, in the 1940s. Green chile cheeseburgers are their main claim to fame, though they offer other typical diner food; Bob considers their chocolate malt to be the best in the city. Your visit starts with a bowl of those brothy beans, which are topped with green chile, and a couple packets of saltine crackers. One day, I was thinking of those beans at home, and I thought the addition of meat, onion, and some extra seasonings would be a great idea. Turns out it was. This is one of the easiest recipes in this cookbook, and it will truly give you a delicious taste of New Mexican cuisine.

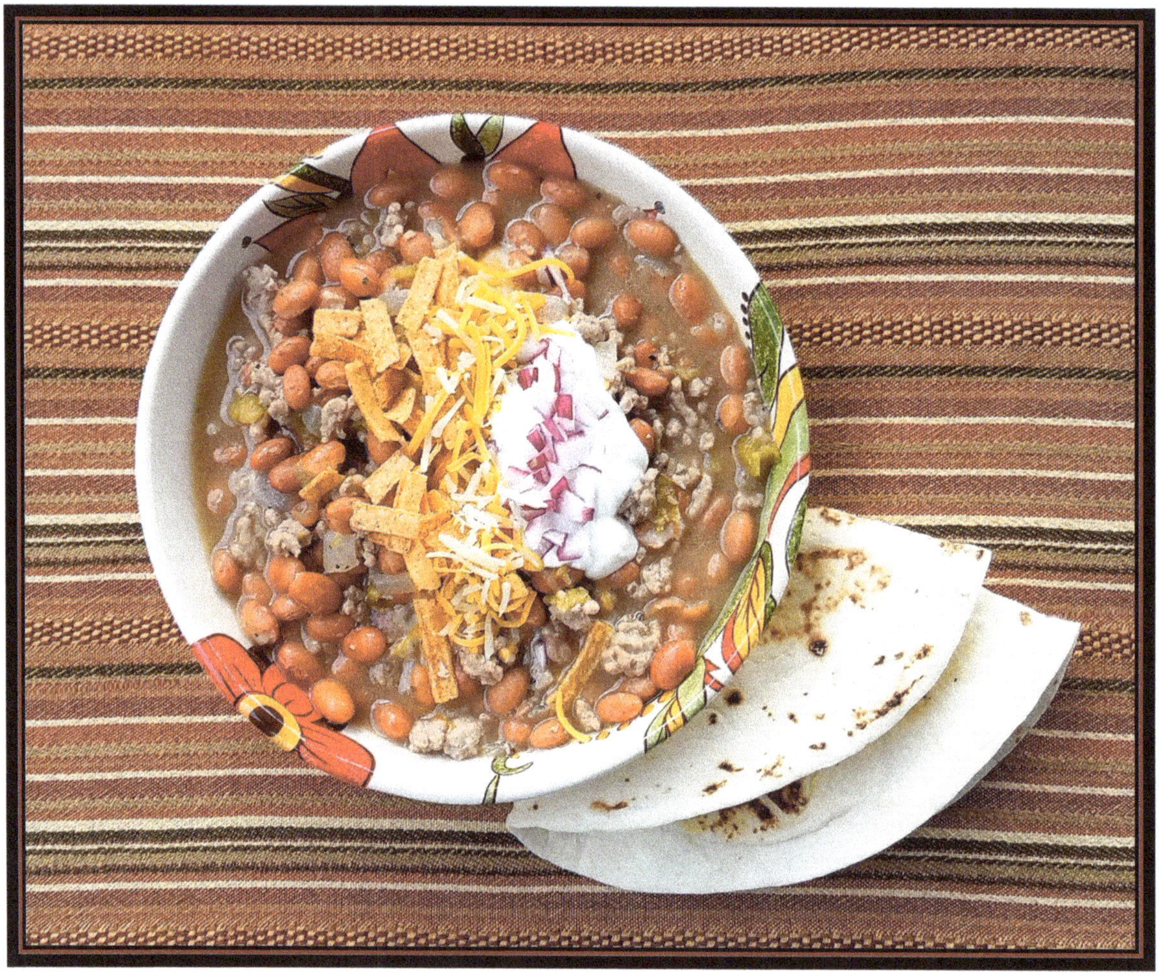

1 tablespoon vegetable oil
1½ pounds ground pork
1 cup onion, coarsely chopped
4 (15.5-ounce) cans pinto beans, drained and rinsed
   (about 5-6 cups of cooked pinto beans)
8 ounces roasted and chopped green chile, with juice
2 (14.5-ounce) cans low-sodium chicken broth
1 teaspoon garlic salt
1 teaspoon onion salt
½ teaspoon black pepper
½ teaspoon dry oregano (1-2 tablespoons fresh, minced)

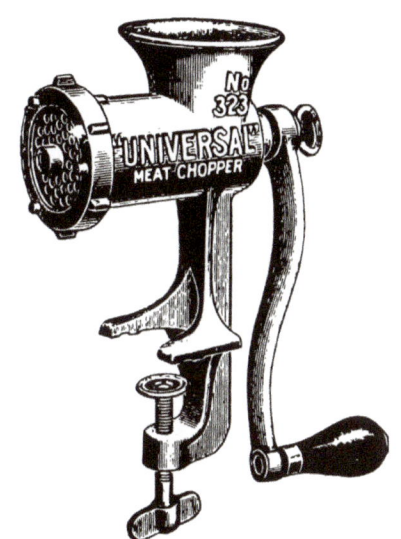

OPTIONAL GARNISH:

Crispy chips (most any variety will work)
Chopped red onion
Finely shredded Fiesta blend cheese
Sour cream or crème fraîche
Do you have some favorites from either the **NICE NEW MEXICAN & MEXICAN GARNISHES** list or the **CHARMING CHILI GARNISHES** list? Use them here.

COAT a 6-quart saucepan with cooking spray. Heat the oil over very high heat; add the pork and onion and fry until the pink is gone, breaking up the meat. Add the remaining ingredients and bring to a boil. Cook on a gentle boil over a medium/low heat, uncovered, 30 minutes. Stir a couple of times. Season, if desired. Garnish, as desired. Cover and chill leftovers. Serves 6-8.

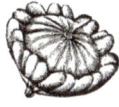 All you need to do is omit the meat and use two extra cans of beans. You could use a different variety of beans, such as black or cannellinis. Or use your favorite ground meat substitute, of course.

Any ground meat (see disclaimer below) will do in this recipe!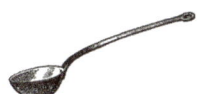

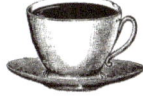 *Tecolote is one of quite a few Spanish words for "owl." In absolutely NO WAY am I suggesting that you use owl meat in this recipe, however.*

Chapter Three: Pork & Seafood   99

Funky Artichoke Bisque

This recipe came about because of my obsession with Costco, which is sort of a holy shrine for me. One day long ago, as I was cruising the aisles on my quest for good deals, I spied a reasonably priced package containing two 33-ounce jars of artichoke hearts packed in water. I thought, fabulous; these will be really handy to have around to put in… well, something…

And then a year passed while the jars continued to sit on my pantry shelves. At least a year; my life can be a blur sometimes. I suppose if they had been marinated hearts, I would have used them up in salads or antipasto lunch plates. Their presence only served to remind me that I'm better off NOT stocking my pantry with too many items (especially bulky ones), in the hope that they will come in handy eventually. Y2K happened many years ago, and who buys artichoke hearts for emergencies, anyway?

They were still within their sell-by date, however, so I finally got around to doing something with them. This recipe turned out to be quite delicious, a creamy, comforting, easy-to-prepare soup that is perfect as an appetizer, or paired with your favorite bread product for more of a meal.

Lesson learned: make a point of using your groceries sooner, rather than later.

Then I was hemming and hawing about a good name for the recipe, though I've always called it "Funky Artichoke Bisque." Finally, I said to myself, well, that's the destined name; it ended up fitting perfectly with the garnish I later made up to go with it: FAB Crostini. You could double the butter recipe from the FAB Crostini and use it whenever you need a garlicky spread.

1 rather large head of garlic
½ teaspoon olive oil
33-ounce jar artichoke hearts in water, or 3 (13.75-ounce) cans
    (whole or quartered; any size)
14.5-ounce can low-sodium chicken broth
2 anchovy fillets (or 1-2 teaspoons anchovy
    paste)
1 cup onion, coarsely chopped
½ teaspoon black pepper
½ teaspoon fennel seeds
¼ teaspoon crushed red pepper flakes
¾ cup heavy cream
2 ounces fresh Parmesan and/or Romano cheese, finely shredded

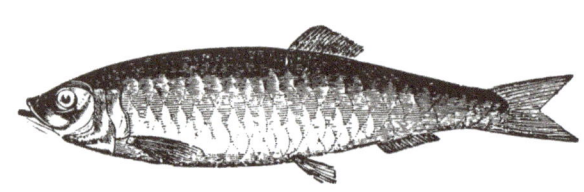

OPTIONAL GARNISH:

FAB Crostini (see recipe below, or use some prepared croutons or other toasts)
Additional shredded fresh Parmesan and/or Romano cheese
Additional crushed red pepper flakes
Minced fresh basil

FOR THE FAB CROSTINI:

¼ cup very soft salted butter
1 tablespoon dry Parmesan cheese
    (Parmesan and/or Romano is fine)
2 teaspoons minced garlic
½ teaspoon crushed red pepper flakes
½ teaspoon dry parsley
½ teaspoon dry Italian seasoning
½ teaspoon black pepper
½ teaspoon garlic powder
French or Italian bread, cut into (16) ½" slices
    (from a slim baguette; don't use the heels,
    only cut from the middle of the loaf)

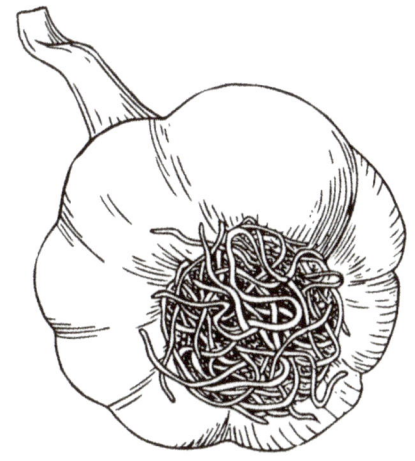

PREHEAT oven to 450°. Cut off the top ¾" of the garlic and place, root side down, on a 12" square of regular aluminum foil. Drizzle with olive oil and enclose loosely. Place on a small baking sheet and roast 35 minutes. Let stand 30 minutes on the pan, still wrapped in the foil. When cooler, squeeze the cloves into a 4-quart saucepan. Add artichokes with liquid, broth, anchovies, onion, pepper, fennel seeds, and the crushed red pepper and bring to a boil. Cook on low, covered, 40 minutes. Stir twice.

MEANWHILE, make the FAB Crostini: Preheat oven to 400°. Combine the soft butter, cheese, garlic, and the 5 seasonings in a small bowl. Spread the butter mixture evenly on each bread slice, then place them on a large (18" by 13") baking sheet. Bake 8 minutes. Remove to doubled paper towels and let stand until ready to serve with the soup. Cover and chill leftovers.

IN 2 batches, puree soup completely. Strain into a 3-quart saucepan. Using a wooden spoon, mash the soup in the strainer to squeeze out as much liquid as you can. Discard the remaining solids. Add the cream and cheese and cook on medium heat, uncovered, 5 minutes. Stir a few times. Season, if desired (but watch it! Your artichokes might already have enough sodium). Garnish, as desired. Cover and chill leftovers. Serves 3-4.

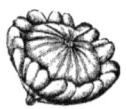 Omit the anchovies and change your broth to either vegetable or even just water.

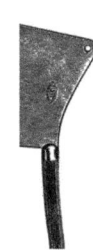

If you love those salty fillets, add one or two more. If you want to add other meats, I would use about a cup of lighter cooked meats, chopped finely (perhaps you have some leftover roasted chicken or shrimp around).

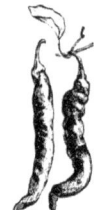 The crushed red pepper flakes can be increased if you like, or you can add the usual half-cup of roasted and chopped green chile, with juice.

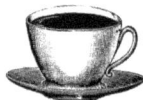

This is a rather intensely flavored soup—hope you love garlic as much as I do! Your artichokes will probably be made with some citric acid and the lemony flavor might increase while cooking. If your artichokes lack this acid, you might add a touch of lemon juice to the soup. Having trouble locating water-packed artichoke hearts? Fear not—a trip to the Amazon will be successful, of course. Hate artichokes? You could substitute the same amount of canned asparagus, tips and spears. Preparation is the same.

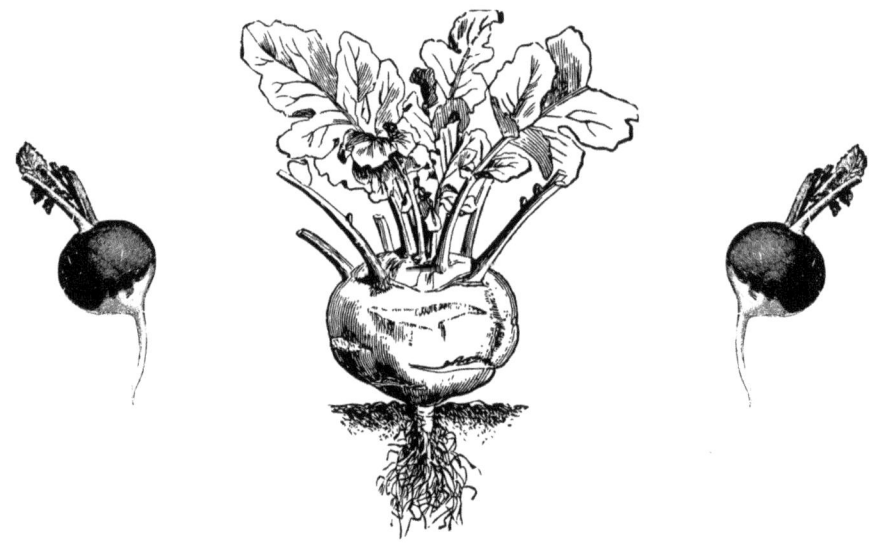

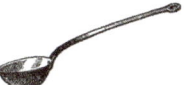
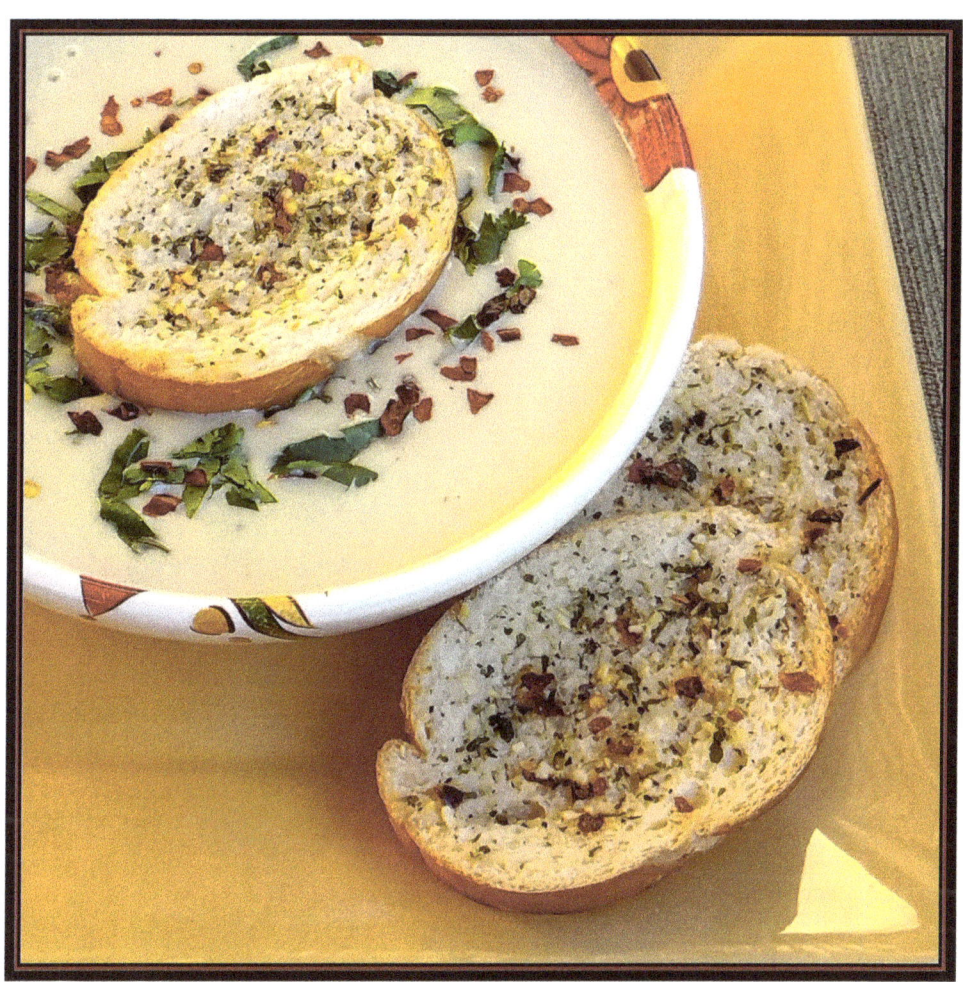
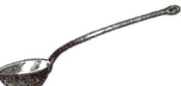

Bob Hates Cauliflower Soup

Since childhood, Bob has hated many types of vegetables, having been a victim of various-stinky-vegetables-cooked-to-death-in-pressure-cookers syndrome. But once in awhile, I'm really in the mood for some of those particular vegetables. So I combined three of his least favorites—cauliflower, zucchini, and lima beans—into a hearty soup. You could substitute peeled turnips and/or rutabagas for the cauliflower; Bob would probably run screaming out of the house if I subjected him to those particular cooking odors.

2 tablespoons olive oil
1 tablespoon minced garlic
½ teaspoon fennel seeds
1 cup carrot, peeled and thinly sliced
1 cup celery, thinly sliced
1 cup red onion, coarsely chopped
1 pound cauliflower, cut into 1" florets
4 ounces zucchini; partially peeled, cut off the ends,
    quarter lengthwise, then cut into ¼" slices
1 quart low-sodium chicken broth
1 cup dry white wine, such as Chardonnay
½ tablespoon lemon juice
½ teaspoon salt
½ teaspoon black pepper
¼ teaspoon cayenne pepper
2 tablespoons prepared pesto sauce, any variety
2 ounces small pasta (such as elbows,
    tiny shells, or ditalini)
½ cup frozen lima beans
6 ounces diced ham
½ cup half-and-half

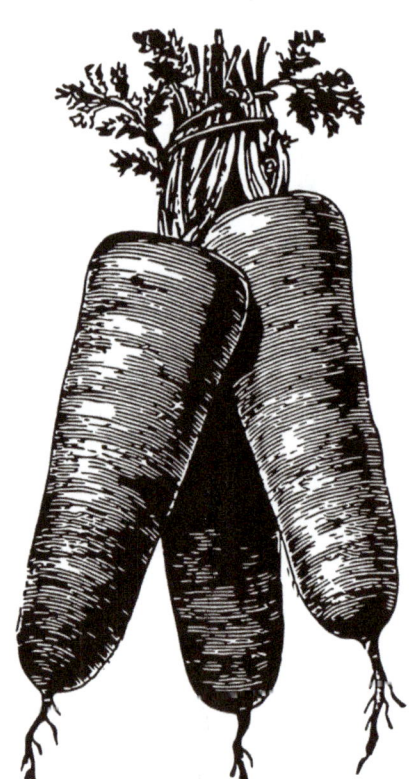

OPTIONAL GARNISH:

Fresh herbs, such as parsley, basil, or oregano
Croutons, any flavor
Parmesan cheese crisps

CO AT a 4-quart saucepan with cooking spray. Sauté the oil, garlic, fennel seeds, carrot, celery, and onion over rather high heat for 5 minutes. Add the cauliflower, zucchini, broth, wine, lemon juice, and the 3 seasonings and bring to a boil. Cook 15 minutes on medium heat, uncovered; stir a couple of times. Add the pesto, pasta, lima beans, and ham and cook another 15-20 minutes on a medium rolling simmer, uncovered. Stir a few times, until the pasta and vegetables are tender. Add the half-and-half. Puree 3 cups, then add back to the pot. Season, if desired. Garnish, as desired. Cover and chill leftovers. Serves 4-6.

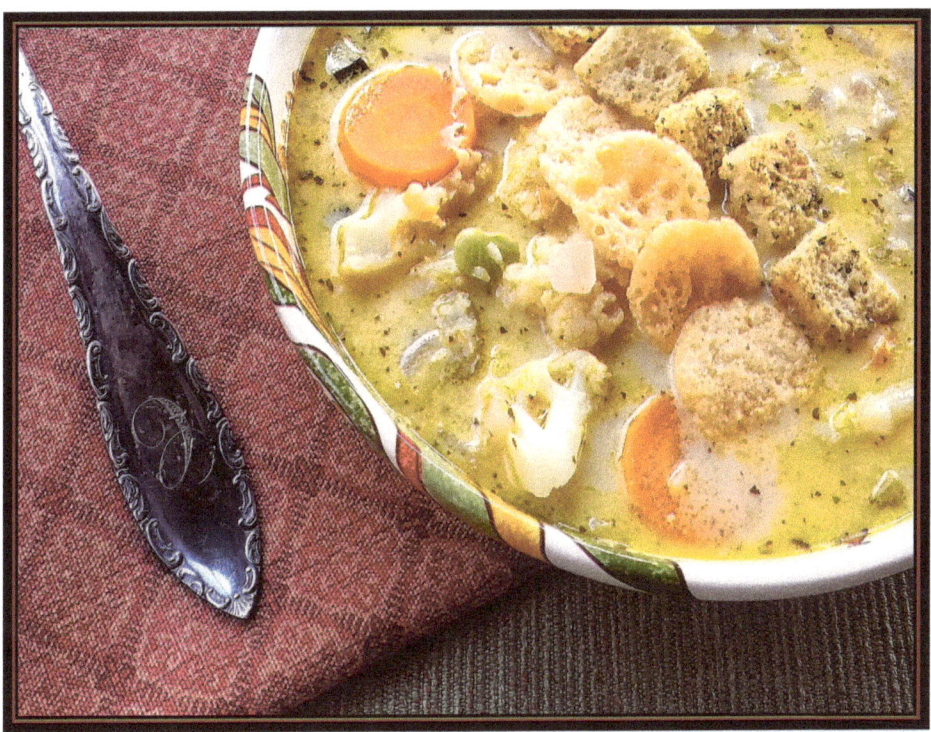

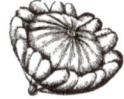 Change to vegetable broth and simply increase your zucchini to half a pound and the lima beans to a cup.

Other cooked meats will work well.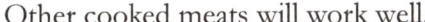

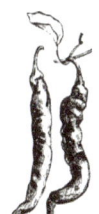 Increase the cayenne to your liking, or add half a cup of green chile or salsa. A teaspoon or so of crushed red pepper flakes would add a real kick.

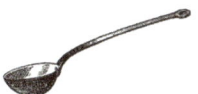

Chapter Three: Pork & Seafood

Tater Ham Chowder

You can use any kind of potatoes you like here. Another nice variation is to use sweet potatoes, or a combination of white and sweet. This is definitely a hobbity soup, so I used the Middle-earth word for potato (see Westron, or the Common Speech...).

1 tablespoon salted butter
1 tablespoon olive oil
4 ounces cooked ham, diced
2 cups carrot, peeled and coarsely chopped
2 cups celery, coarsely chopped
2 cups red onion, coarsely chopped
1½ pounds potatoes, cut into ½" cubes
    (peeled or not; it depends on the variety of potato you use)
3 cups cabbage, coarsely chopped
1 quart low-sodium chicken broth
1¼ teaspoons salt
1¼ teaspoons marjoram
    (2-3 tablespoons fresh, minced)
1 teaspoon black pepper

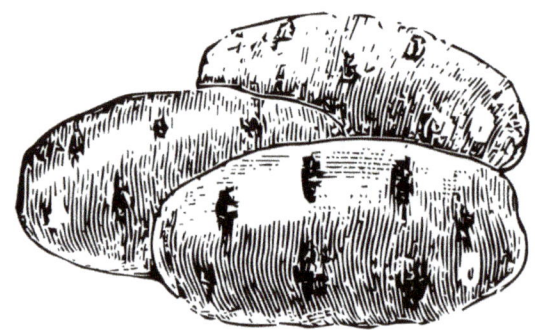

OPTIONAL GARNISH:

Minced fresh chives
Cooked and crumbled bacon
Sour cream or crème fraîche

COAT a 4-quart saucepan with cooking spray. Melt the butter and olive oil over rather high heat. Add the ham, carrot, celery, and onion and sauté 10 minutes, stirring often. Add the remaining ingredients and bring to a boil. Cook on low heat 15-20 minutes, covered, until vegetables are tender. Stir a couple times. Puree 3 cups of the soup, then add it back to the pot. Season, if desired. Garnish, as desired. Cover and chill leftovers; don't freeze. Serves 4-6.

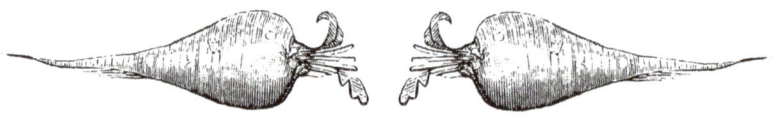

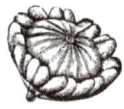 Change the broth and substitute about a quarter-pound of diced turnip, rutabaga, or parsnip (all should be peeled). Or you could simply increase each of the required vegetables.

Green Chile? Of course. I'd recommend about 4 ounces. Salsa would also be delicious.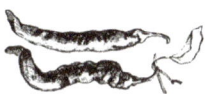

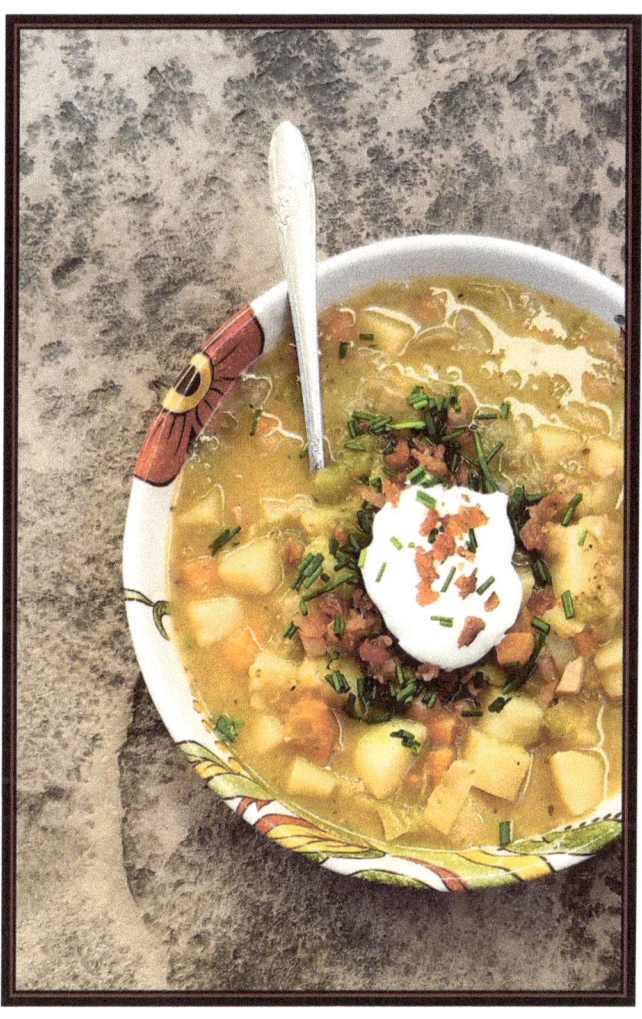

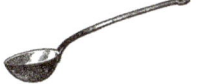

Chloë's Kale-apalooza

Sometimes I push the adjective creation a little too far, I guess. Nevertheless, I've named this after my eldest daughter, because she and her husband like to make smoothies with frozen and fresh fruit and a bunch of kale. They then serve this to their children, who seem to be fine with drinking their vegetables, as long as the fruit flavor masks the flavor of the kale. Sneaky.

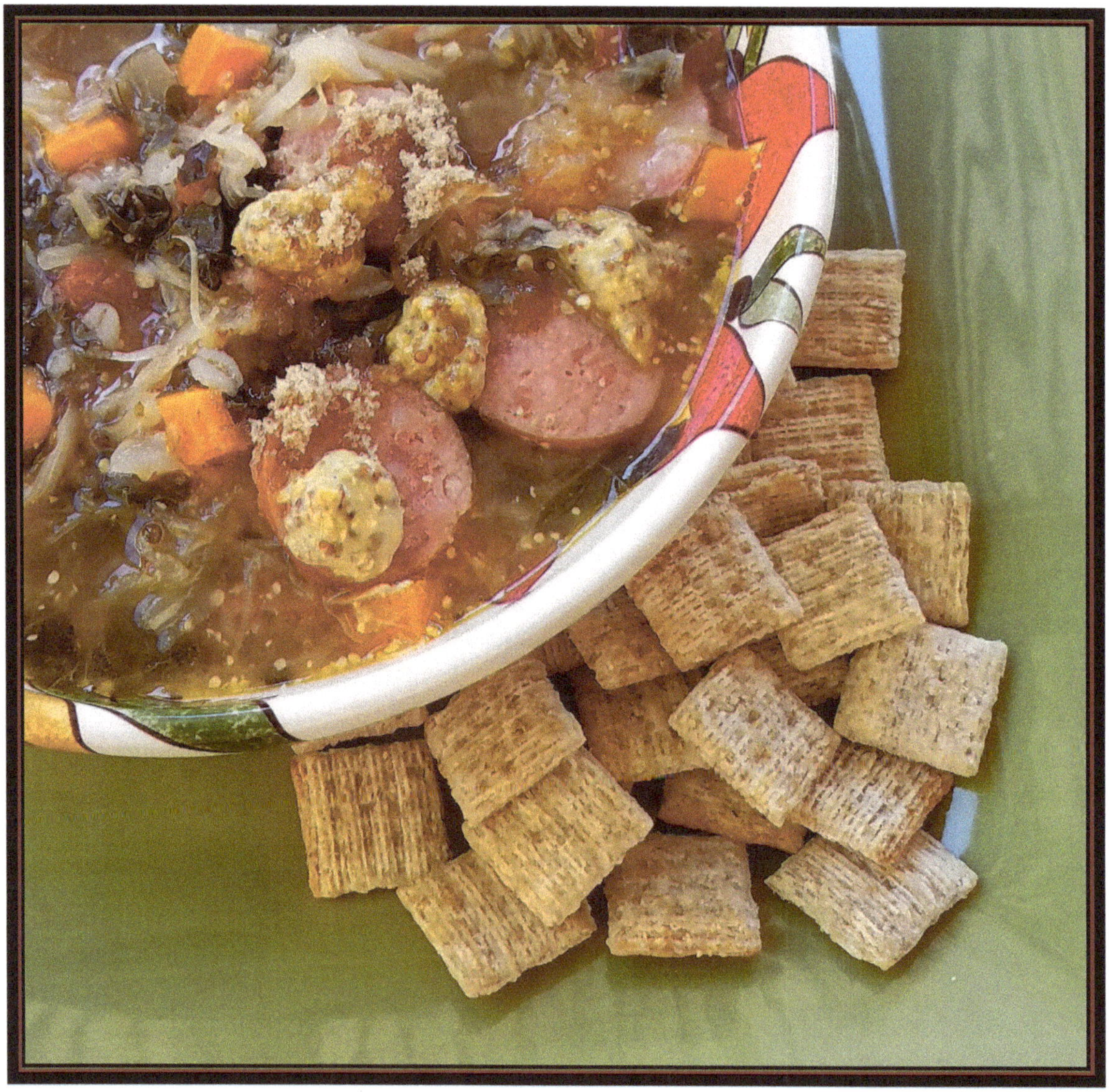

2 tablespoons salted butter
1 tablespoon minced garlic
1 cup onion, coarsely chopped
1 cup carrot, peeled and coarsely chopped
¼ cup stone ground mustard
2 tablespoons packed golden brown sugar
¾ teaspoon salt
¾ teaspoon black pepper
¾ teaspoon dry marjoram (1-2 tablespoons fresh, minced)
14.5-ounce can diced tomatoes, with juice
4 cups cabbage, finely chopped or shredded
5-6 ounces fresh baby kale
   (and/or fresh baby spinach),
   coarsely chopped
6 cups low-sodium chicken broth
1 pound smoked sausage, cut into ¼" slices
½ cup quick barley

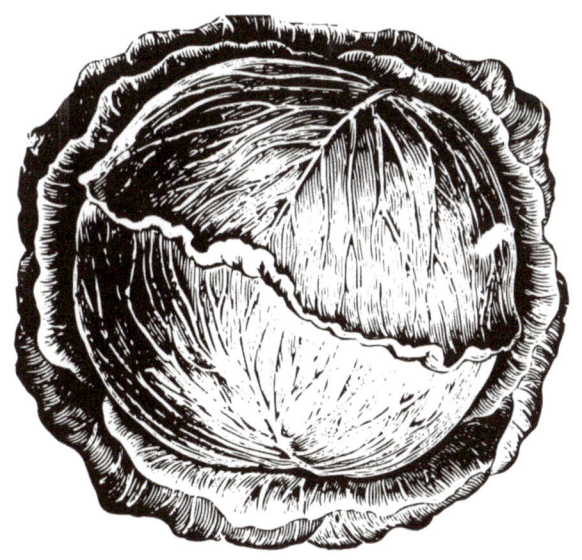

OPTIONAL GARNISH:

Sour cream or crème fraîche
Fresh minced chives
Small dollops of stone ground mustard
An extra sprinkling of brown sugar

COAT a 6-quart saucepan with cooking spray. Melt the butter over moderately high heat, then sauté the garlic, onion, and carrot 5 minutes. Add mustard, brown sugar, the 3 seasonings, tomatoes, cabbage, kale, broth, and sausage and bring to a boil. Cook, covered, on low heat for 15 minutes. Stir a couple times. Add the barley and raise heat a notch. Cook another 15-20 minutes on medium/low (a rolling simmer), uncovered. Stir a few times until the barley and vegetables are tender. Season, if desired. Garnish, as desired. Cover and chill leftovers. Serves 6-8.

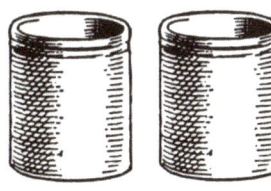

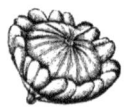 A change of broth to vegetable or water, and a pound of sliced mushrooms would be a delicious variation.

A pound of cooked and diced chicken or turkey would reduce the fat content of this soup quite a bit, if that's important to you. Though the sausage is SO good here… Compromise by using turkey sausage! Bob thinks twice as much sausage would be good in this soup, but I think that is rather excessive. It's up to you, however, if you want to increase the meat to two pounds.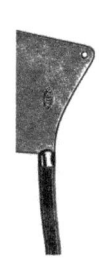

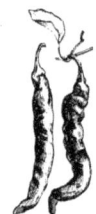 Maybe, though the mustard adds a kick already, and makes this an incredibly comforting Germanic-type of soup.

I was originally going to make this with homemade dumplings, but they sort of overwhelmed the soup. Then I was thinking of cheese-filled tiny tortellini or even miniature gnocchi, but the barley really added the right type of subtle carbohydrate touch to this recipe. So if you hate barley (for some reason), you could substitute these pasta-type carbohydrate options in small amounts; for example, four ounces of tiny tortellini or miniature gnocchi. To me, it's hardly worth the effort to make homemade dumplings in such a small amount. A half a cup of rice would also work, come to think of it.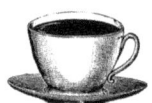

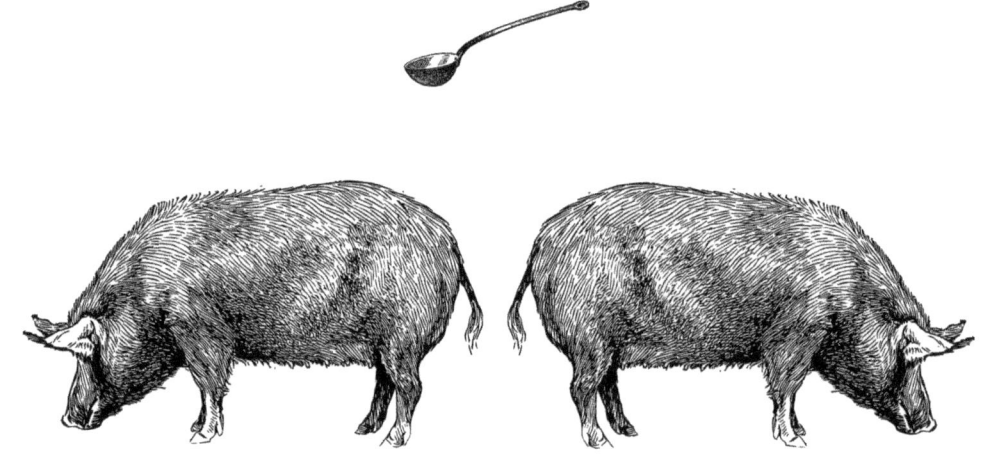

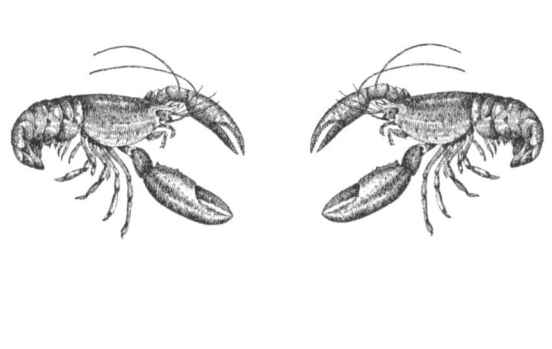

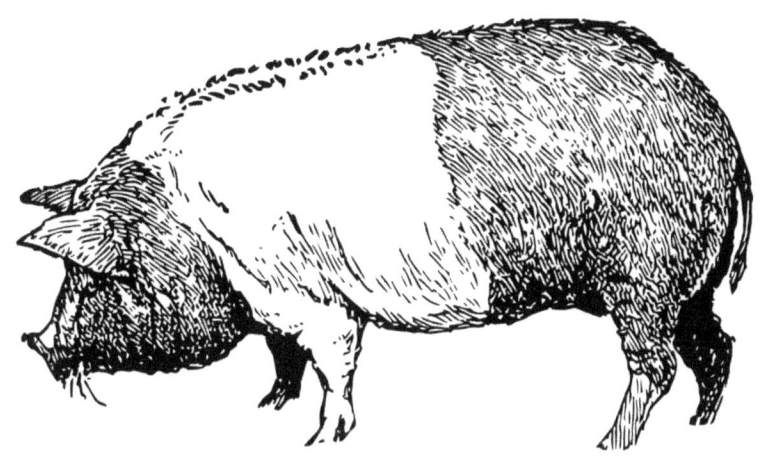

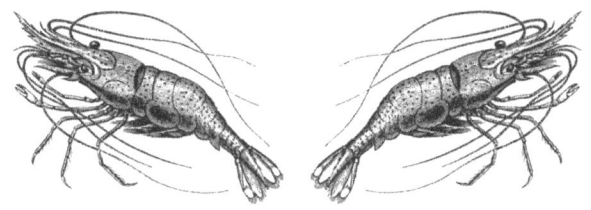

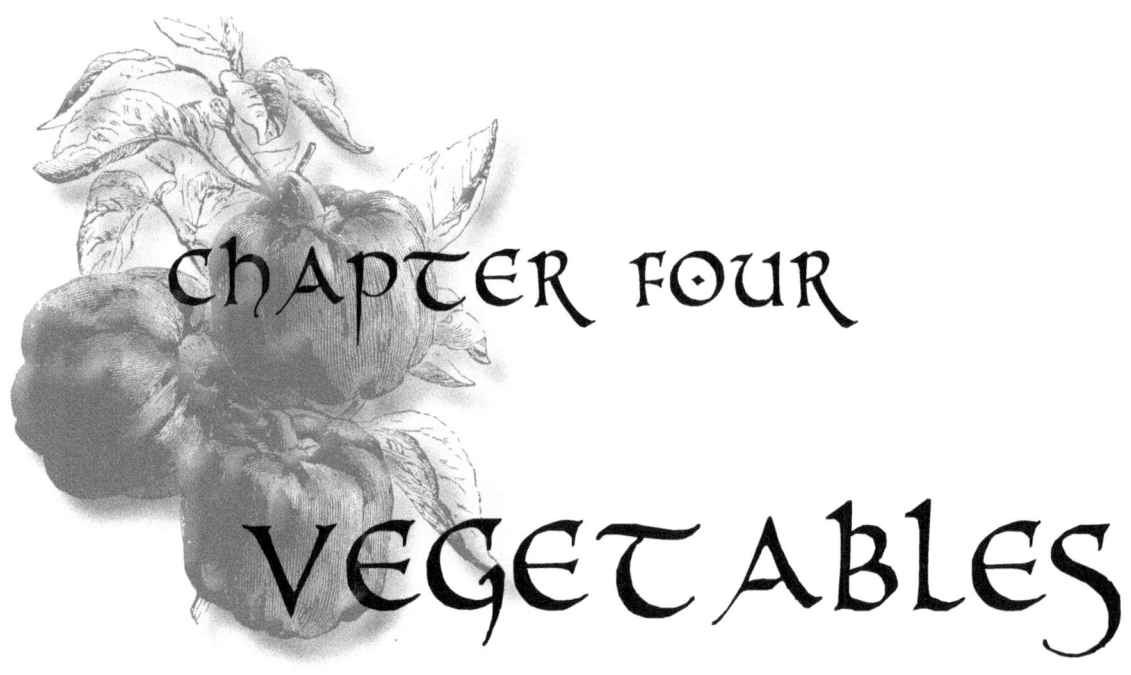

CHAPTER FOUR

VEGETABLES

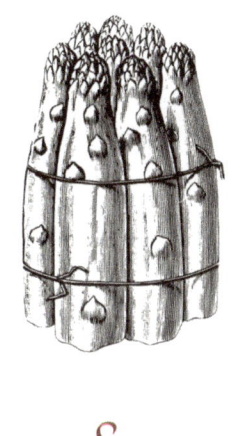

Creamy Vegetable Posole
Onion Soup C'est Magnifique
Warren Asked for Seconds (!) Tomato Soup
Mom's Masher Soup
Little Squash: Little Stew
William Said This Was His Favorite Soup
Enchanted Forest Soup
Baba Yaga Borscht
Sopa del Diente Quebrado
Ellen's Exotic Cauliflower Bisque
Savory Mushroom Soup
Saffron Madness Soup
My Darling Minestrone
Elfryda's Strawberry Soup

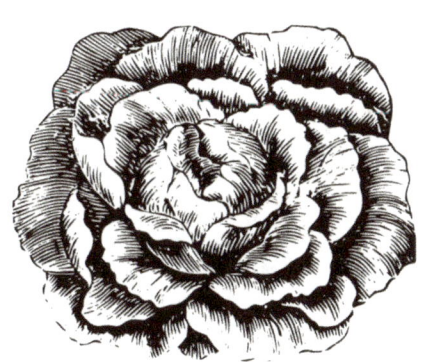

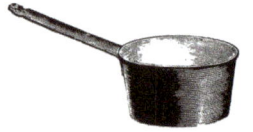 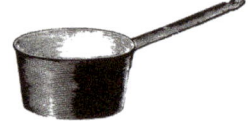

Chapter Four—Vegetables

Some of the recipes included here might happen to start with chicken or beef broth as their base. I will suggest substitutes accordingly; however, I have listed the preferred broth/stock first in the ingredient list. I guess I use the term "vegetarian" more loosely, simply meaning that there are no pieces of meat within the recipe. If you'll recall, I haven't designed the recipes to be vegan, but if you happen to be vegan, you are probably used to making adjustments. Sometimes all you will need to do is substitute oil for butter and change your broth to vegetable or water. I will also make suggestions for the meat lover.

Creamy Vegetable Posole

My final posole gets a touch of creamy richness. This is chock-full of vegetables and quite filling.

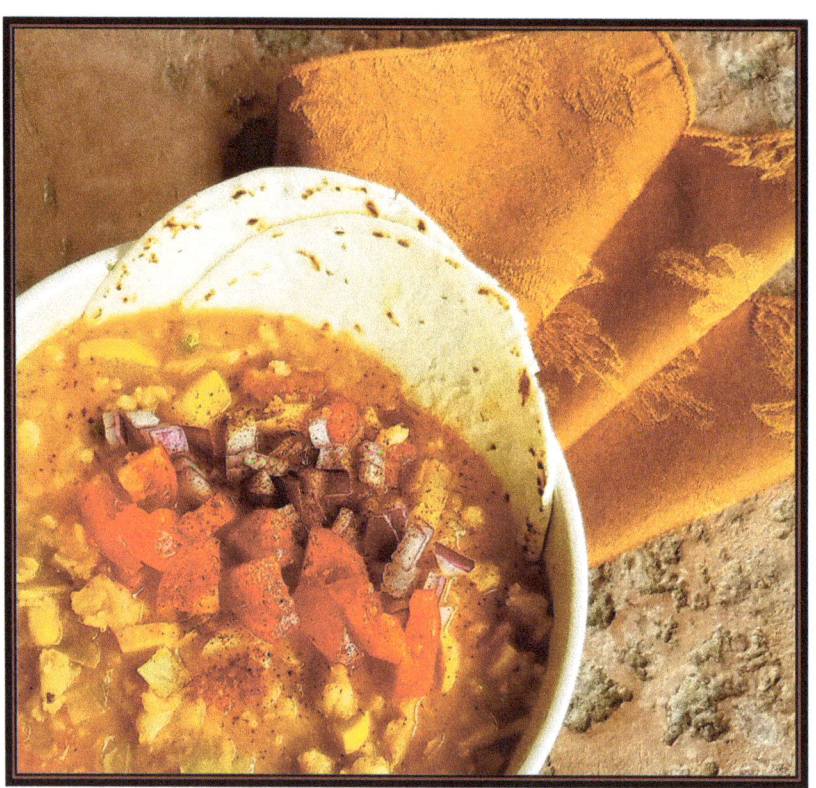

2 tablespoons salted butter
¾ cup shallots, coarsely chopped
8 ounces summer squash; cut off ends, cut into quarters
	lengthwise, then cut into ¼" slices
2 cups cabbage, finely chopped or shredded
½ cup frozen peas
½ cup frozen corn
14.5-ounce can diced tomatoes, with juice
4 ounces roasted and chopped green chile, with juice
2 (15.5-ounce) cans white hominy, drained and rinsed
	(if you like, or 3 cups cooked hominy;
	yellow hominy is also fine)
3 cups water
1½ teaspoons salt
1 teaspoon white pepper
1 teaspoon cumin
1 teaspoon chili powder
½ cup half-and-half
¼ cup heavy cream
2 tablespoons all-purpose flour

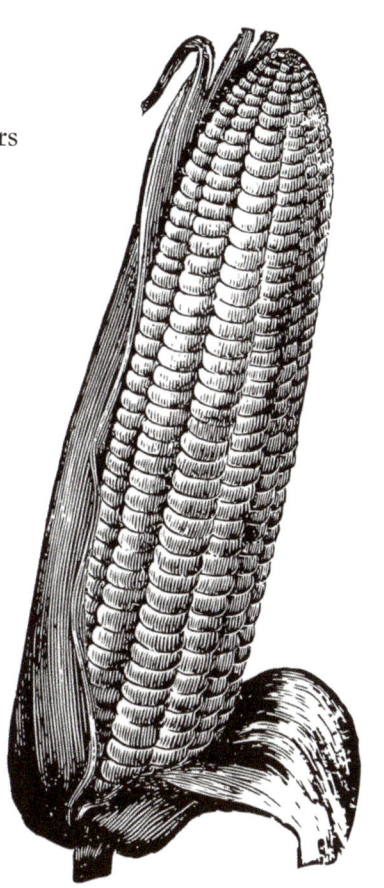

OPTIONAL GARNISH:

Coarsely chopped tomatoes
Diced red onion
Chili powder
I'm sure you have almost memorized the items in the **NICE NEW MEXICAN & MEXICAN GARNISHES** section by now!

COAT a 6-quart saucepan with cooking spray. Melt the butter over moderately high heat. Add the shallots and sauté for 3 minutes. Add squash, cabbage, peas, corn, tomatoes, green chile, hominy, water, and the 4 seasonings and bring to a boil. Cover and cook on medium/low heat for 20 minutes. Stir a few times. Whisk half-and-half, cream, and flour in a 2-cup glass measuring cup. Add ½ cup of hot cooking liquid to this and whisk well; add this to the pot and cook on low heat, uncovered, 4-5 minutes or so, until the squash is tender and it thickens a bit; stir a few times. Season, if desired. Garnish, as desired. Cover and chill leftovers. Serves 4-6.

You can add a cup or so of any diced, cooked meat near the end of cooking.

Chapter Four: Vegetables

Onion Soup C'est Magnifique

Redolent with plenty of onions, herbs, and cognac; topped with ginormous cheesy toasts. These will count as your garnish. See the garnishing option and anecdotal material at the end of the recipe for other ideas.

¼ cup salted butter
1 tablespoon sugar
1 tablespoon minced garlic
2 teaspoons dry thyme (3-4 tablespoons fresh, minced)
3 pounds onions (preferably on the smaller side),
	cut into ¼" rings
¼ cup all-purpose flour
6 cups low-sodium beef broth (or vegetable broth)
¼ cup cognac
2 tablespoons Worcestershire sauce
1½ teaspoons salt
1½ teaspoons black pepper

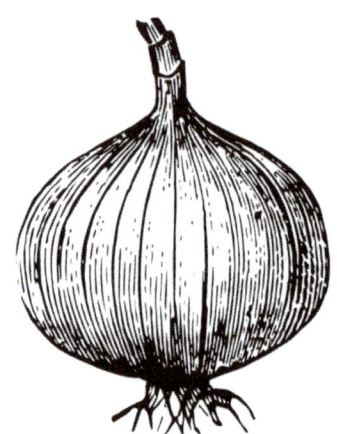

OPTIONAL GARNISH:

Ginormous Cheesy Toasts (see ingredients below—these are easy and worth making!)
If you decide not to make the toasts, sprinkle some ready-made croutons on top; then sprinkle a generous amount of shredded Gruyere cheese over them. You could broil your bowl for a few minutes, if you like; be sure to use broiler-safe bowls.

FOR THE GINORMOUS CHEESY TOASTS:

A loaf of French bread (Italian or sourdough will also work; about 1 pound)
8 ounces Gruyere cheese, sliced from a 1-pound block (Swiss or Jarlsberg are also fine)

In a 6-quart saucepan, melt the butter over moderately high heat. Add the sugar, garlic, and thyme and mix in. Add the onions and sauté over moderately high heat 10 minutes. Stir often and break up the rings as necessary. Turn heat to lowest setting and continue cooking for another 10 minutes, uncovered. Stir frequently. Add flour and mix in well. Add remaining ingredients and bring to a boil. Cover and cook on a low simmer 15 minutes. Stir occasionally, scraping up any browned bits. Raise heat to medium and cook, uncovered, on a gentle boil another 10 minutes; stir a few times.

MEANWHILE, prepare the Ginormous Cheesy Toasts. Preheat oven to 450°. Coat a large (18" by 13") baking sheet with cooking spray or grease lightly. Cut the bread into 8 slices, each about 1¼" thick. Don't use the heels of the bread. Lay on prepared sheet. Thinly slice cheese and distribute 1 ounce on each bread slice. Bake 9 minutes. Let stand on pan. Cover and chill leftovers. Makes 8.

TO SERVE: divide soup evenly between 4 bowls, preferably rather shallow ones. Place 2 toasts on each. Season, if desired. Garnish, as desired. Cover and chill leftovers. Serves 4.

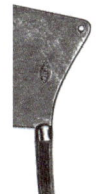

Change the broth to vegetable and the Worcestershire to soy sauce.

This is a soup I really feel should be left vegetarian. But I suppose if you really must add meat, I would keep it minimal, just for a taste. Something like a quarter-pound of cooked chicken or roast beef; just a few strips of cooked bacon crumbled up should be fine.

Green chile? Of course Bob thinks this would be a good idea, but he would put green chile in everything except dessert. So, you've got your typical 4-8 ounces of roasted and chopped chile as a suggestion.

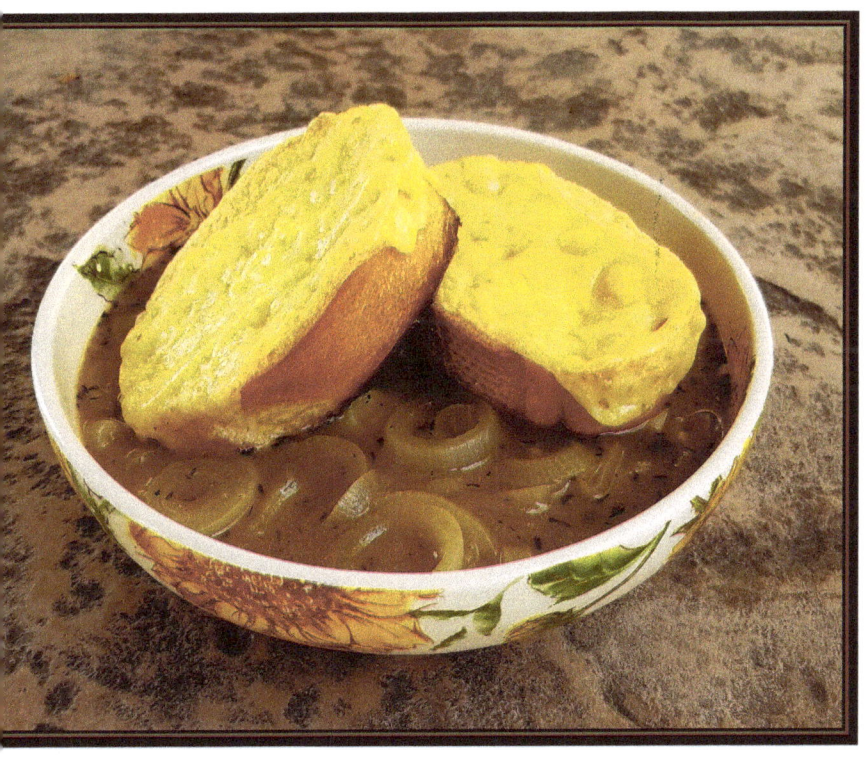

I've had many versions of French Onion Soup that are merely glorified dish water. I think it's because people shy away from the onions, for some reason. Why is that? This is ONION soup! I never much liked having to broil my bowls of soup to melt the cheese on top, so I figured some toasty cheesy bread would be a delicious way to top it off. You can make all of the soup at once and make half of the toasts, if you like; that way, you can make fresh ones the next time you serve the soup.

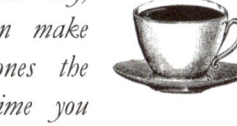

Chapter Four: Vegetables

Warren Asked for Seconds (!) Tomato Soup

This is a chunky tomato soup, though you could puree the entire recipe after you have cooked it and before you have added the cream and basil. Or you could simply puree the whole thing, especially if you are feeding it to people (children) who are sensitive about foods such as fresh herbs. I made this one day and took a chance on feeding it to my toddler grandsons, mainly because I am determined that their entire diet should **NOT** consist of PB&Js, chicken nuggets, and boxes of macaroni and cheese. I was shocked—**SHOCKED**—when one of them asked for a second bowl. And—he actually ate it **WITHOUT** it being pureed. This is why you have to keep exposing children to new foods; you never know when something will appeal to them.

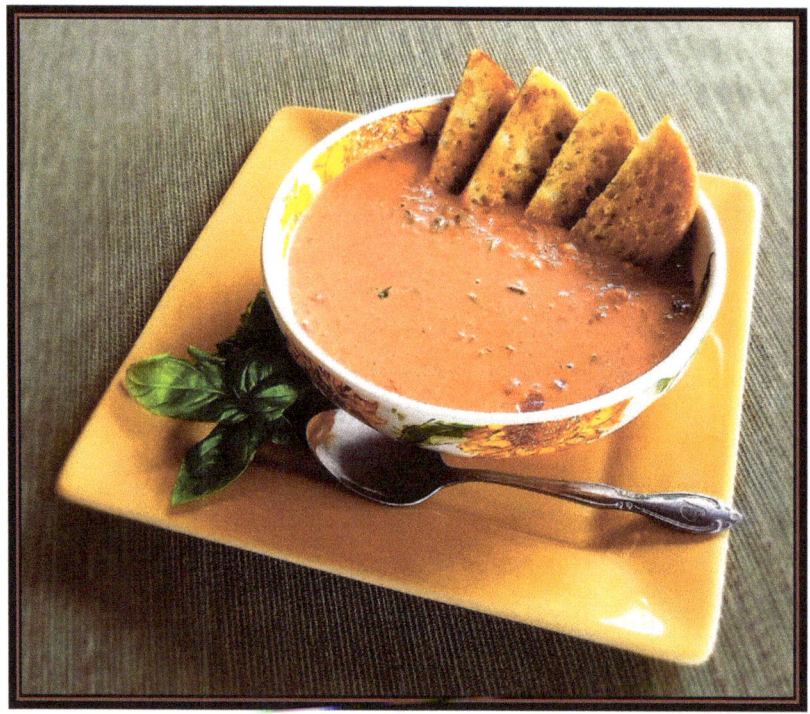

2 (29-ounce) cans stewed tomatoes
2 tablespoons minced garlic (or use 6-8 large cloves)
2 (14.5-ounce) cans low-sodium chicken broth (or vegetable broth)
2 cups onion, finely chopped
1 teaspoon pepper
1 cup heavy cream
1 cup loosely packed fresh basil, cut into slivers

OPTIONAL GARNISH:

More fresh slivered basil
Crazy Croutons (see ingredients below, or fry up your basic grilled cheese sandwich for dunking, if you prefer)

FOR THE CRAZY CROUTONS:

6 English muffins
½ cup olive oil
Coarse kosher salt

DRAIN 1 can of stewed tomatoes over a 6-quart saucepan. Press down on the tomatoes to release as much juice as possible. Chop these tomatoes into ¼" bits and add them to the pot. Puree the garlic and the other can of tomatoes, with the juice, completely; add this to the pot. Add the broth, onion, and pepper and bring to a boil. Cover and cook on a low heat, 30 minutes. Stir a couple times. Raise heat to medium/low setting and cook another 30 minutes, uncovered. Stir a few times.

MEANWHILE, make the Crazy Croutons. Split the English muffins into halves and set aside. In a large skillet, heat the olive oil over rather high heat until it sizzles a little; swirl the pan to coat thoroughly. Fry 4 halves of the muffins, placing the outside part down first. Fry about one minute. Using forks, turn all over and fry another minute. They should become golden brown. Place on doubled paper toweling, with the interior side up. Sprinkle lightly with salt, about a pinch on each. Repeat with the remaining halves, 4 at a time. Let stand on the paper towels. To serve, cut each in half and serve on the side of the soup. Cover and keep leftovers at room temperature.

MEASURE the cream in a 2-cup glass measuring cup. Add ½ cup of hot soup to the cream, then add this back to the pot. Cook, uncovered, another 3 minutes on medium heat. Add the basil and cook another minute. Mix and serve. Season, if desired. Garnish, as desired. Cover and chill leftovers. Serves 4-6.

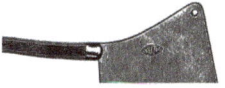 Your best bet is about a half a cup or so of cooked, crumbled, crispy bacon.

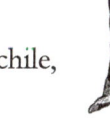

This soup lends itself to any kind of spice you might desire; Sriracha, green chile, salsa, hot sauce, etc.

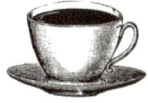 *If you have oil leftover from the croutons, feel free to use it within a few days to sauté some other items, or to start another soup. It will have some English muffin crumbs in it, but that's okay.*

Chapter Four: Vegetables

Mom's Masher Soup

My Norwegian mom was a potato connoisseur; she loved experimenting with different varieties, from teeny-tiny reds to fingerlings to purple Peruvians. We often had leftover mashed russet potatoes, which she usually converted to pancakes. But I discovered that whipping up a super-simple soup is a classic Scandinavian treatment as well. Peeled Russets and Yukon Gold varieties are your best bets here, if you are making your taters from scratch.

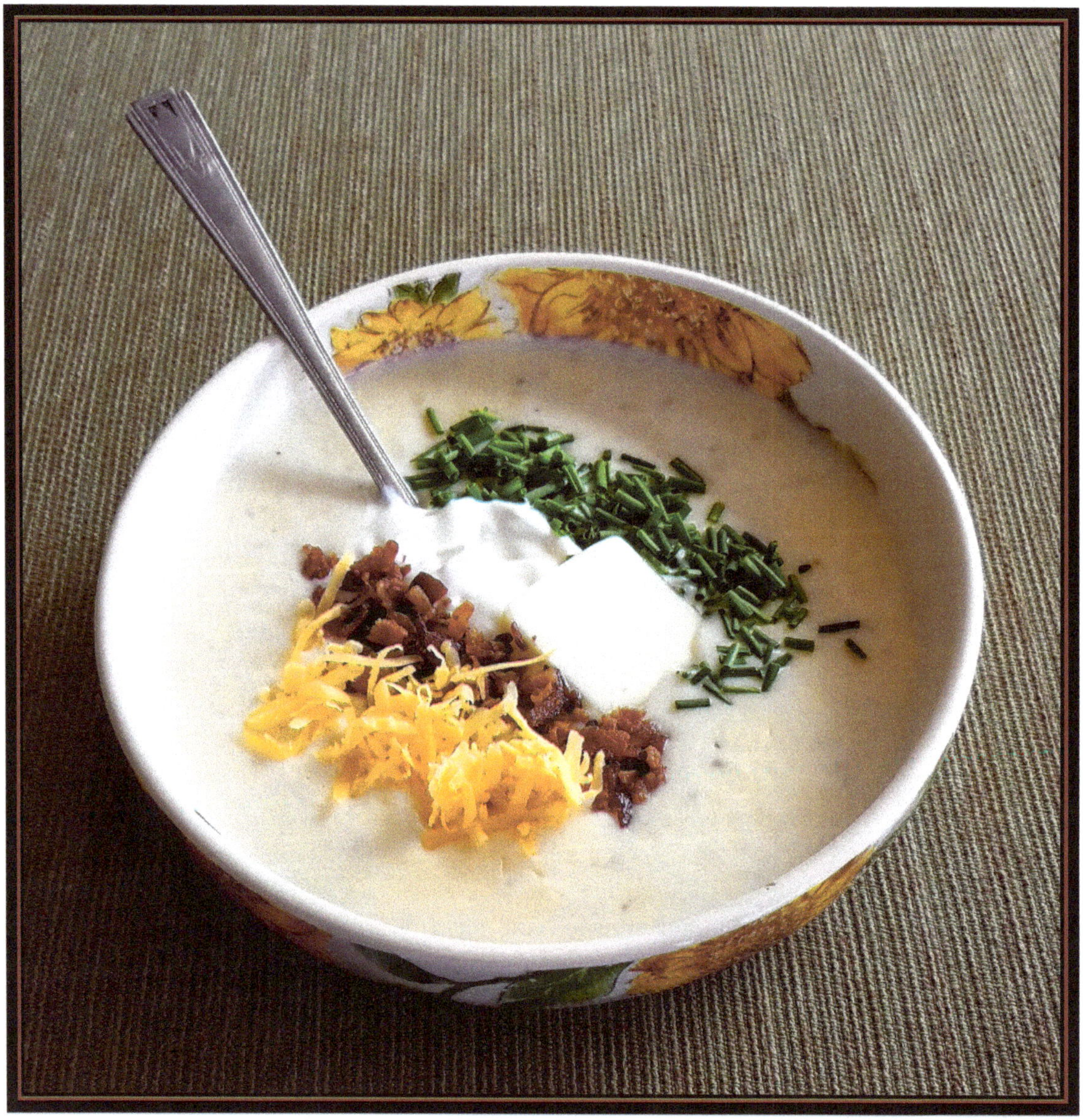

3 cups leftover, seasoned mashed potatoes (be sure to use peeled potatoes, or a 24-ounce container of ready-made potatoes will also work)
14.5-ounce can low-sodium chicken broth (or vegetable broth)
¼ cup heavy cream
¼ cup half-and-half
¼ teaspoon salt
¼ teaspoon black pepper
¼ teaspoon nutmeg (or allspice)

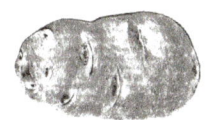
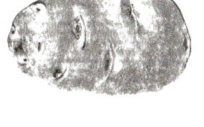
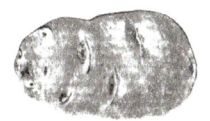

OPTIONAL GARNISH:

Shredded Cheddar cheese, any degree of sharpness you like
Bacon bits
Sour cream or crème fraîche
A pat of butter
Minced chives or thinly sliced scallions

PLACE the potatoes and broth in a 3-quart saucepan. Whisk well to combine. Bring to a gentle boil. Add the remaining ingredients and boil gently again. Cook, uncovered, on a medium/low heat, 10 minutes. Maintain a gentle simmer. Stir a few times. Season, if desired; your seasoning will depend on how well seasoned your mashed potatoes were. Garnish, as desired. Cover and chill leftovers; don't freeze. Serves 2-3.

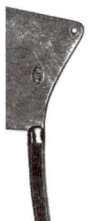

Just give in to the bacon garnish, or slice or dice some smoked sausage and turn this into a heartier meal; as little as a quarter pound should do it.

Always an option; whatever spice you like.

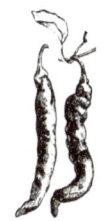

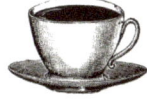

Skip the bowl and the garnish and just serve this in mugs—perfect for sipping on a cold night.

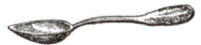

Chapter Four: Vegetables   121

Little Squash: Little Stew

A long while ago, I became tired of the usual side dishes when I used to order Mexican/New Mexican entrées. Refried beans and rice—that was usually it. Then I discovered you could sometimes substitute "calabacitas" for beans and rice. This is a low-carb/low-calorie alternative I could enjoy, especially since summer squash is one of those vegetables I don't serve too often, because of Bob (of course). Not every version of *calabacitas* is great; it really depends on the individual restaurant. *Calabacitas* (or "little squash") is quite similar to zucchini, though with a milder flavor and a pale green skin, marked by subtle striping. If you can't find any, zucchini and yellow squash are perfectly fine to use. I like it so much, I decided to convert it into a filling vegetable stew. I make a rather small pot of it, since I'm the only one who usually eats it, but it's easy to double the recipe. If you use zucchini and it turns out to be bitter, give it a partial peeling.

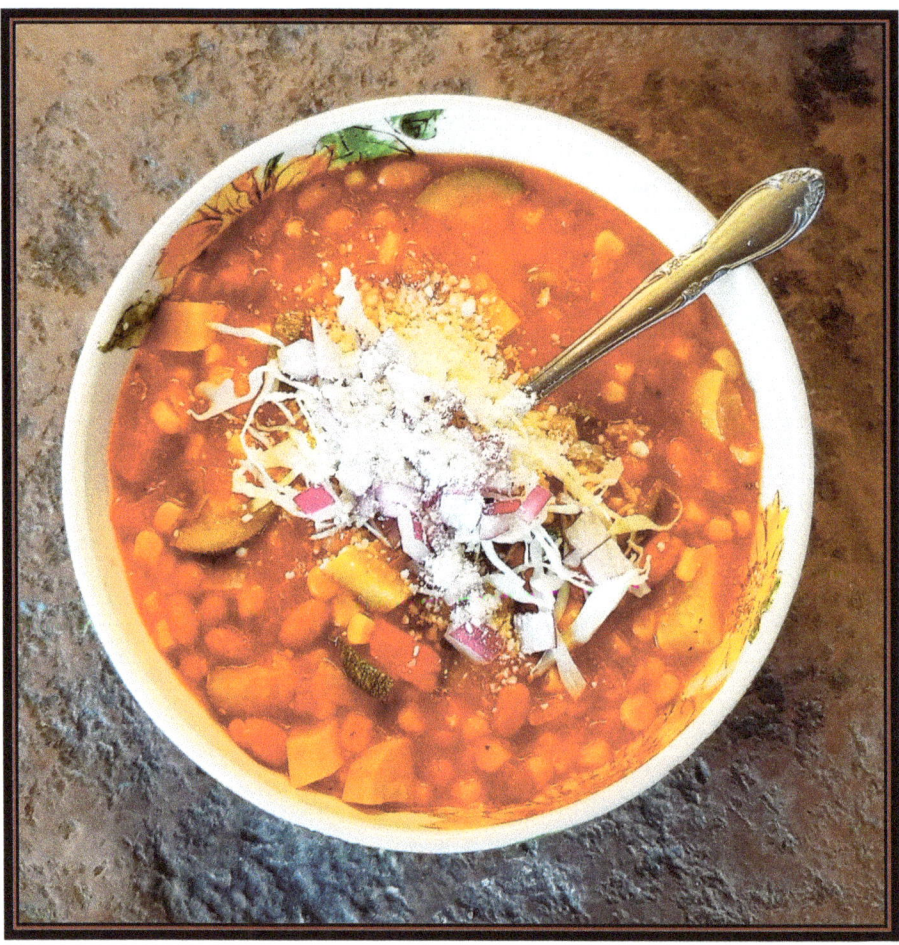

1 pound *calabacitas* (or any type of summer squash; you may mix your varieties)
1 tablespoon salted butter
1 tablespoon minced garlic
½ cup red onion, coarsely chopped
8-ounce can tomato sauce
10-ounce can diced tomatoes and green chilies, with juice (such as Ro*Tel)
15.25-ounce can corn, with juice
4 ounces roasted and chopped green chile, with juice
2 cups water
2 tablespoons cornmeal
15.5-ounce can pinto beans, drained and rinsed
½ teaspoon salt
½ teaspoon black pepper
½ teaspoon cumin
½ teaspoon dry oregano (1-2 tablespoons fresh, minced)

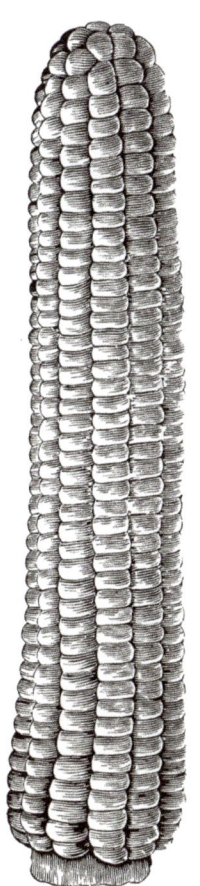

OPTIONAL GARNISH:

Shredded cabbage
Diced red onion
Crumbled Cotija cheese
Use your favorite items from the **NICE NEW MEXICAN & MEXICAN GARNISHES** list.

CUT off the ends of the *calabacitas*. Quarter lengthwise, then cut into ¼" slices; set aside. Coat a 4-quart saucepan with cooking spray. Sauté the butter, garlic, and onion over rather high heat 3 minutes. Add the *calabacitas* and sauté another 3 minutes. Add the remaining ingredients and bring to a boil. Cook, uncovered, on a medium heat (a rolling simmer) 25 minutes, until the squash is tender. Stir a few times. Season, if desired. Garnish, as desired. Cover and chill leftovers. Serves 4-6.

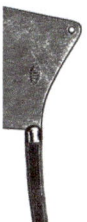

This is a great place to throw a cup or so of any kind of cooked meat, if you like. Or sauté half a pound of diced, raw chicken breasts or thighs (either option should be boneless and skinless) with the garlic and onion.

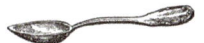

Chapter Four: Vegetables

William Said This Was His Favorite Soup

If you happen to make this in the summertime, you might want to use fresh tomatoes from your garden, if you end up with a bumper crop. If so, you'll need about a pound of tomatoes. You can peel them if you like by submerging them in some boiling water for a few minutes; cool them off, then peel and cut them into small chunks. You'll also want to add ½ teaspoon each of dry basil and dry oregano (or 1-2 tablespoons of minced fresh herbs—maybe you have some of these in your garden, as well).

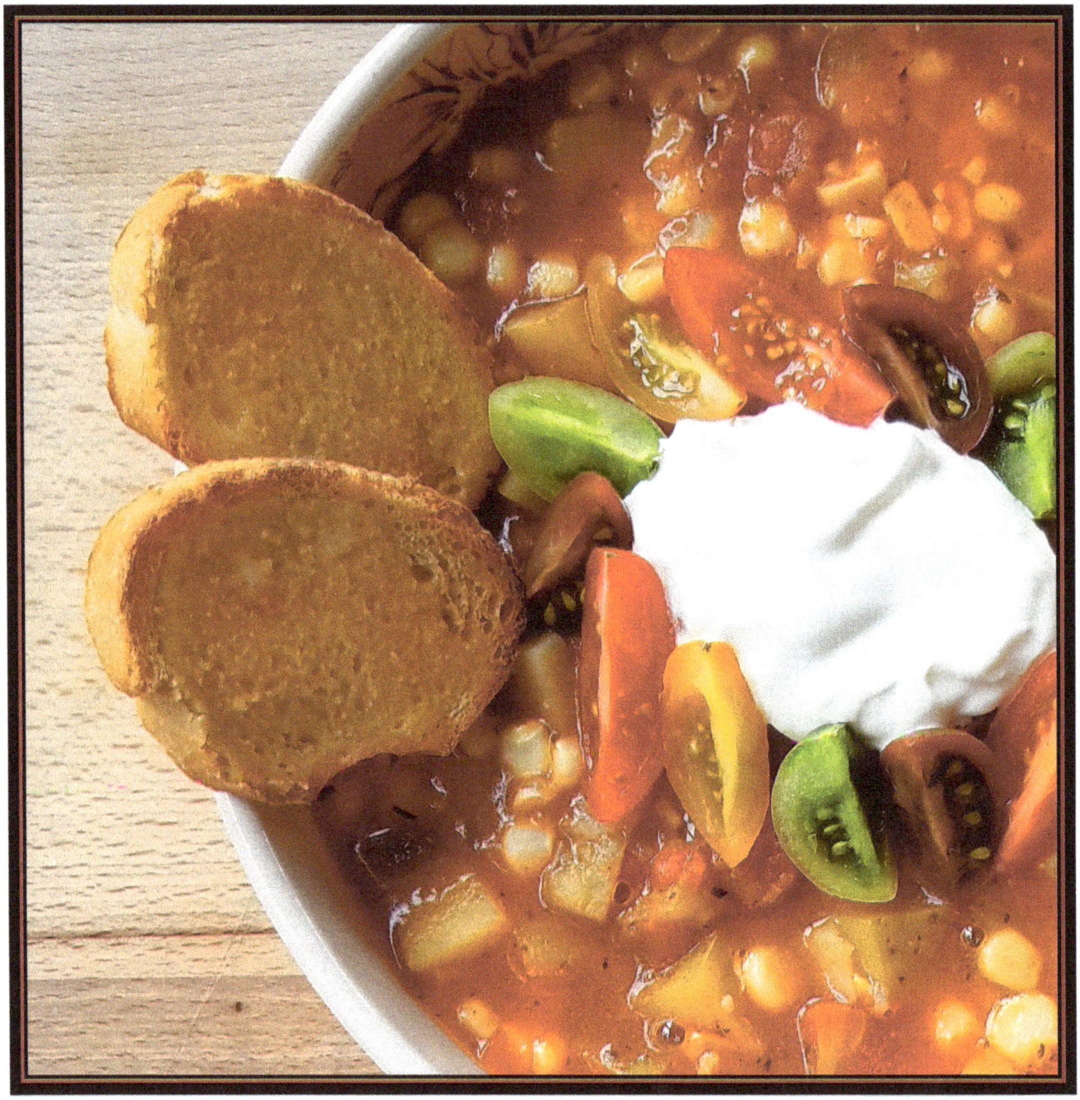

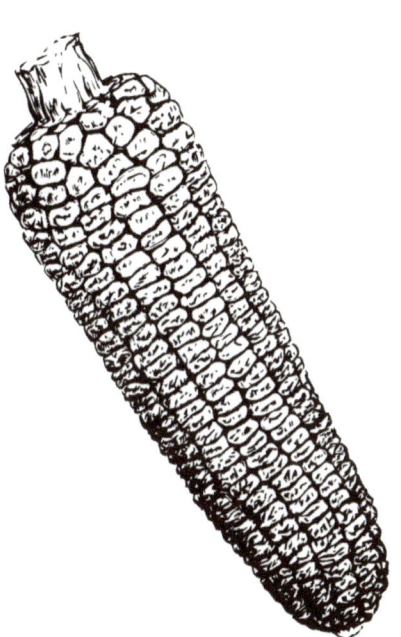

2 tablespoons olive oil
¾ cup shallots, coarsely chopped
1 tablespoon minced garlic
1 teaspoon salt
1 teaspoon black pepper
2 teaspoons Herbes de Provence
1 quart low-sodium chicken broth (or vegetable broth)
1 pound Yukon Gold or red potatoes, unpeeled,
    cut into ½" chunks
3 cups fresh corn kernels (or 3 cups frozen corn,
    or 2 (15.25-ounce) cans of corn, drained)
14.5-ounce can stewed tomatoes; with juice, cut into ½" bits

OPTIONAL GARNISH:

Some fresh tomatoes, sliced or diced
Sour cream or crème fraîche
A sprinkling of other fresh herbs, such as basil or oregano

COAT a 4-quart saucepan with cooking spray. Sauté the oil, shallots, garlic, salt, pepper, and Herbes de Provence over a rather low to moderate heat 5 minutes, stirring frequently, until the shallots start browning. Add the broth and potatoes and bring to a boil. Cook, covered, over low heat (a rolling simmer), 10 minutes. Add the corn and tomatoes and bring to another boil. Cook over medium heat, uncovered, 10-15 minutes, until the vegetables are tender. Stir a few times. Season, if desired. Garnish, as desired. Cover and chill leftovers; don't freeze. Serves 3-4.

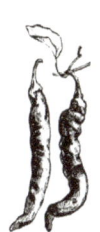

Add one or two cups of cooked, chopped meat near the end of cooking. Chicken is a good bet here; or try crumbled bacon, ham, or sausage.

A half cup of whatever salsa you like is a great addition, or the usual suggestion of roasted and chopped green chile.

You never know what a young child will like, do you? I had one grandchild who loved this soup (hence the name) and another who couldn't even bring himself to take a single bite. Yet he asked for a second bowl of my chunky tomato soup… Well, maybe when he's older he'll give this corn chowder a try. But for now—guess it will be another PB&J.

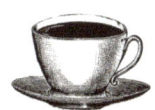

Chapter Four: Vegetables   125

Enchanted Forest Soup

Use a hearty extra-sharp Cheddar, either yellow or white, for this comforting soup. I'm usually not a fan of Velveeta, but if you can purchase that variety of cheese already shredded, you won't regret it. You can't beat its meltability. And for a radically different version, substitute cauliflower for the broccoli and a mellow, nutty cheese for the Cheddar—Gruyere, Swiss, or Jarlsberg will work well, or perhaps you'd prefer something like a Monterey (Pepper) Jack.

    I was originally going to call this by the rather pedestrian title Classic Broccoli Cheese Soup, but the daughter of one of my recipe testers suggested this whimsical name. She liked this soup quite a lot and associated chunks of broccoli with tiny trees; she was probably reminiscing about her younger days when dinosaur-shaped chicken nuggets were always more fun to eat with miniature broccoli trees.

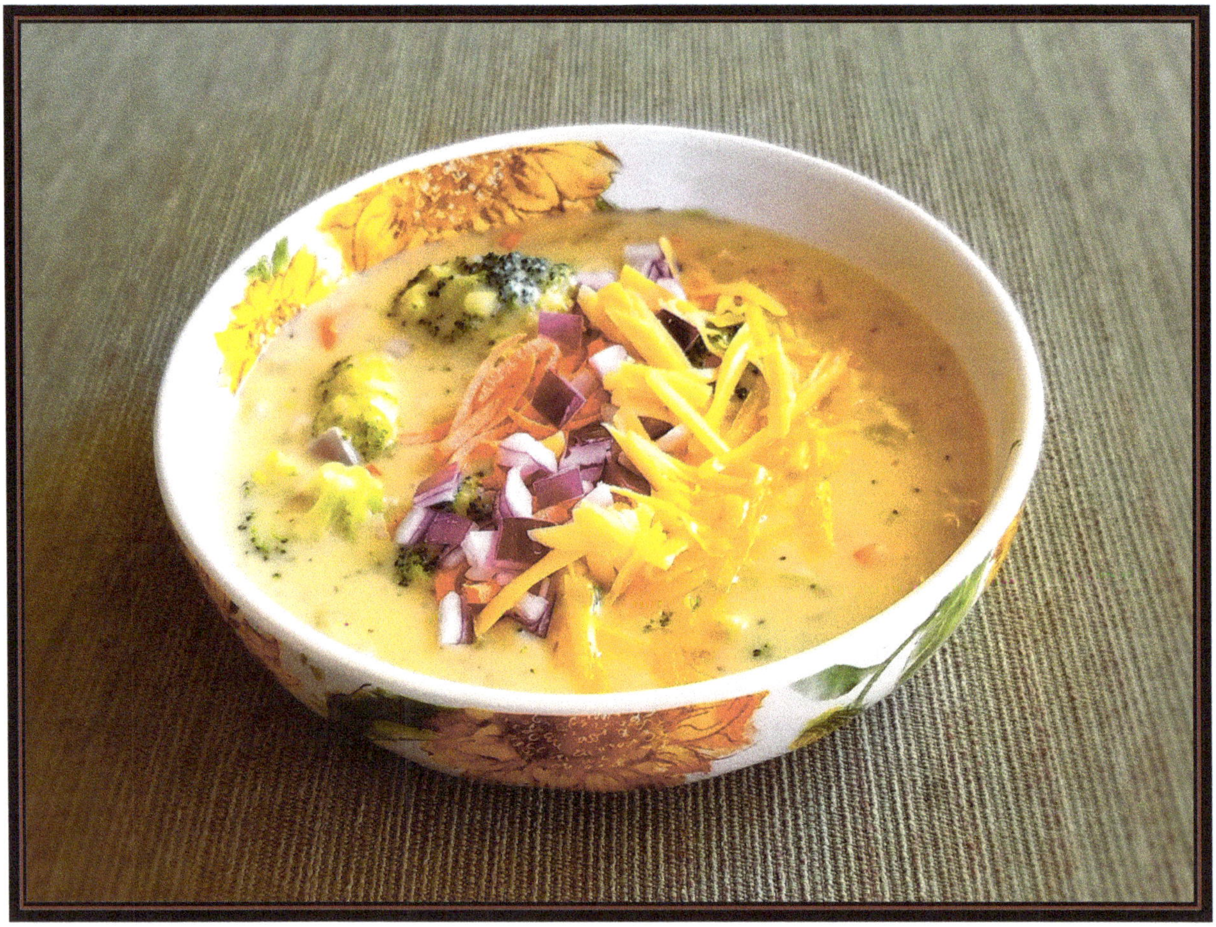

2 tablespoons salted butter
¾ cup carrot, peeled and coarsely chopped
¾ cup celery, coarsely chopped
¾ cup shallots, coarsely chopped
1 quart low-sodium chicken broth
   (or vegetable broth)
¾ teaspoon salt
¾ teaspoon black pepper
12 ounces fresh broccoli florets
8 ounces shredded extra-sharp Cheddar cheese
   (or Velveeta)
½ cup all-purpose flour
1 cup half-and-half

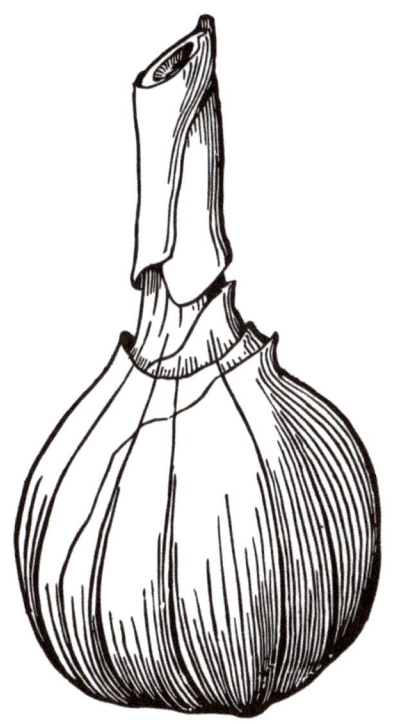

OPTIONAL GARNISH:

Shredded carrot
Diced red onion
More shredded Cheddar cheese

COAT a 4-quart saucepan with cooking spray. Melt butter over rather high heat. Add carrot, celery, and shallots and sauté 5 minutes. Add broth, salt, pepper, and broccoli and bring to a boil. Cover and cook over moderately low heat for 20 minutes. Stir a few times. Gently break up any larger broccoli florets near the end of cooking. Combine cheese and flour in a medium bowl and set aside. Add half-and-half to the soup. Then add the cheese mixture. Raise heat a couple of notches and cook on a medium setting, uncovered, 3-4 minutes, until the cheese has melted and the soup is thicker. Stir a few times. Season, if desired. Garnish, as desired. Cover and chill leftovers. Serves 3-4.

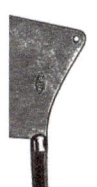
Add a cup or so of cooked, chopped meat near the end of cooking (e.g., chicken, ham, sausage, bacon…).

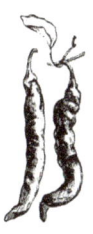
A half cup or so of green chile or salsa will work nicely here.

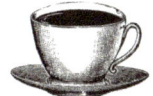
This is my version of the soup I usually get whenever I visit my local Panera in the cold months of the year; however, now I usually only get one particular salad and it's a half order at that. I still usually get a cookie, but I bet one day I'll have to give that up, too.

Chapter Four: Vegetables   127

Baba Yaga Borscht

You know how you see a small jar of borscht next to the beets in the canned goods section of your market? It's merely some magenta-colored broth with a few bits of beets in it. I thought it needed an upgrade. Roasting fresh beets is not as hard as you might think, but if you are pressed for time, you may certainly use a 15-ounce can of sliced beets. Drain, then chop them into rather small chunks. You would also ignore the instructions about the greens, which is a shame; beet greens are underrated.

For the garnish, you would need to make the crème fraîche at least 24 hours before you want to use it. Sour cream is acceptable, though it has a tendency to break down once it touches hot liquid.

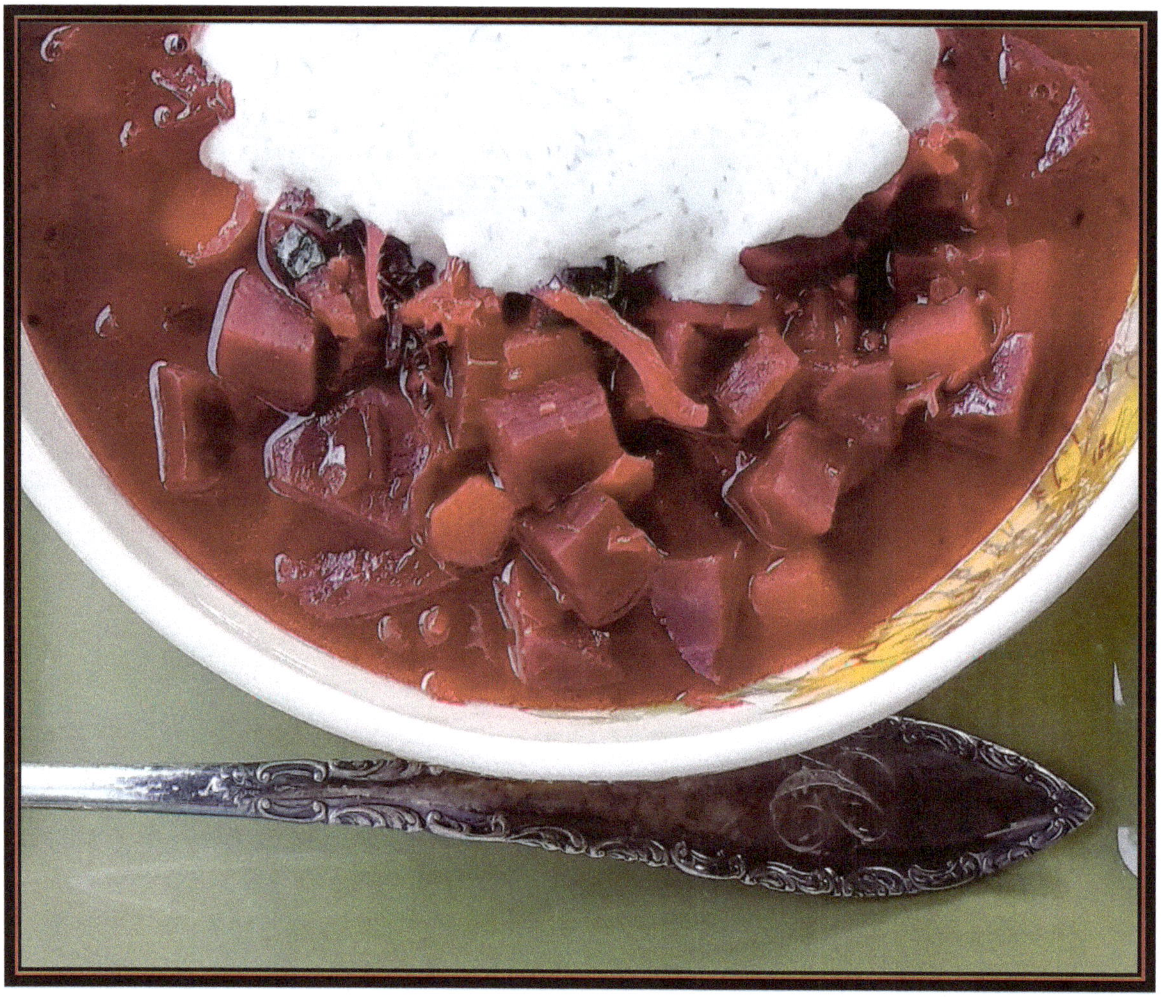

1-1½ pounds of fresh beets (about 3 medium ones)
3 tablespoons salted butter, divided
1 tablespoon minced garlic
½ cup carrot, peeled and thinly sliced
½ cup celery, thinly sliced
½ cup red onion, coarsely chopped
1¼ teaspoons salt, divided
¾ teaspoon white pepper, divided
½ teaspoon dry thyme (1-2 tablespoons fresh, minced)
1 quart low-sodium beef broth (or vegetable broth)
8 ounces potato; peeled and cut into ½" bits
3 cups cabbage, finely chopped or shredded
3 tablespoons red wine vinegar
1½ tablespoons packed golden brown sugar
1 bay leaf

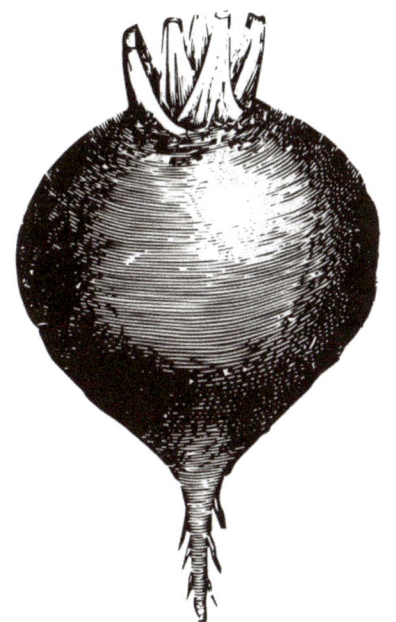

Optional Garnish:

1 cup Crème de la Crème Fraîche (see recipe on page xviii and prepare in advance, or use light sour cream)
2 teaspoons dry dill weed (2-3 tablespoons fresh, minced)
½ teaspoon salt
¼ teaspoon white pepper

AT least 3 hours before needed: Preheat oven to 400°. Cut the stems and roots of the beets down to 1". Place the greens back in your plastic grocery bag or in a covered container and store in the refrigerator for later use. Wash the beets well and enclose loosely in heavy duty foil. Bake 60-90 minutes, until they are sharp knife tender. The total time will depend on the relative size of the beets; you might need to remove smaller beets earlier. Let stand in foil for an hour or so. Cut off the stems and roots and peel them. Cut into ½" cubes and set aside.

COAT a 3-quart saucepan with cooking spray. Melt 2 tablespoons butter over medium heat. Add garlic, carrot, celery, onion, 1 teaspoon salt, ½ teaspoon pepper, and thyme and sauté on a medium heat 8-10 minutes, stirring often. Add the broth, potato, cabbage, vinegar, sugar, and bay leaf and bring to a boil. Cook 20 minutes on low heat, covered. Stir a few times. Add the reserved beets and cook another 25 minutes on low, covered, until the vegetables are very tender.

MEANWHILE in a medium bowl, combine the crème fraîche and the following 3 seasonings well, with a whisk. Cover and chill until ready to use.

AFTER you add the beets to the soup, start your greens preparation. Break off the stems right below the start of the green leaves; discard the stems. Wash leaves well and shake off excess water. Cut into ½" slices. Coat a medium skillet with cooking spray. Melt the remaining 1 tablespoon butter over very high heat. Add the ¼ teaspoon salt and ¼ teaspoon white pepper and mix in. Add the greens. Sauté 2-3 minutes until fully wilted. Shake or stir frequently; don't let it burn. Let it stand in the pan on your stove top.

TO FINISH: add the greens right near the end of cooking. Remove bay leaf. Season, if desired. Garnish with generous dollops of the crème fraîche mixture. Cover and chill leftovers separately; don't freeze. Serves 3-4.

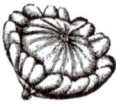 You would only need to change your broth to vegetable.

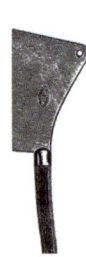

When I originally tasted borscht, it was served cold, with a small amount of flank steak throughout, sliced paper thin. You would only need about 4 ounces of flank steak; I would add it right near the end, so it doesn't overcook. The beef broth really adds enough of a beef flavor to the soup; actual meat is probably unnecessary.

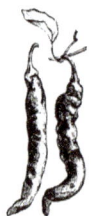 Well, of course you can add spice, but this soup has a wonderful sweet/sour flavor that probably doesn't need the competition.

Occasionally I like to dabble in mythology, so I decided to name this after Baba Yaga, a hideous, deformed female creature of Russian and Slavic mythology. I do like my alliteration, you know; plus sometimes after a hard day, I feel like I might resemble a Baba Yaga—a crazed, cranky old lady who is often accompanied by domestic implements, such as brooms and kitchen utensils. Baba Yaga lives in a hut that stands on giant chicken legs; the hut can walk about on its own in the forest, or maybe B.Y. just takes the whole house with her to the grocery store to buy her beets and cabbage. That might be the coolest residence in mythology; if it's not the coolest, it's at least one of the most unusual. I believe she is rather misunderstood and enigmatic—sort of like this soup.

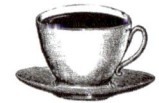

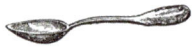

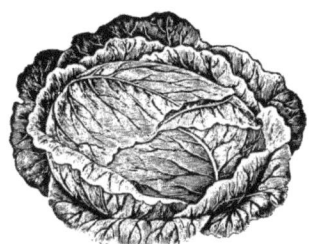
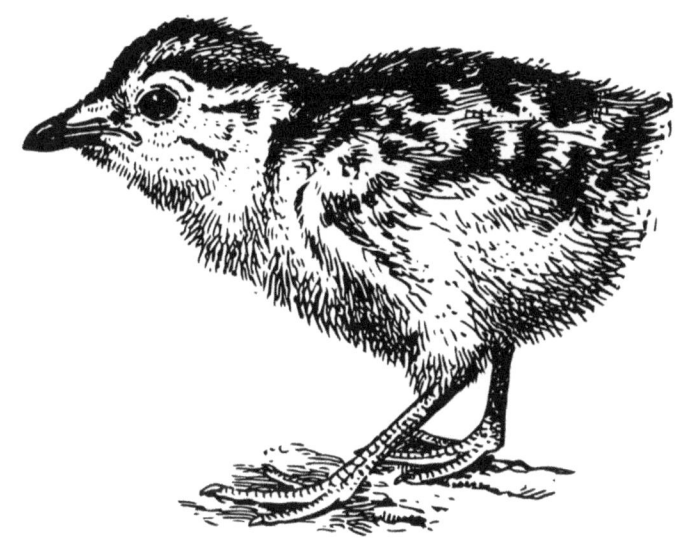
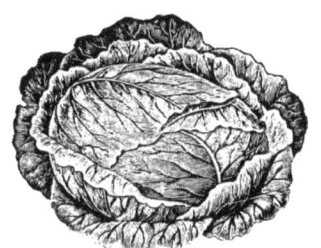

Sopa del Diente Quebrado

(A.K.A. Broken Tooth Soup)

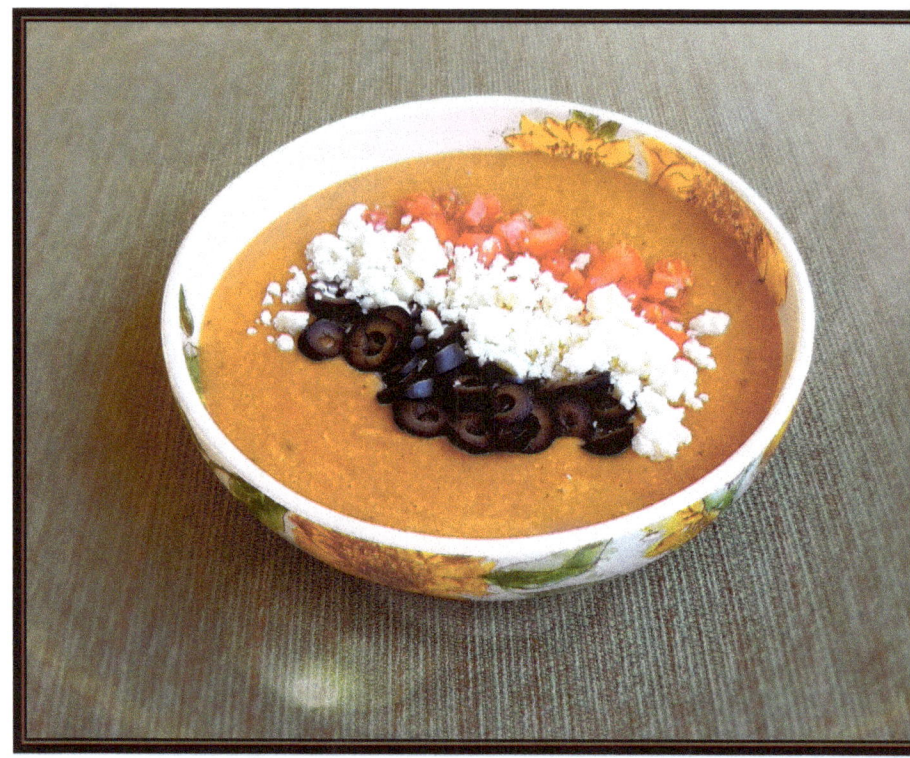

This is a great soup to serve if you are trying to get youngsters to acquire a taste for some spice. They will also be unaware of all the vegetables involved. It is hearty enough for a meal, low fat, and would also serve eight to ten as an appetizer. Double the amount of chile if you really want to knock your socks off. Will this soup break your teeth? Read on…

1 quart low-sodium chicken broth (or vegetable broth)
15.5-ounce can pinto beans, drained and rinsed
15.25-ounce can corn, with juice
14.5-ounce can stewed tomatoes, with juice
4 ounces roasted and chopped green chile, with juice
2 tablespoons minced garlic
1 tablespoon lime juice
1 cup carrot, peeled and coarsely chopped
1 cup celery, coarsely chopped
1 cup onion, coarsely chopped
4 corn tortillas (6-7" diameter),
    cut into 1" pieces

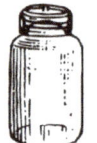 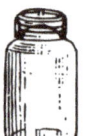 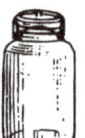

2 teaspoons dry oregano (2-3 tablespoons
    fresh, minced)
1 teaspoon cumin
1 teaspoon salt
1 teaspoon black pepper
½ cup half-and-half

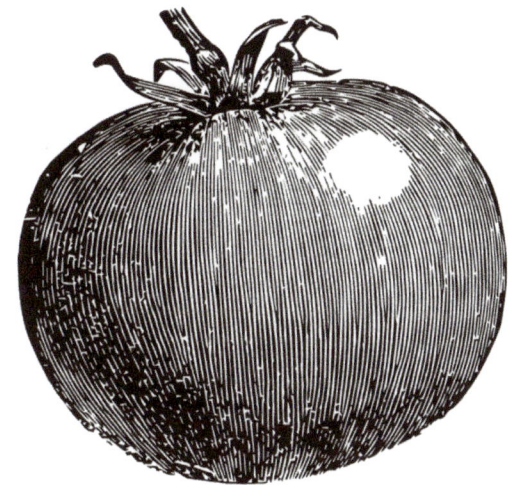

OPTIONAL GARNISH:

Sliced black olives
Diced tomatoes
Crumbled Cotija cheese or shredded Cheddar cheese
Any of the **NICE NEW MEXICAN & MEXICAN GARNISHES** or even the **CHARMING CHILI GARNISHES** will work, unless you really do have a broken tooth—then you should just pick out the softer types, of course. No Fritos for you!

COMBINE the broth, beans, corn, tomatoes, chile, garlic, lime juice, carrot, celery, and onion in a 4-quart saucepan. Bring to a boil, then cook on a low simmer, covered, 30 minutes. Stir a few times. Add the tortillas and the 4 seasonings and cook on a medium heat (a gentle boil), uncovered, 20 minutes. Stir a couple times. Mix in the half-and-half. Puree to complete smoothness in 2 or 3 batches and pour into a 3-quart saucepan. Season, if desired. Garnish, as desired. Cover and chill leftovers. Serves 4-6.

You could use any sort of meat-based broth you would prefer. If you decide to add some (a cup or two) leftover cooked meat, such as chicken or beef, you can puree it along with the vegetables. Conversely, you could add some cooked ground or diced meat after the final puree.

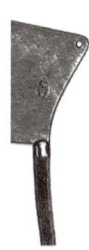

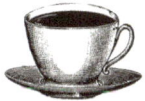

So, will this soup break your teeth? Definitely not. In August 2010, Bob was eating his beloved graham cracker/peanut butter snack in the middle of the afternoon. And he broke a tooth. That must have been some tough cracker. We were all set to go out for a steak dinner as a monthly date night sort of thing (steak for him, probably a salmon fillet for me). He had been looking forward to it all week. Rather than face the disappointment of going out and not being able to order something enjoyable, we decided to stay home. I figured I must have something hanging around the house that would produce something edible, at the least. A look at my pantry shelves and freezer suggested this soup. Except for all of the garnishes, I actually had all of these ingredients on hand (I usually use chicken broth), and it turned out to be a very comforting soup.

Ellen's Exotic Cauliflower Bisque

My husband, as you may have learned by now, hates a few particular vegetables and various unusual flavors, so I used to cheekily call this recipe "Bob Gets Two Hot Dogs Tonight Soup" (or two tamales, or a can of chili; whatever is around). But then my sister decided she loved this soup, so it is now much more appropriately named in her honor.

Cauliflower is Bob's least favorite vegetable in the entire universe and he will NEVER consume it, either raw or cooked. I love it either way, so when I do bother to cook with it, I usually produce rather small quantities. This recipe makes about five and a half cups of soup and is lovely served with some naan bread on the side, either plain or try my Naughty Naans on page 158.

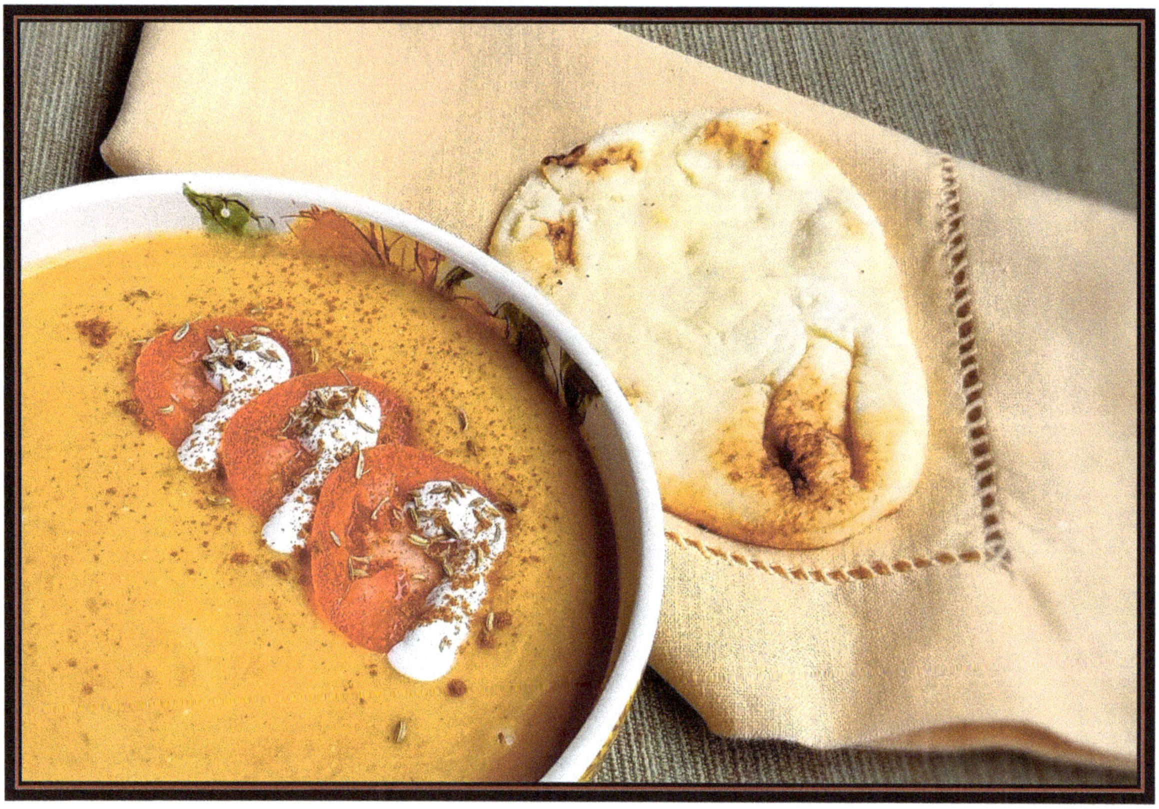

1 quart low-sodium chicken broth (or vegetable broth)
1 pound cauliflower, cut into 1" florets
8 ounces onion, coarsely chopped
8 ounces fresh tomatoes, coarsely chopped (any variety)

1½ teaspoons pink Himalayan salt
1 teaspoon smoked paprika
1 teaspoon cumin seeds
1 teaspoon packed golden brown sugar
½ teaspoon fennel seeds
½ teaspoon mustard seeds
½ teaspoon coriander seeds
½ teaspoon white pepper
½ teaspoon cinnamon
½ teaspoon ground cumin
¼ teaspoon ground cardamom
¼ teaspoon turmeric
6 ounces plain yogurt (2/3 cup), room temperature (light sour cream or crème fraîche will also work)

OPTIONAL GARNISH:

Extra plain yogurt or light sour cream, thinned with a little cream and drizzled over soup
Fennel seeds
Cinnamon
Sliced or diced fresh tomatoes

COMBINE broth, cauliflower, onion, tomatoes, and the 12 seasonings in a 4-quart saucepan. Bring to a boil and cook, covered, on lowest heat for 30 minutes. Then cook on medium heat, uncovered, 30 minutes. Stir a few times. Puree completely and place back in the pot. Whisk in the yogurt well. Season, if desired. Garnish, as desired. Cover and chill leftovers. Serves 3-4.

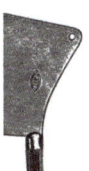
A change of broth to seafood or clam juice and perhaps a bit of cooked shrimp could be added, but it's a nice vegetarian puree on its own.

Maybe, maybe not… it has quite a lot of flavor already.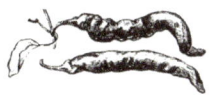

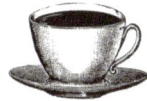
This is one of the lowest calorie soups in the cookbook. Shocking. Oddly enough, however, I find it to be quite filling. It would also make a nice appetizer soup.

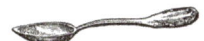

Savory Mushroom Soup

This recipe packs a punch you certainly won't get in your average can of cream of mushroom soup. Please read the anecdotal material for the rather amusing Narnian provenance of this substantial soup.

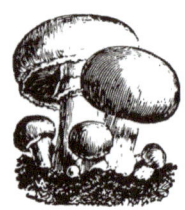

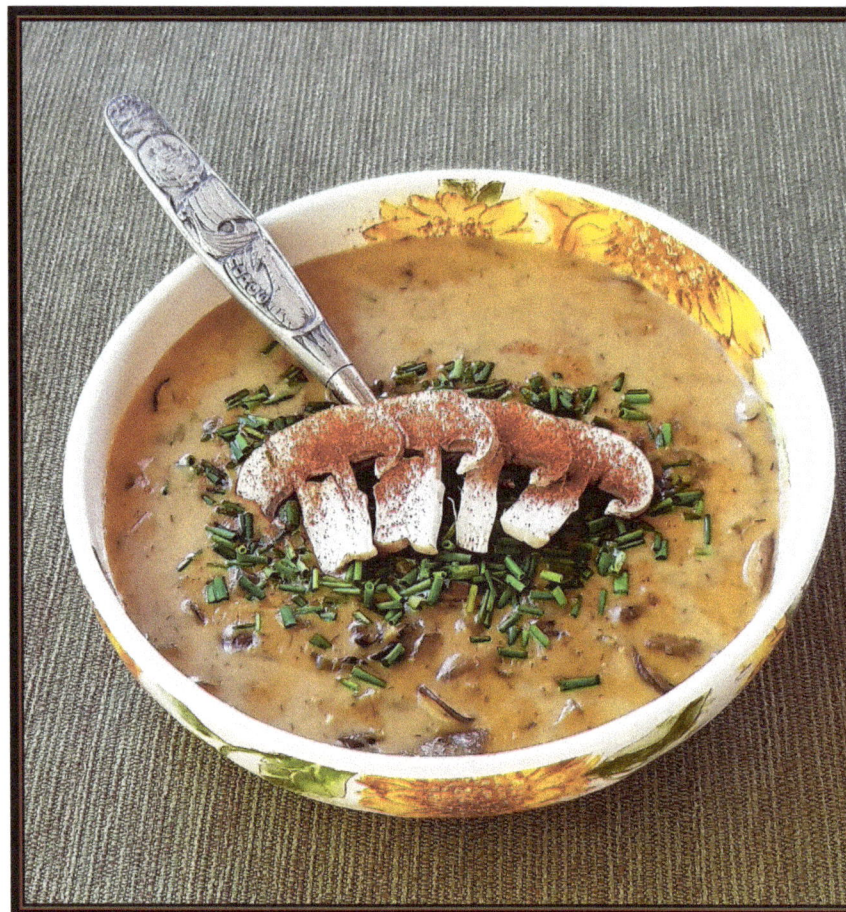

2 tablespoons salted butter
2 tablespoons olive oil
1 tablespoon minced garlic
2 teaspoons dry mustard
2 teaspoons smoked paprika
2 teaspoons soy sauce
2 teaspoons Worcestershire sauce
1½ teaspoons dry dill weed (2-3 tablespoons fresh, minced)
½ teaspoon salt
½ teaspoon cayenne pepper
1 cup celery, thinly sliced
1 cup onion, coarsely chopped
1 pound cremini mushrooms (baby portabellas), thinly sliced
½ cup all-purpose flour
1 quart low-sodium chicken broth (or vegetable broth)
1 cup heavy cream

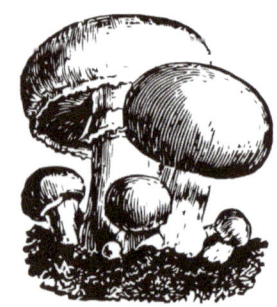

OPTIONAL GARNISH:

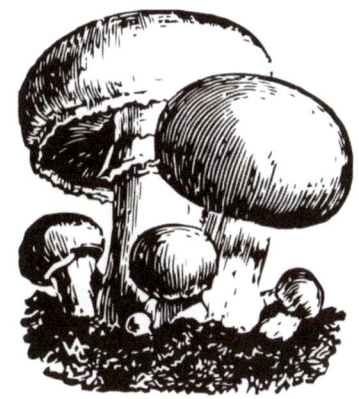

Sour cream or crème fraîche
Minced fresh chives
Additional fresh mushrooms,
   sliced paper thin
An extra sprinkling of smoked paprika

MELT the butter and oil in a 6-quart saucepan over moderately high heat until melted. Add the garlic and the next 7 seasonings and mix in well. Add the celery and onion and sauté for 5 minutes, stirring frequently. Add mushrooms and sauté another 5 minutes over rather high heat. Stir frequently and scrape up any browned bits. Add the flour and mix in. Add the broth and mix in. Bring to a boil, then simmer 35 minutes, covered, on lowest heat. Stir a few times. Pour the cream in slowly and mix in. Raise heat to medium/high and cook 5 minutes, uncovered. Stir a few times. Season, if desired. Garnish, as desired. Cover and chill leftovers. Serves 4.

About a cup or so of cooked meats could be added at the end of cooking; chicken or shrimp would be great. A few strips of cooked and crumbled bacon would also be tasty.

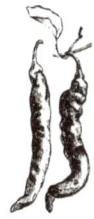

This soup already has a bit of a pleasant bite, but you can always add salsa or green chile, if you like; about half a cup would be good. Or increase the cayenne; that will wake you up!

In The Voyage of the "Dawn Treader," *Lucy, Edmund, and Eustace share a meal prepared and served by some mysterious and invisible creatures who they later learn are called Dufflepuds. It was... well, interesting, to put it mildly. It was also particularly messy, since their invisible hosts "progressed up the long dining-hall in a series of bounds or jumps. [...] When the dish contained anything like soup or stew the result was rather disastrous." Then, of course, there were the conversations: "What I always say is, when a chap's hungry, he likes some victuals," or "Getting dark now; always does at night," or even "Ah, you've come over the water. Powerful wet stuff, ain't it?"*

Actually, to me, these sound like corny jokes you'd hear from your dad or grandpa; it wouldn't surprise me in the least to hear my husband use one of those lines on our grandsons, merely substituting "guy" for "chap" and "food" for "victuals." Regardless, the children are served a "good meal," though Eustace regretted drinking any mead. The Dufflepuds serve a mushroom soup and other assorted items. Try not to jump very high when you serve it, however.

Chapter Four: Vegetables   137

Saffron Madness Soup

"I'm just mad about Saffron / Saffron's mad about me"

Quite rightly, you will (probably) love this mellow yellow soup. It is one of my own favorites! If you would prefer a different flavor, try a tablespoon (or even two) of curry powder or chili powder; both will be fine. You can even use a 1-pound bag of cauliflower crumbles here; it will resemble rice after it has been cooked.

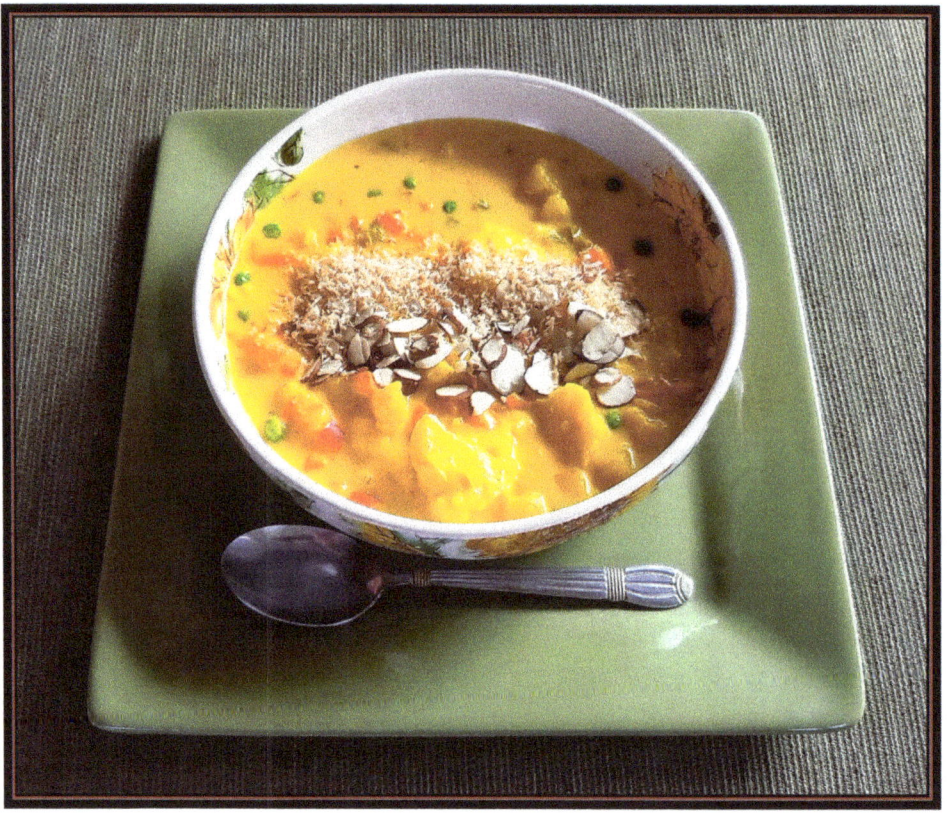

2 tablespoons salted butter
1 teaspoon saffron threads, crushed
½ teaspoon salt
½ teaspoon white pepper

1 cup carrot, peeled and finely chopped
1 cup celery, finely chopped
1 cup red bell pepper, cored and finely chopped
8 ounces potato, peeled and cut into ½" bits
1 pound cauliflower, cut into 1" florets
1 quart low-sodium chicken broth
    (or vegetable broth)
½ cup frozen peas
½ cup heavy cream
¼ cup water
1/3 cup all-purpose flour

OPTIONAL GARNISH:

Lightly toasted sliced almonds
Lightly toasted unsweetened coconut

COAT a 4-quart saucepan with cooking spray. Melt the butter over rather high heat. Sauté the saffron, salt, pepper, carrot, celery, red pepper, potato, and cauliflower 5 minutes, stirring frequently. Add the broth and bring to a boil. Reduce heat to medium and cook 15 minutes, uncovered. Stir twice. Add the peas and cook another 3 minutes.

IN a 2-cup glass measuring cup, whisk the remaining ingredients well. Pour ½ cup of hot soup into this and combine. Pour all back into the pot and cook over a medium heat 4-5 minutes, until the vegetables are tender and the soup thickens. Stir a few times. Season, if desired. Garnish, as desired. Cover and chill leftovers (don't store in plastic; saffron will stain it). Don't freeze. Serves 3-4.

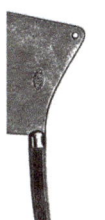

I think your best bet here would be a few small or even medium-sized shrimp, maybe 4-8 ounces, added near the end of cooking. If you must.

Green chile? NO. Don't do it. Are you surprised? You don't want to overpower that expensive saffron, do you?

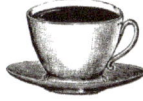

Bob hates cauliflower as you know by now, whereas I love it no matter how it is prepared. So when I make this, I'm (usually) the only one who gets to eat it. I NEVER add meat or spice to it; however, the cauliflower gives the illusion of a meaty texture.

Chapter Four: Vegetables

My Darling Minestrone

It's a darling, because it's probably the most versatile soup ever. A minestrone starts with a few humble ingredients, then builds itself with whatever happens to be in season or in your freezer or pantry.

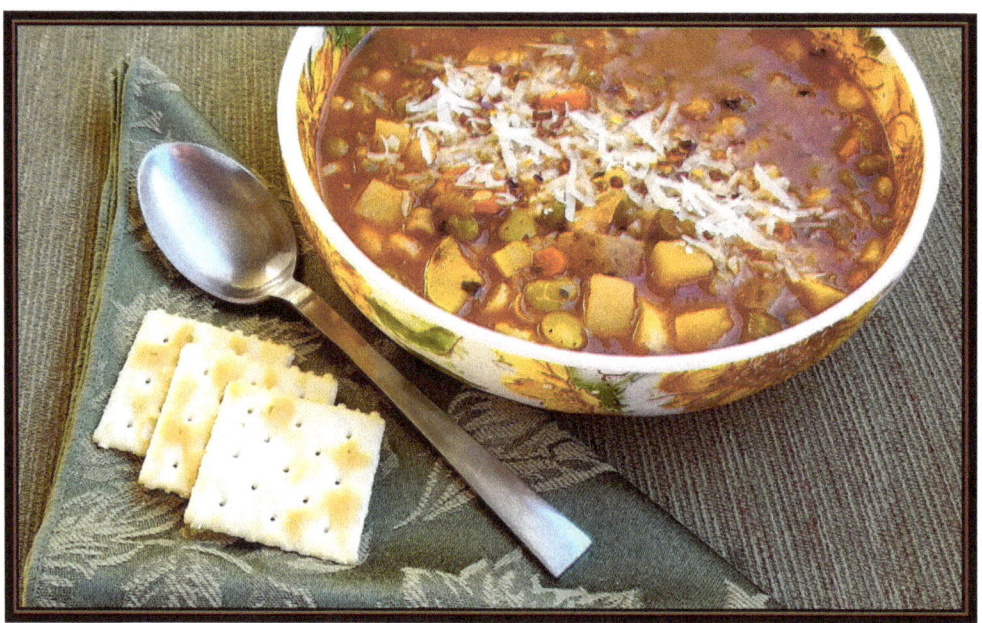

1 tablespoon olive oil
1 tablespoon minced garlic
½ cup carrot, peeled and thinly sliced
½ cup celery, thinly sliced
½ cup onion, coarsely chopped
1 quart low-sodium chicken broth (or vegetable broth)
8-ounce can tomato sauce
15.5-ounce can cannellini beans, with juice (other beans will work, too)
4 ounces yellow summer squash, unpeeled, cut into ½" bits
   (zucchini is fine; peel or partial peel, if it seems bitter)
4 ounces red potato, unpeeled, cut into ½" bits
½ teaspoon salt
½ teaspoon black pepper
½ teaspoon crushed red pepper flakes (optional)
½ teaspoon dry oregano (1-2 tablespoons fresh, minced)

2 cups assorted fresh or frozen vegetables (whatever is convenient or in season; cut into small chunks, as needed)
¼ cup prepared pesto sauce (any variety)
2 ounces small pasta (such as elbows or ditalini—or break spaghetti into 1" long pieces)

OPTIONAL GARNISH:

Shredded fresh Parmesan and/or Romano cheese
Minced fresh herbs
More crushed red pepper flakes

COAT a 4-quart saucepan with cooking spray. Sauté the oil, garlic, carrot, celery, and onion on rather high heat, 5 minutes. Add the broth, tomato sauce, beans, squash, potato, the 4 seasonings, and the 2 cups of vegetables and bring to a boil. Cook on medium heat, uncovered, 15 minutes. Stir a few times. Add the pesto and pasta and cook another 18-22 minutes on medium heat, uncovered, until the pasta is cooked to your liking and the vegetables are very tender. Stir a few times, especially at the bottom of the pot. Season, if desired. Garnish, as desired. Cover and chill leftovers; don't freeze. Serves 4-6.

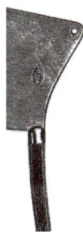

Add a cup of chopped, cooked meat near the end of cooking. Most any type of meat will work well with this soup, and you could even change your broth to beef or seafood (or clam juice).

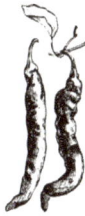

Of course, the green chile/salsa option will work well; about half a cup or so. Or you could simply increase the crushed red pepper flakes.

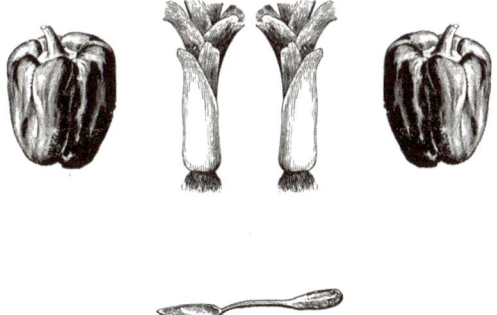

Chapter Four: Vegetables

Elfryda's Strawberry Soup

(A.K.A. Elfryda's Söt Suppe)

Finally, here's a dessert! For my last soup recipe, I figured I'd go with something a bit unusual. In Norway, this would be called Sot Suppe (alternatively spelled Söt Suppe), which means "sweet soup." It's a classic recipe that you can vary according to your tastes, meaning you can substitute nutmeg or cardamom for the cinnamon. You can even omit any spice, if you want to keep it simple so more of the fruit flavors will shine through. I like to make it in the summer and serve it cold, though it can be served hot, warm, or even at room temperature. It'll keep for at least a week, so you can enjoy a little cup of it after quite a few meals. Children will probably like it, too; at least my grandkids do. Bob thinks cold soups are weird, but he will eat this one. Occasionally he has poured it over vanilla ice cream. Try garnishing it with dollops of Sweet Crème Dream (see page xx), for a tart and creamy finish.

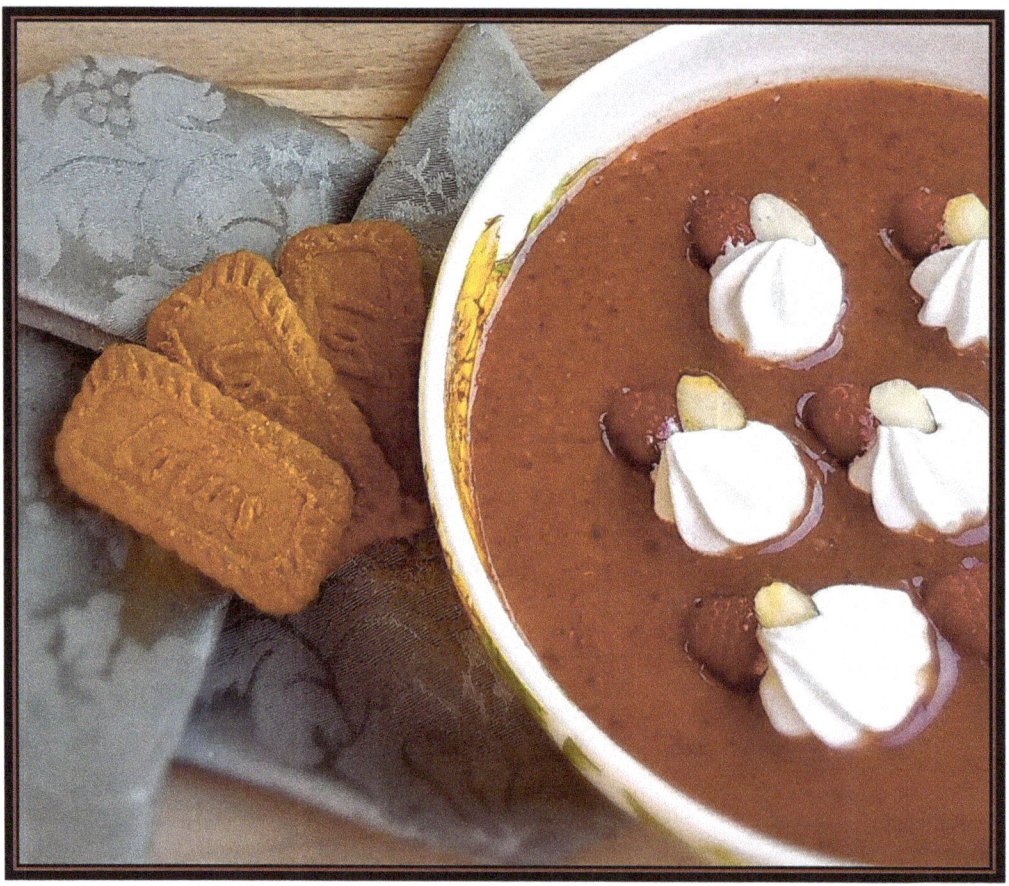

6 cups water
4 ounces raisins
4 ounces dried apricots
6 ounces fresh raspberries
1 pound fresh strawberries
½ cup sugar
¼ cup minute tapioca
1 teaspoon cinnamon
½ teaspoon salt

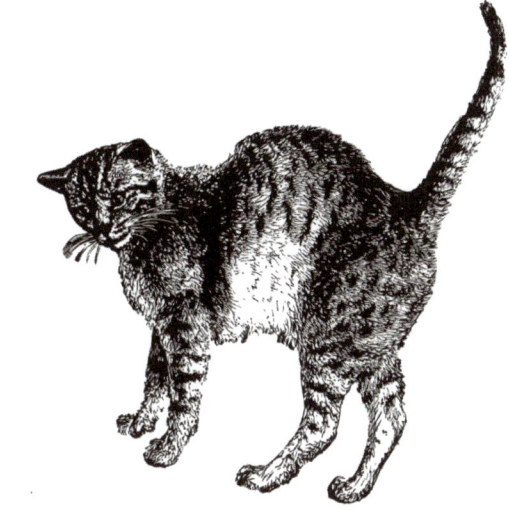

OPTIONAL GARNISH:

Dollops of whipped cream (a squirt from a can will work, too!)
Sliced or slivered almonds, lightly toasted, if you like
Shredded sweetened coconut, lightly toasted, if you like
A few perfect little raspberries

PLACE the water, raisins, and apricots in a 4-quart saucepan and soak 1 hour, covered. Drain over a 4-cup glass measuring cup. Reserve 4 cups water and discard the rest. Place this fruit in a blender; add the raspberries and 2½ cups of the reserved water. Puree well and pour back into the saucepan. Wash and stem strawberries. Break or cut the bigger ones in half and place in the blender along with the remaining 1½ cups water. Puree well, then add to the saucepan. Bring to a boil. Whisk in the remaining ingredients. Reduce heat to the lowest setting and cook, covered, 30 minutes, whisking occasionally, especially at the bottom of the pot. Uncover and raise heat one notch. Cook, uncovered, another 30 minutes. Whisk a few times. Serve immediately as a hot soup, if desired. You may set the soup aside until the desired temperature is reached, or chill it when it cools off a bit. Garnish, as desired. Cover and chill leftovers; stir it up before serving. Serves 6-8.

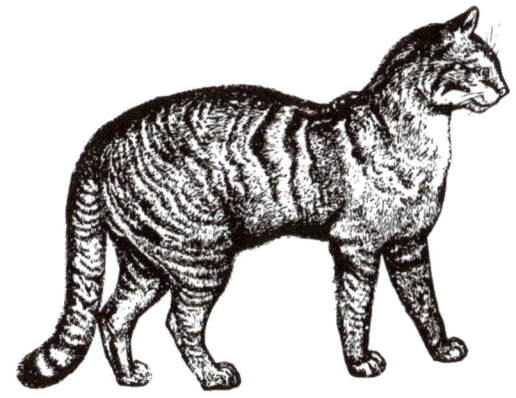

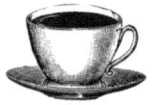 *I have named this for my maternal grandmother. Elfryda Egeland Aslaksen, one of nine children, was born in Brooklyn, New York, in 1895. She moved to Farsund, Norway, when she was an infant. Elfryda traveled back to New York with one of her big sisters when she was 14. On this voyage, she got her period for the first time and thought she was going to die. Homesick, she returned to Norway and went to nursing school in Bergen (maybe because of her rather traumatic menarche experience traveling to New York). She met Asbjorn on a blind date at a dance held on May 17, 1918—this date is celebrated as the Norwegian Independence Day and, coincidentally, the same day my mother died, in 2012.*

My sister and I always called Elfryda Mama. She was a private nurse and a stamp collector/dealer. She and Asbjorn lived in South Ozone Park, in Queens, New York, for a few years in the 1920s, then they built a house in Lindenhurst, on Long Island. Here, Mama was able to keep many pets, dogs, cats, chickens. After retiring to New Mexico in 1969, she spent much of her time swimming in their apartment complex. Oddly enough, my current house is about one mile away from this apartment complex, so I always think of my grandparents when I pass by.

After working as a nurse for so many years, she ended up with back problems and always wore a corset—even while swimming. After Asbjorn died, she moved into my bedroom and I moved into our den until she died in 1978. I didn't mind; I ended up with a much bigger room.

My favorite story about Mama came from my mom. My mom, Esther, had a long-time fear and hatred of cats which apparently originated from an encounter with a rather nasty Siamese cat when she was a child. She thought they were "mushy." Meaning, when you pick up a dog, it is a rather solid animal; when you pick up a cat, however (which she obviously would have never done; she was only making observations about other people picking up cats), they are limber and flexible. It freaked her out, and we certainly never owned cats, only dogs.

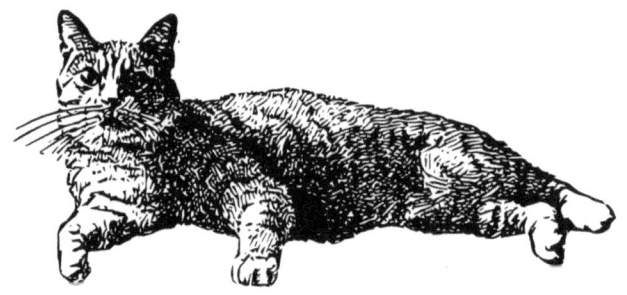

Anyway, around 1950, Mama had a black cat with a white star on his chest, who was named Snowflake. He was rather the king of the household and his chosen resting place was always on my mother's bed. The oblique rays of the sun would shine down upon him from the window and it was a quiet place for important feline reflection. Snowflake also knew that my mom hated him for sleeping there. Cats always knew my mom hated them; whenever we would visit a house with a cat, inevitably they sought her out and rubbed against her legs. Ellen and I always thought this was quite amusing.

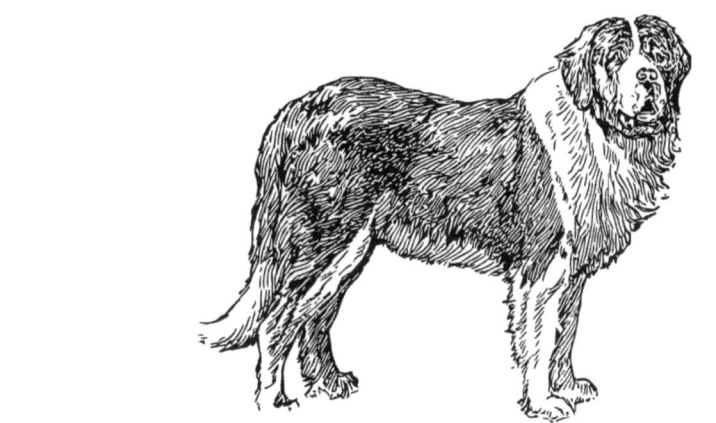

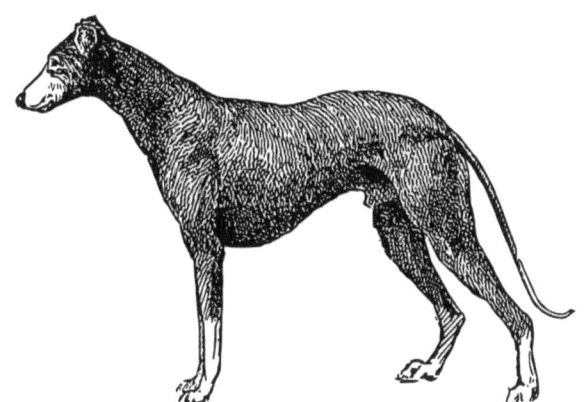

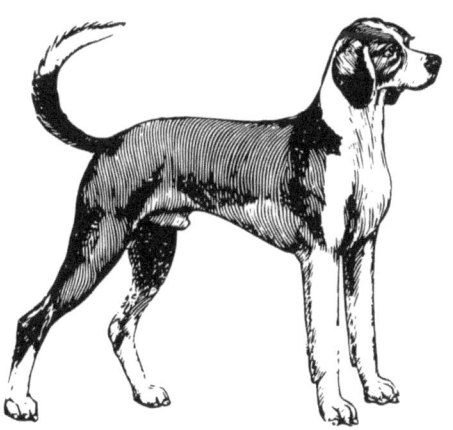

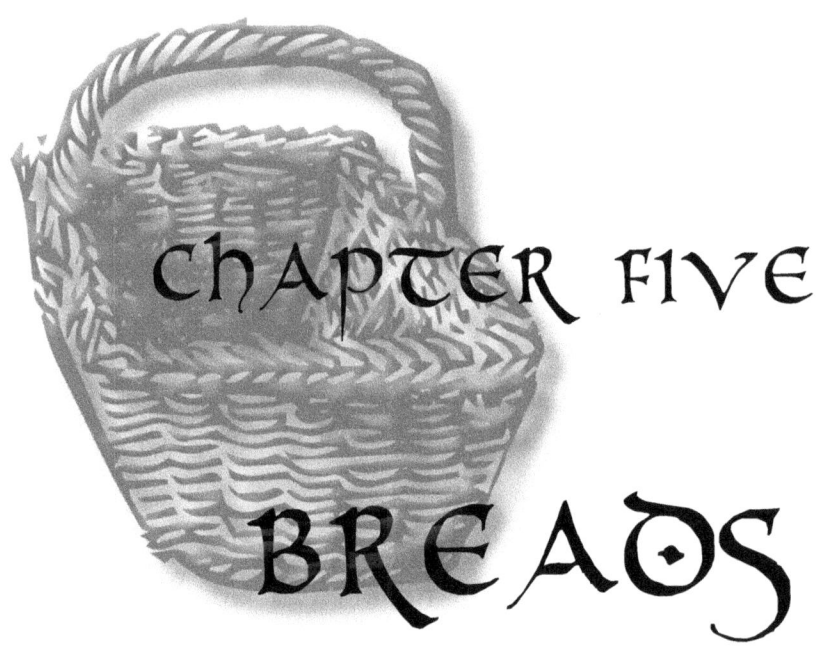

Chapter Five
Breads

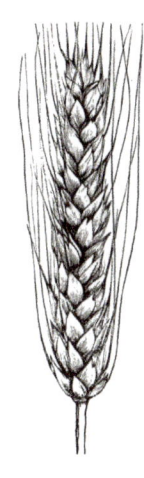

Toasty Muffin Bread
Buffins
Bill's Table Tortillas
Naughty Naans
Cottage Dill Bread
Oaten Cake with "Narnian" Wheat

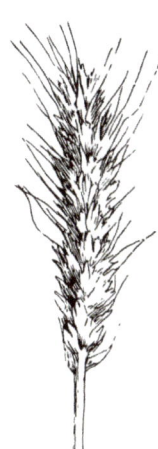

Bran's Brans
Game of Scones
Lovely Artisan Loaf
Nifty "Narnian" Biscuits
Easy Focaccia
Epic Iron Skillet Cornbread
Land of Enchantment "Lembas"
with Spicy Honey Butter

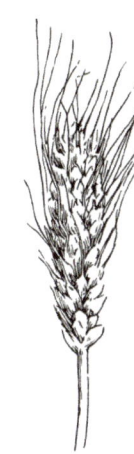

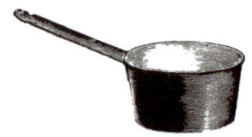 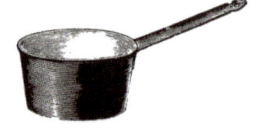

Chapter Five—Breads

(PLUS SUGGESTIONS FOR GOOD PAIRINGS)

Man (or woman…) apparently does not live by bread alone. But wouldn't you like to try doing so? Bagels, bialys, biscuits, brioche, buns; challah, ciabatta, crumpets; focaccia, fry bread; lavash, lefse; panettone, proja; scones, sopaipillas, sourdough… why, oh why, do carbs have to be so comforting and delicious? Naan… mmm… naan…

Here's an assortment of baked goods you can mix and match with your soups, stews, and chilis. Check out the **GOOD PAIRINGS** section at the end of each recipe for two to four suggestions; however, you might find many more options. I didn't want to suggest 30 items to go with the Toasty Muffin Bread, though probably 30 recipes would definitely go well with it.

Baking bread at home can sometimes be challenging, since your home kitchen is more subject to the whims of weather, altitude, and your mood. If you don't already have one, an oven thermometer is a handy gadget to use, especially if your oven is having problems regulating its temperature. Sometimes I wonder if ovens are susceptible to changes in weather, or if they get moody… probably not…

Professional bakeries usually put out consistent products (and they often have access to mysterious ingredients not commonly available to the typical home baker), but your favorite bread recipe can sometimes betray you by not rising much at all or by strangely oozing out of the pan, like some yeasty lava flow. I have found that mutant bread is usually still quite edible, as long as it isn't moist and doughy inside. You can chalk your loaf up to the capricious yeast gods, slice it, then slather some butter and jam all over it. That's better. And remember not to apologize.

REGARDING BAKING: my own personal baking time is right in the middle, if I list a range. Your oven rack should be in the middle, unless I specify a different level. When I require buttermilk in a recipe, I am referring to fresh liquid buttermilk, as opposed to the powdered variety. However, I have found that if you mix buttermilk powder with milk instead of water (as directed on the package), the finished product works out fairly well. I'm also baking in a conven-

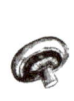

tional oven at a mile-high altitude—you might need to adjust proportions sometimes, but maybe not. I have baked plenty of recipes that ended up needing no adjustments, so you never know. I also added approximate preparation times just for these bread products, so you can bake accordingly; because sometimes you really want the bread to be fresh out of the oven. These times reflect the whole process from assembling ingredients, mixing, rising, baking, and cooling. Remember, these are approximations only; your rising times might vary according to variables such as weather and altitude, or how fast you are at assembling ingredients.

REGARDING THE MICROWAVE: all microwave melting is done on HIGH setting, unless I specify a different setting, which I never do.

REGARDING VOCABULARY: some products might be known by different names in various other countries and even in various parts of the United States of America. All-purpose flour is apparently known as plain flour in Australia; an extra-fine sugar is sometimes known as castor (or caster) sugar. When I refer to sugar, I mean just regular white sugar commonly sold in America, not the extra-fine variety. I'm hoping that my terms are rather standard or easily researched in case of confusion. One day, you could entertain yourself by conducting an Internet search for the word sugar and you would be surprised at how many different terms describe that sweet demon stuff.

REGARDING LUBRICATION: this might sound naughty, but I am merely referring to your pans. Do you like to use cooking spray, or do you prefer to go old school and use butter or some other shortening to grease your baking pans? Do you always use parchment paper? Do you always use paper cups for your muffins? Do you prefer to use silicone baking mats? It's tough to predict what every kitchen is equipped with, and after doing some research into all of these products, I'm going to have to conclude that we all have our preferred methods and they all have their advantages and disadvantages, as well as their environmental issues. I guess I would hope that you won't become bogged down in pan preparations, because the recipes are not intended to be that rigid in their presentation.

REGARDING MIXING: I have a KitchenAid stand mixer, and some of the items within were made with it. Many items are merely mixed up in a bowl with your hands or a different utensil (wooden spoon or spatula; I use both), or you can use a hand mixer. In case you don't have a stand mixer, however, that doesn't mean you can't replicate the results with a very large bowl and a pair of strong arms. Kneading bread dough can be therapeutic. So, don't fret about not having a particular small appliance such as a stand mixer around; you can adapt the recipes to fit your situation. What about bread machines? Can you mix up the Toasty Muffin Bread in a machine? I can't help you there; I've never had one. My neighbor had one and I always thought it was strange that each loaf she shared with us had a hole in the bottom. Don't get me wrong—the loaf tasted good. Perhaps TOO good; we would probably end up with too much bread in the house if I had one of those machines. Plus, I was always thinking that a bread machine would end up being another one of those small trendy appliances that take up much-needed space in the kitchen, at least around our house.

REGARDING VARIOUS OTHER ITEMS OR SUBSTITUTIONS: I use golden brown sugar (light brown), but the darker variety will be fine to use. I use a double-acting baking powder. If you have trouble finding buttermilk, you could substitute the powdered form (mix with milk, not water) or make your own by using the proportion of one cup of milk combined with one tablespoon either of lemon juice or white vinegar; whisk it together and let it stand for 15 minutes or so. This will curdle the milk and become an acceptable substitute for buttermilk. All measurements should be level, unless otherwise specified. When I say "room temperature" I mean that the item (usually eggs and dairy products) should be taken out of the refrigerator for about an hour or so before use, just to take the chill off. Many of the following recipes can be modified according to your tastes; for example, you might want to throw a couple teaspoons (or tablespoons) of some dried herbs into the breads or biscuits, or a few tablespoons (or a quarter cup, or even half a cup) of minced fresh herbs. You might want to experiment with adding garlic or chili powder. You might even want to add some well drained roasted and chopped green chile to the cornbread. Pretty much most of the recipes can handle creative changes such as these.

Regarding eggs: in my first cookbook, all the eggs were extra large and purchased from Costco. But then Costco went crazy (as they are wont to do occasionally) and decided to carry only large eggs, so all of these recipes were designed to utilize large ones. Now the difference between an extra large egg and a large egg is rather small. You can probably get away with using two large eggs, even when a recipe might call for two extra large ones. Perhaps you could add a bit more liquid, if your dough seems dry. If you are using mediums, however, you would definitely need to calculate some conversions in your measurements.

Then suddenly—out of the blue—Costco started carrying extra large eggs again.

I'm obviously going to have to get over my Costco obsession, especially now that it's just two of us living in this house. Though I've become quite adept at figuring out the smallest portions I can manage to buy from them, and we simply don't visit as often as we did when we had kids around the house, so that's an improvement. We must change with the times, mustn't we? Always forward.

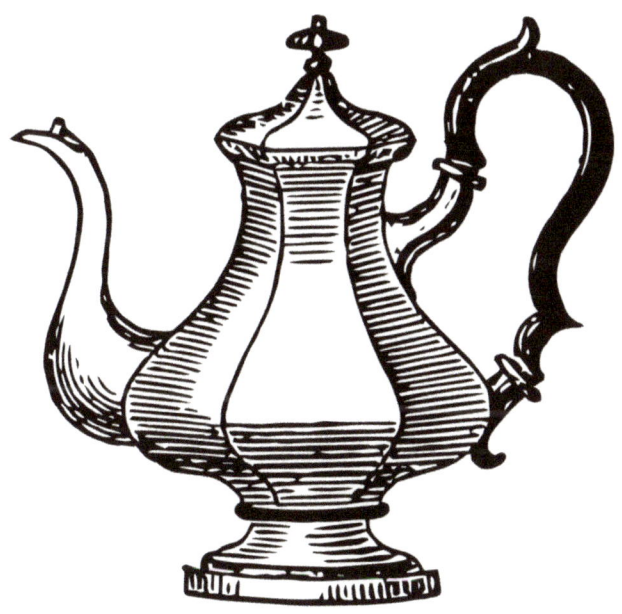

Toasty Muffin Bread

This particular basic white bread lends itself to anything you might want to put on it—meats, cheeses, butters, jams, honey. It is perfect to slice and perfect to sandwich. Though freshly tender when you first bake it, I like to toast it to a golden brown on the next day. It sort of resembles an English muffin when you do this. When I want to serve this at exactly 6:00 p.m., I start making it right around 3:45 p.m. Obviously, you can make it earlier if you like; or you could go nuts—double the recipe and freeze one for later.

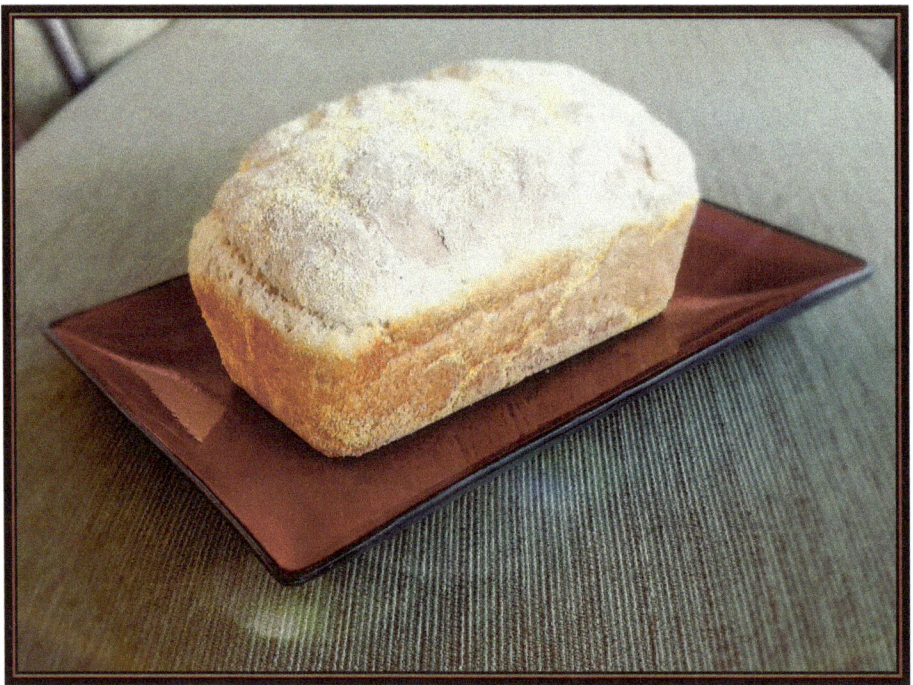

Total preparation time: approximately 2 hours and 15 minutes

¾ cup water
¾ cup fresh buttermilk
3¼ cups all-purpose flour, divided
1 tablespoon sugar
1 (¼-ounce) packet active dry yeast (2¼ teaspoons)
1¼ teaspoons salt
¼ teaspoon baking soda
1½ tablespoons cornmeal, divided
Additional all-purpose flour

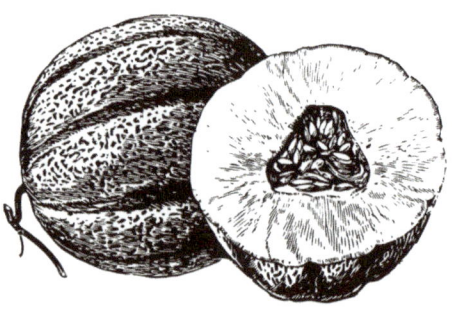

COMBINE the water and buttermilk in a 2-cup glass measuring cup. Microwave on HIGH 1 minute; let stand. Combine 2¼ cups flour, sugar, yeast, salt, and baking soda in a large stand mixer. Add the water mixture and combine on low speed until combined, about 1 minute. Add the remaining 1 cup flour and mix on low speed 2 minutes.

WHILE the dough is mixing, coat an 8½" by 4½" loaf pan with cooking spray or grease lightly. Sprinkle 1 tablespoon cornmeal into the pan and shake pan to distribute on the bottom and most of the sides. Press dough into pan; use floured fingers to press it down relatively evenly. Sprinkle remaining ½ tablespoon cornmeal over the top evenly. Cover with a towel and let rise in a relatively warm, draft-free place for 40-45 minutes.

PREHEAT oven to 400°. Bake 30 minutes. Place pan on a rack and let stand 10 minutes. Remove from pan and set on rack 30 minutes before cutting. Cover and keep leftovers at room temperature or in the refrigerator; it freezes well. 10-12 slices.

Good Pairings:

★ Cheeseburger Soup
★ Esther's Manhattan Clam Chowder
★ Asbjorn's New England Clam Chowder

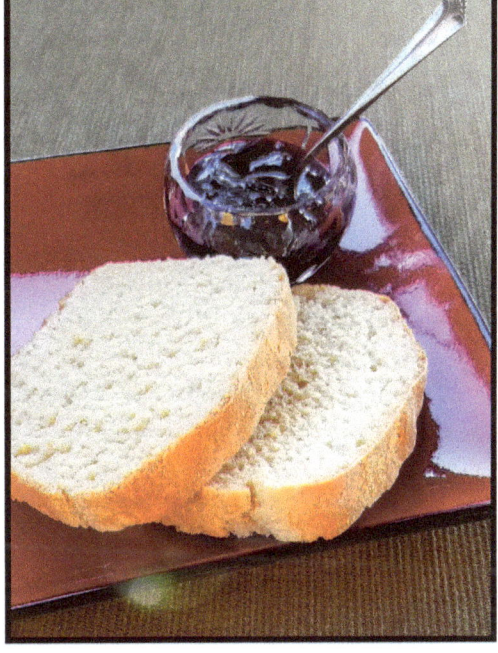

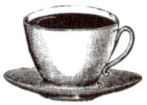 *My grandsons think this is one of the most special things they can eat at my house. However, I think my younger daughter Callista will always associate this recipe with the time when I had an emergency gallbladder removal; I had baked one the day before I ended up in the hospital, so I think she and Bob finished up the loaf while I was gone. Good times…*

After my surgery, I came home and had a .25¢ package of beef ramen. It was SO delicious.

This particular recipe was also invented for my Narnian writings; it was originally called "Mr. Tumnus's Toasty Muffin Bread." In The Lion, The Witch and The Wardrobe, *the faun, Mr. Tumnus, served buttered toast, sardines on toast, and toast with honey to Lucy Pevensie before he betrayed her to the White Witch. He also served her a lightly boiled brown egg and some sugar-topped cake. After all that food, no wonder Lucy let her guard down and fell fast asleep.*

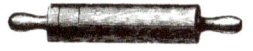

Chapter Five: Breads

Buffins

Originally I called these Biscuit Muffins, but my smart-ass daughters started messing around with some wordplay just to tease me as teenagers are often known to do. I explained I was going for a sort of hybrid between a biscuit and a muffin, so one said, "Why don't you call them 'Miscuits'?" The other said, "How about 'Buffins'?" I thought Buffins sounded positively hobbitish, so there you are.

> "Oh, Miss Buffins, would you like some of these delightfully herby treats to go with your mushroom and bacon casserole?"
>
> "Yes, please; but do hurry, or I'll be late for my foot-brushing appointment... I'll also take a few to go for my second breakfast tomorrow. Mmm... better make that a dozen..."

Total preparation time: approximately 30 minutes

1½ cups all-purpose flour
2 tablespoons whole wheat flour
2 tablespoons cornmeal
3 tablespoons dry Parmesan cheese (Parmesan and/or Romano is fine)
1½ tablespoons baking powder
1½ teaspoons salt
1 tablespoon Easy Herbes de Provence (see page xxix for a recipe; other dried herbs are also fine, or use 3-4 tablespoons of fresh, minced herbs)
¾ cup fresh buttermilk, room temperature
¼ cup vegetable oil
2 large eggs, room temperature

PREHEAT oven to 450°. Coat 9 regular size muffin cups with cooking spray, grease lightly, or use papers. Combine the 2 flours, cornmeal, cheese, baking powder, salt, and herbs in a large bowl. In a 4-cup glass measuring cup, combine the buttermilk, oil, and eggs well with a whisk. Add the egg mixture to the bowl and mix just until combined. Divide evenly into the prepared cups. Bake 10 minutes. Let stand in pan 5 minutes before serving. Keep leftovers covered at room temperature. Makes 9.

GOOD PAIRINGS:

- ☆ Casbah-Rockin' Chicken Stew
- ☆ Chloë's Kale-apalooza
- ☆ Notorious CSC

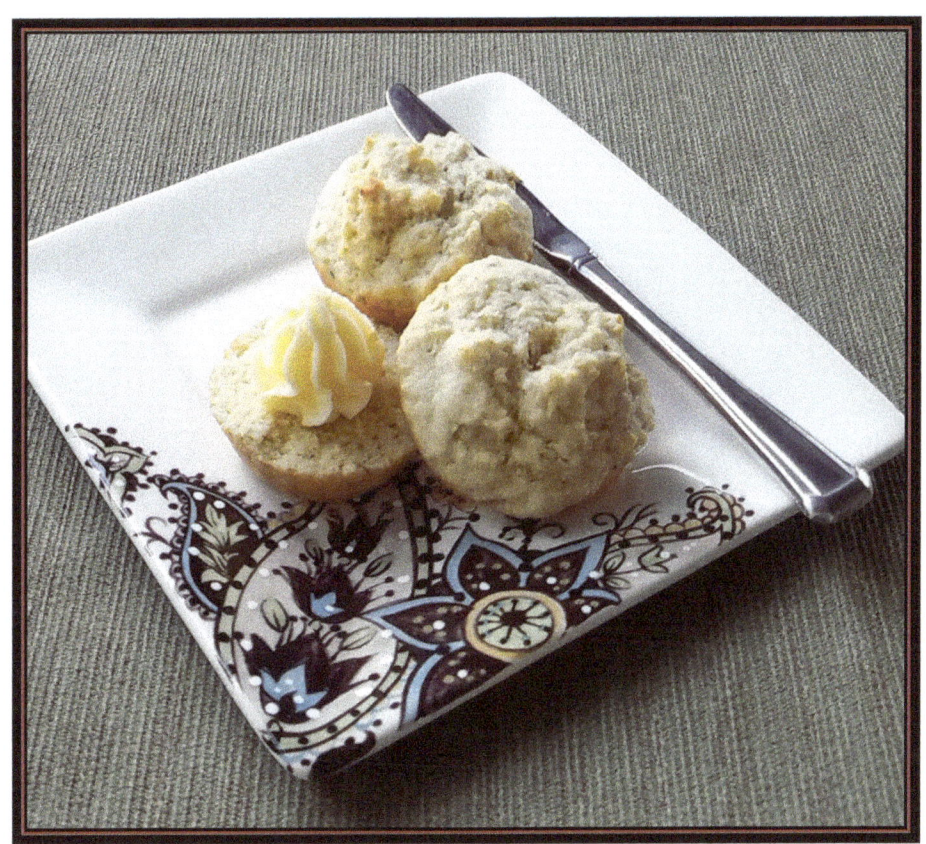

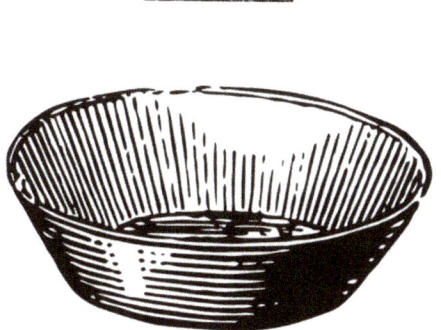

Chapter Five: Breads

Bill's Table Tortillas

Homemade tortillas, so warm and soft; you just want to cover your face with them and absorb that carby goodness right through your pores. If you prefer, you could make eight larger tortillas, instead of 12. These will end up thicker than your average store-bought flour tortillas, so they are more appropriate for dunking in a bowl rather than wrapping as a burrito. They are great as a substantial accompaniment to many of the soups, stews, and chilis included in the cookbook, but you can also butter one up and sprinkle cinnamon sugar all over it.

When it comes to mixing up a tortilla dough, I've been favoring an old-school approach and simply combining it completely by hand in a large bowl. You can certainly throw it in a stand mixer or processor, if you prefer, but sometimes using your hands feels right.

Total preparation time: approximately 1 hour and 15 minutes

3 cups all-purpose flour
2 teaspoons salt
2 teaspoons baking powder
¼ cup soft lard (a traditional ingredient, but you can use vegetable shortening)
1 cup very warm tap water (about 110° F.; you can touch it without burning yourself)

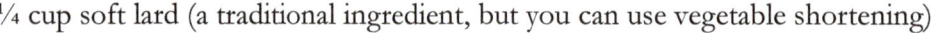

COMBINE the flour, salt, and baking powder in a large bowl. Add the lard and mix it in with your hands until crumbly (you can use a pastry blender, if you prefer). Add the water and mix it in with your hands until thoroughly combined (you can use a wooden spoon or spatula, if you prefer). In the bowl, gather the dough together into a ball or a flattened disc. Cover bowl with a kitchen towel and let the dough rest 30-40 minutes.

SET towel aside and knead the dough a few times, until smoother. You shouldn't need much extra flour; it should end up being a smooth dough (but flour surface as needed). Cut into 12 portions. Roll each into a ball and place on half of the towel. Cover with the other half of the towel.

HEAT a medium skillet over rather high heat. It is ready when a few drops of water sizzle on it. Meanwhile, start rolling out each ball into circles that measure about ⅛" thick and about 6-7" diameter. Fry one side about a minute; flip over and fry the other side. Both sides should have light golden brown spots to indicate doneness. You might lower the heat a smidge if it seems to be getting too hot. Stack on a plate and wrap with another towel or cloth napkin to keep warm. Serve immediately. Cover and keep leftovers at room temperature, though you can refrigerate or freeze them as well. Makes 12.

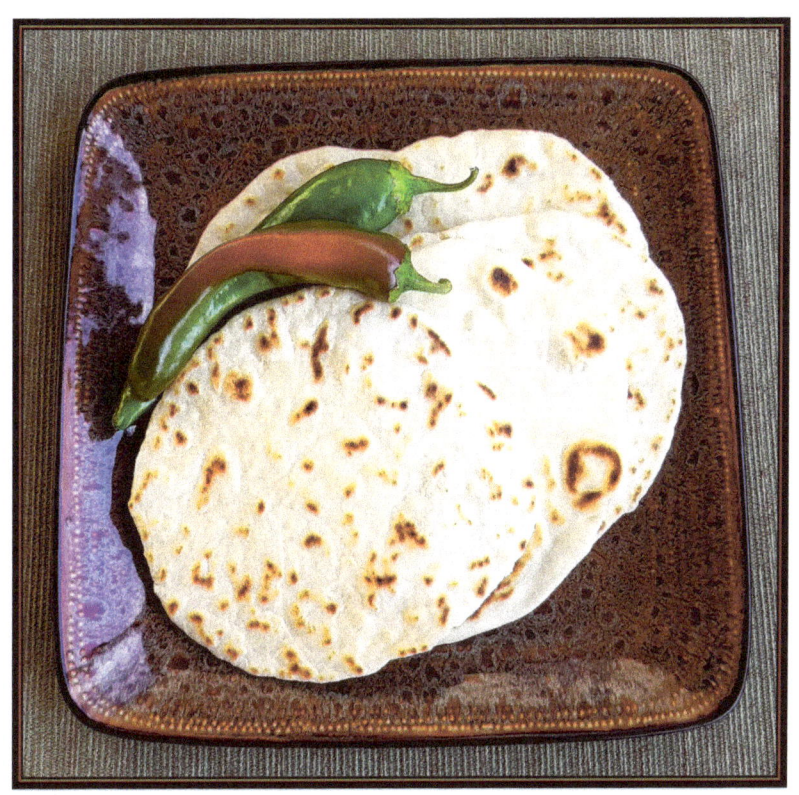

GOOD PAIRINGS:

☆ Oh, so many… all the posoles!
☆ All the chilis!
☆ Carpe Caldillo!
☆ Sopa de los Burqueños! (sorry for all of the exclamation points!!!)

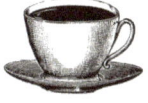
As you fry them, some tortillas might develop bubbles. These are fine and you don't have to pop them, unless they really get out of hand and start resembling a pillow. If a tortilla grows an unruly bubble, simply give it a little poke with a sharp knife. Your tortillas will probably not all be perfectly circular, either, because you are not a machine. I've never bothered to buy a tortilla press; in my kitchen, I'm afraid it would end up being another one of those kitchen gadgets taking up much-needed space in my cabinet.

These are named for my brother-in-law, who died unexpectedly in January, 2018. Bill was an enthusiastic lover of most Mexican and New Mexican foods. He was a quirky, life-long bachelor, who often came to our house for some old-fashioned home cooking.

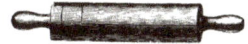

Naughty Naans

Super simple and super fast; wonderfully cheesy and spicy. You might just want to make them all on their own and skip serving some soup. These are also good served with a salad. If you have trouble locating naan, you could substitute pita bread—then you can call them "Pistol-Packin'-Pitas," if you like.

Total preparation time: approximately 20-25 minutes

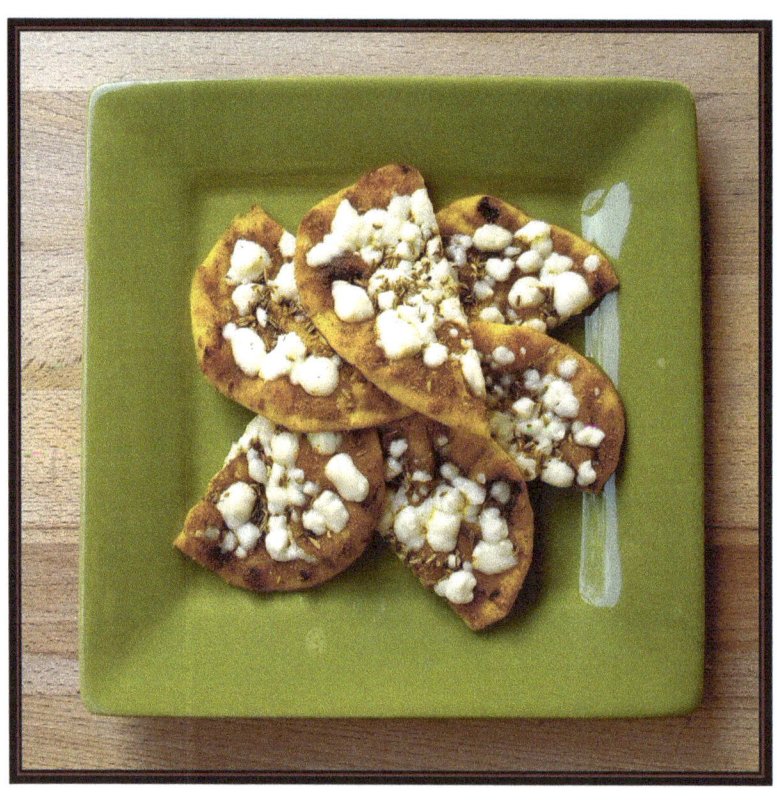

6 miniature naans (or 3 large ones, to be cut in half after baking)
¼ cup salted butter
2 teaspoons hot Madras curry powder
2 teaspoons garam masala
1 teaspoon garlic powder
½ teaspoon cayenne pepper
6 ounces crumbly white cheese (such as Paneer or Feta, or use Mexican varieties
    such as queso Panela, Fresco, or even Cotija)
1½ teaspoons fennel seeds

PREHEAT oven to 400°. Place naans on a large (18" by 13") baking sheet. Place the butter in a small glass bowl and microwave just until it melts. Whisk the 4 seasonings in well. Brush butter mixture evenly all over the naans. Crumble the cheese into small chunks (not too small) and sprinkle evenly all over each. Sprinkle the fennel seeds evenly over each. Bake 8 minutes. Let stand on pan 5 minutes before serving. Serve whole, or cut into halves or wedges. Cover and chill leftovers. Makes 6.

GOOD PAIRINGS:

- ★ Nothing Wrong With Mulligatawny
- ★ Ellen's Exotic Cauliflower Bisque
- ★ Coconut Beef Stew

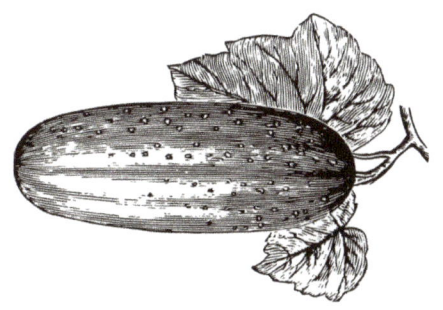

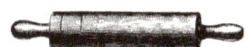

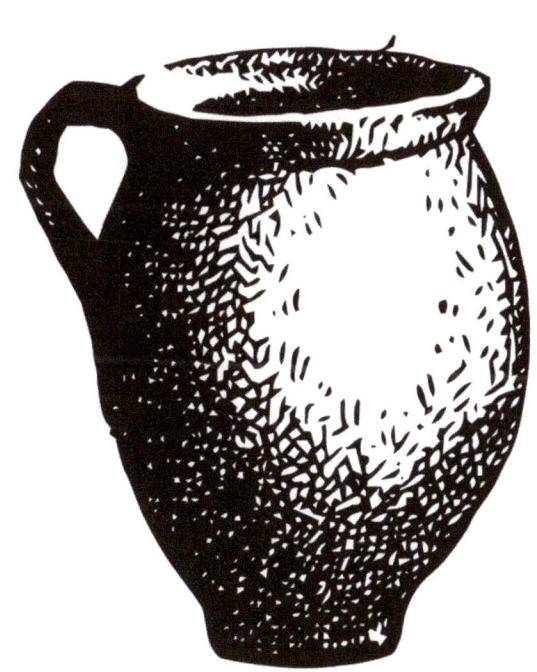

Chapter Five: Breads 159

Cottage Dill Bread

This bread has a northern European flavor, perfect for your favorite spread of butter, margarine, or even jam. Maybe not Nutella, but you never know. If you dislike dill, try substituting cumin (ground and seeds). This will create more of a south-of-the-border flavor. Other varieties of chopped onions are also fine to use, if you prefer.

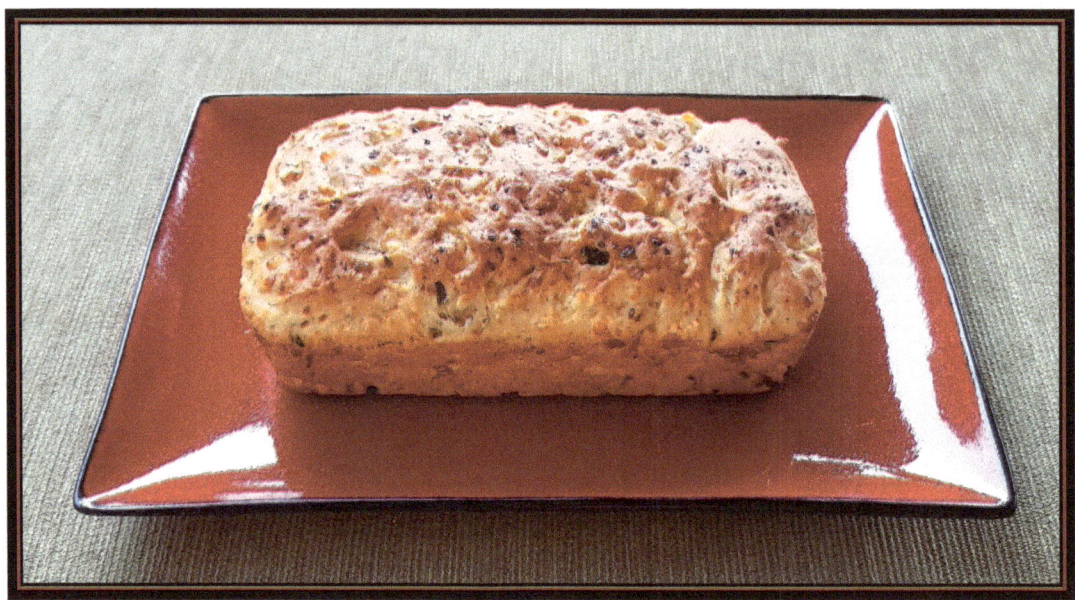

Total preparation time: approximately 2 hours and 25 minutes

2 tablespoons salted butter
1 tablespoon dill seeds
1 teaspoon dill weed (2-3 tablespoons fresh, minced)
½ cup scallions, thinly sliced
½ cup water
2 teaspoons coarse kosher salt
¼ cup sugar
12-ounce container low-fat cottage cheese (1½ cups)
3 cups all-purpose flour, divided
1 (¼-ounce) packet active dry yeast (2¼ teaspoons)
½ teaspoon baking soda
2 large eggs, room temperature

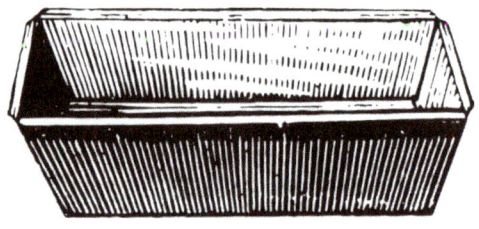

MELT the butter in a 2-quart saucepan over moderately high heat. Add the dill seeds, dill weed, and scallions and sauté on low heat for 5 minutes. Add the water and bring to a boil. Take off heat. Add the salt, sugar, and cottage cheese and whisk in well. Let it stand while you prepare the next step.

COMBINE 1 cup flour, yeast, and baking soda in a stand mixer. Add the eggs and cottage cheese mixture and beat on medium speed for 1 minute. Add the remaining 2 cups flour and mix on low 30 seconds or so, then medium for another few seconds, until completely combined. It will be sticky. Coat **TWO** 8½" by 4½" loaf pans with cooking spray or grease lightly. Divide the dough evenly between the prepared pans. Cover with a towel and let rise in a relatively warm, draft-free place for about 1 hour.

PREHEAT oven to 375°. Bake 30 minutes. Set pans on racks 10 minutes. Turn out onto the racks and let cool 30 minutes. Slice and serve. Cover and keep refrigerated; it freezes well. 20 slices.

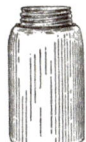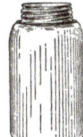

Good Pairings:

- ★ Baba Yaga Borscht
- ★ Savory Mushroom Soup
- ★ Robert the Bruce's Cock-a-Leekie Soup

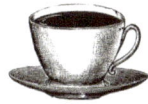 *This flavorful loaf is great freshly baked; but as a leftover, I love to toast it to a crispy golden brown.*

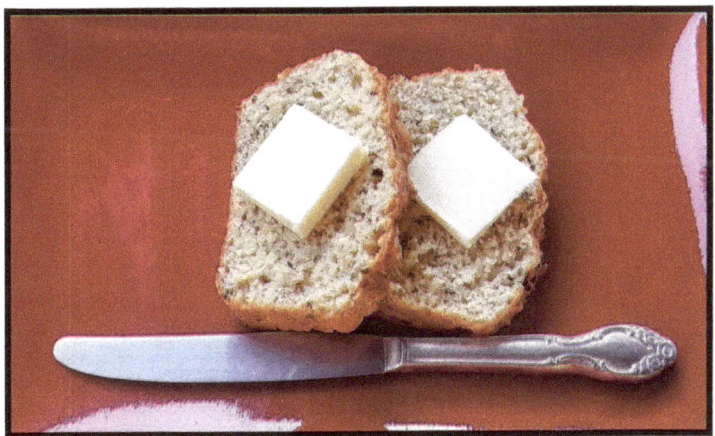

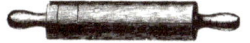

Oaten Cake with "Narnian" Wheat

If you can't locate a magical wardrobe through which you could obtain pure Narnian wheat flour, just substitute whatever brand you can find at your local grocer. If you really want to feed your fantasy desires, King Arthur might be the perfect brand for you to use, although I usually use Gold Medal, all-purpose and unbleached.

    This delicate bread/cake can be served plain, but it also lends itself to butter or margarine, if you like. You might also spoon some jam all over the top of a slice or drizzle with some honey, then it'll be more like a dessert. One recipe tester whipped up some cream and served this with a crisp white wine; another tester thought a cup of chopped apples in the batter would be delicious. I can definitely see some dessert options for you with this cake, if you wanted to veer off in that direction.

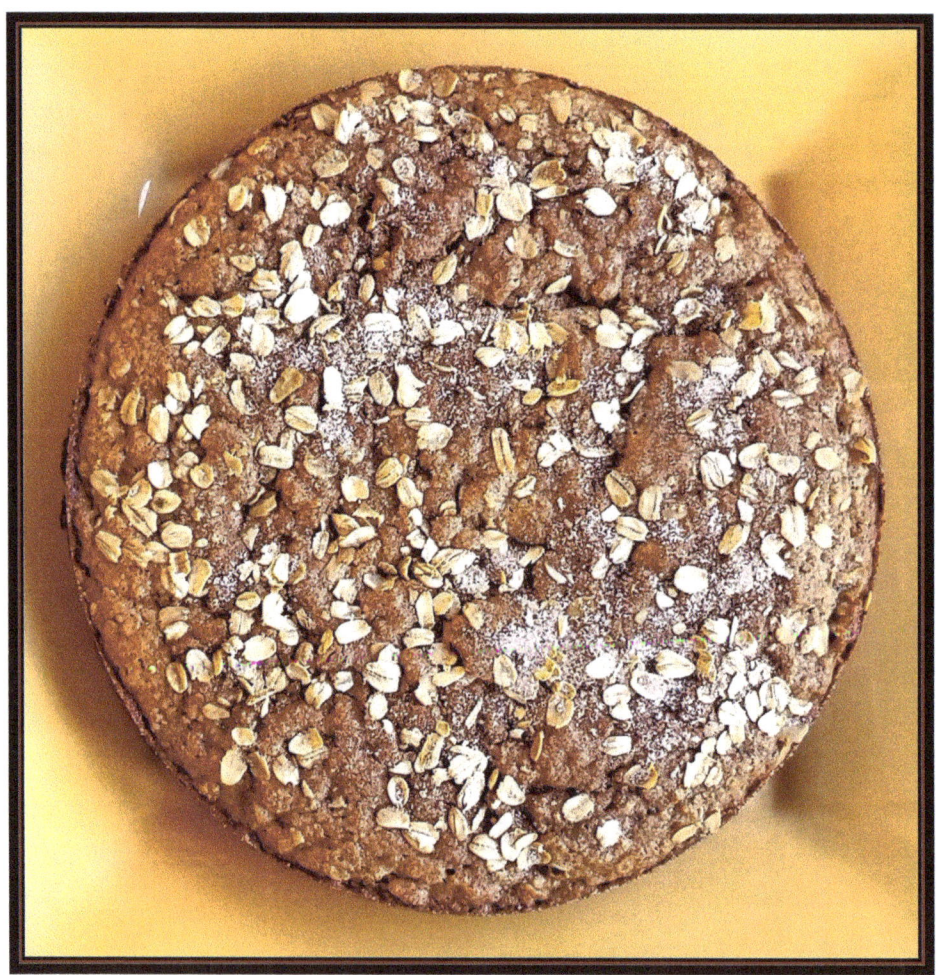

Total preparation time: approximately 1 hour and 20 minutes

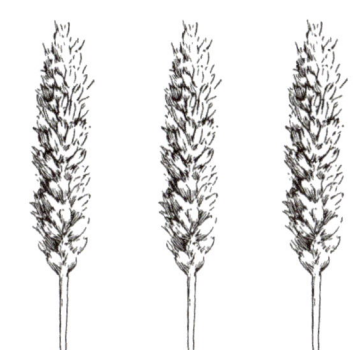

1 cup plus 2 tablespoons old-fashioned oats
1 cup all-purpose flour
¼ cup whole wheat flour
½ cup packed golden brown sugar
2 teaspoons cinnamon
1¼ teaspoons salt, divided
½ teaspoon baking soda
½ cup soft salted butter
1 cup fresh buttermilk, room temperature
1 large egg, room temperature
2 tablespoons cinnamon sugar (5 teaspoons sugar mixed with 1 teaspoon cinnamon)

PLACE 1 cup of oats in a medium skillet. Toast oats over rather high heat, 5-6 minutes. Toss or stir oats frequently until they are lightly toasted and fragrant. Let stand in the pan.

PREHEAT oven to 400°. Coat a 9" springform pan with 2" sides with cooking spray or grease lightly. Combine the 2 flours, brown sugar, cinnamon, 1 teaspoon salt, and baking soda in a large bowl. Add the oats and combine. Mix in the butter with a wooden spoon until crumbly. Whisk the buttermilk and egg in a 2-cup glass measuring cup and add to the flour; mix just until combined. Spread in prepared pan. Combine the 2 tablespoons oats, cinnamon sugar, and ¼ teaspoon salt in a small bowl. Sprinkle evenly over the batter. Bake 30 minutes. Let stand in pan on a rack 30 minutes. Release sides and cut into wedges. Cover and keep at room temperature or refrigerate. Serves 8.

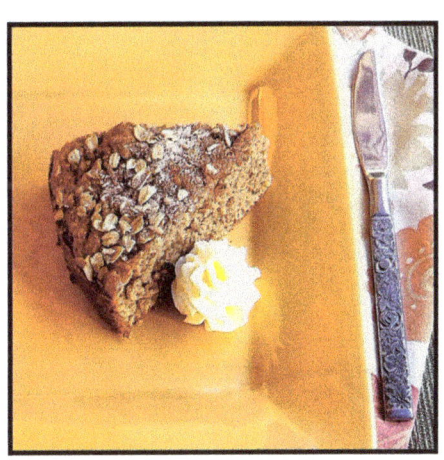

GOOD PAIRINGS:

★ Tater Ham Chowder
★ Butternut Risotto Soup

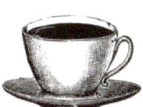

This recipe came about after my last reading of all the Chronicles of Narnia. C. S. Lewis often mentions "oaten meal cakes" or "wheaten cakes." I decided simply to combine the two grains and ended up with this fragile, yet hearty cake, which has a nutty quality to it without actually having any nuts in it. So, it IS sort of magical…

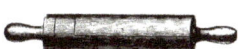

Bran's Brans

These substantial, yet delicate muffins are named for the character of Bran Stark, from *Game of Thrones*. They just seem like a snack that would be consumed in the North area of the fictional land of Westeros especially when winter was coming (which it always is…); plus, they have the added bonus of some healthful fiber. This would probably be an issue for the unfortunate Brandon, one of the earliest victims of the perversely fascinating Lannister family.

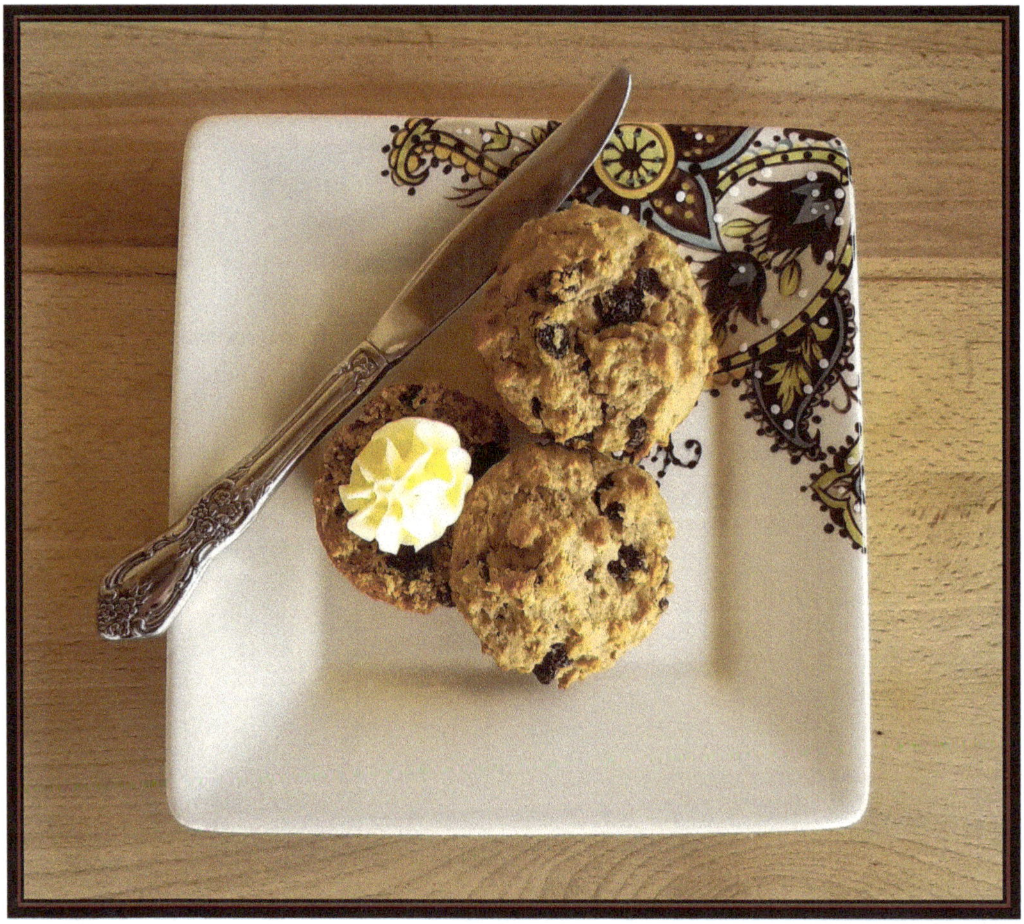

Total preparation time: approximately 40 minutes

¾ cup bran type of cereal (such as Kellogg's All-Bran®)
1¼ cups all-purpose flour
½ cup old-fashioned oats
¼ cup sugar
2 tablespoons wheat germ
1 tablespoon cinnamon
1 tablespoon baking powder
1 teaspoon salt
¼ teaspoon baking soda
¾ cup fresh buttermilk, room temperature
½ cup vegetable oil
1/3 cup applesauce (any flavor; you can use a 3.2-ounce pouch for just the right amount)
1 large egg, room temperature
1 cup raisins
1 cup walnuts, coarsely chopped

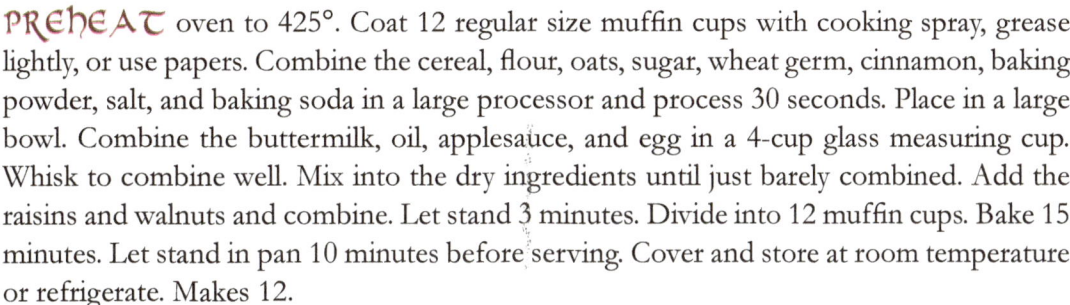

PREHEAT oven to 425°. Coat 12 regular size muffin cups with cooking spray, grease lightly, or use papers. Combine the cereal, flour, oats, sugar, wheat germ, cinnamon, baking powder, salt, and baking soda in a large processor and process 30 seconds. Place in a large bowl. Combine the buttermilk, oil, applesauce, and egg in a 4-cup glass measuring cup. Whisk to combine well. Mix into the dry ingredients until just barely combined. Add the raisins and walnuts and combine. Let stand 3 minutes. Divide into 12 muffin cups. Bake 15 minutes. Let stand in pan 10 minutes before serving. Cover and store at room temperature or refrigerate. Makes 12.

GOOD PAIRINGS:

★ Mom's Masher Soup
★ Bob Hates Cauliflower Soup

I apparently sometimes have a predilection for mixing grains, which I have done here. You may certainly substitute other small dried fruits or other nuts—dried blueberries and pecans would make a nice variation, or how about chopped up dried pineapple and macadamia nuts? You can experiment with combinations. As a leftover, these are nice warmed up in a microwave or toaster oven, served with butter and/or jams. These are not intended to be overly sweet, but you can sprinkle cinnamon sugar or raw sugar (turbinado) all over the tops before you bake them as an added muffin-top treat.

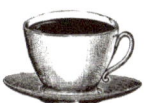

Chapter Five: Breads

Game of Scones

Bob actually came up with the name for these strange and fragile items; he said, "Well, why don't you make something up and call it 'Game of Scones?'" The game consists of this activity: people will take a bite of one of these scones; they'll tilt their head and wonder, just what is the flavor here? You can smirk to yourself about the mystery ingredient, while you see if they can guess what it is.

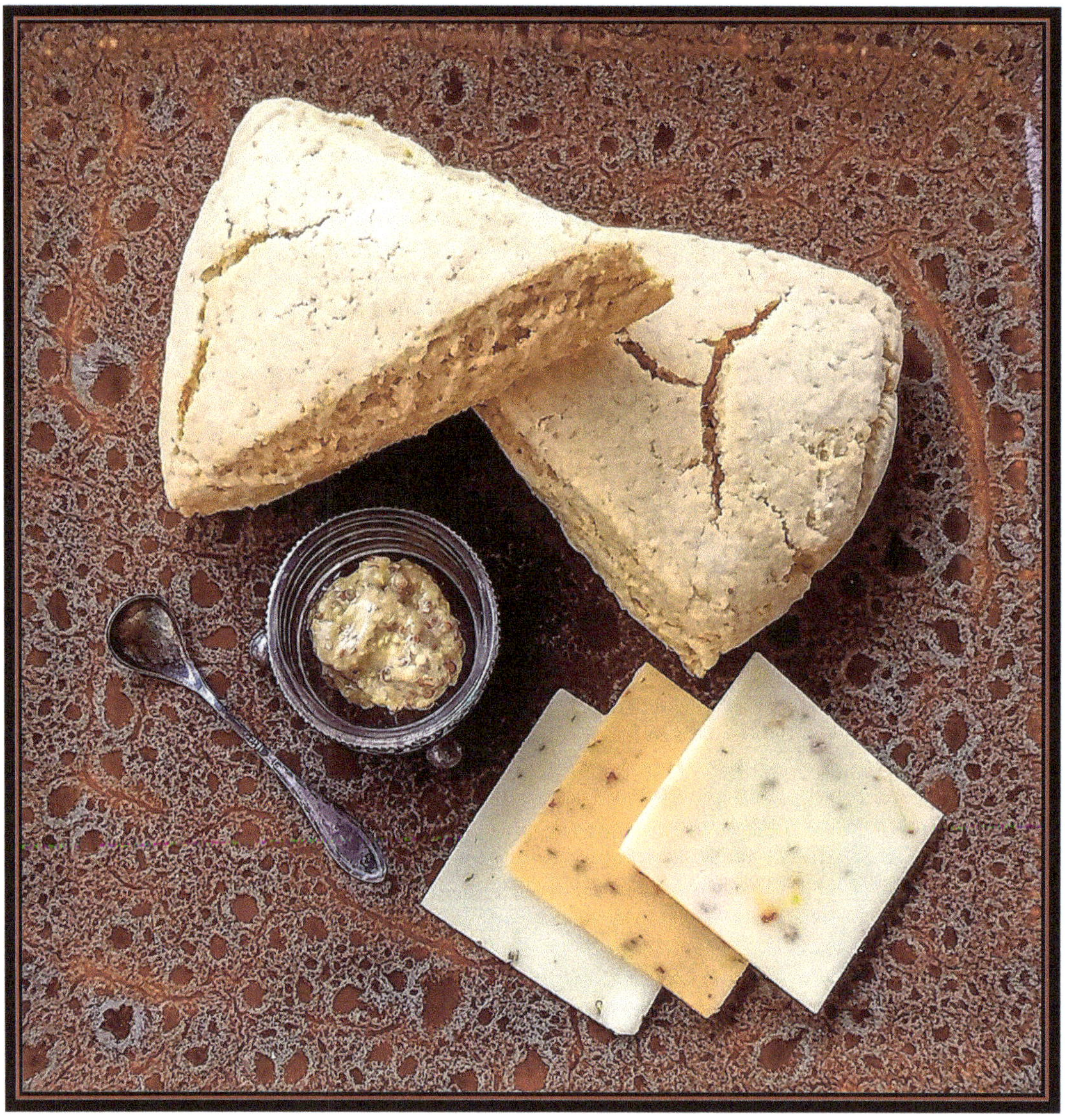

Total preparation time: approximately 35 minutes

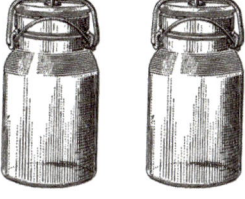
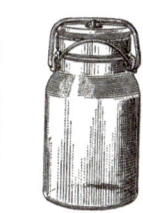

4 ounces Bugles corn chip snack
1½ cups all-purpose flour
¼ cup wheat germ
1 teaspoon baking powder
½ teaspoon baking soda
½ teaspoon salt
½ cup soft salted butter
¾ cup fresh buttermilk, room temperature
1 large egg, room temperature
Additional all-purpose flour

PREHEAT oven to 400°. Coat a large (18" by 13") baking sheet with cooking spray or grease lightly. Place the Bugles, flour, wheat germ, baking powder, baking soda, and salt in a large food processor. Process well. Add the butter and process. Add the buttermilk and egg and process. Knead a few times on a floured surface. Pat dough to a circle, approximately 8" in diameter and 1" thick. Cut into 8 wedges. Lay on the prepared sheet 1" apart. Bake 13-15 minutes, until lightly browned on the bottom. Let stand on pan 5-10 minutes before serving. Cover and store at room temperature or refrigerate. Makes 8.

GOOD PAIRINGS:

- ★ Turkey Black Bean Soup
- ★ Sopa del Diente Quebrado (a.k.a. Broken Tooth Soup)
- ★ Tecolote Chili

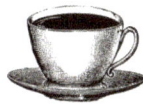

Though these are savory and delicious with butter and assorted cheesy accompaniments, they are also nice with various jams or fruit butters. Play a game and try a different chip to test the taste buds of your diners.

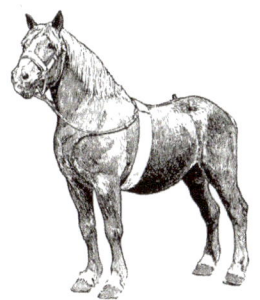
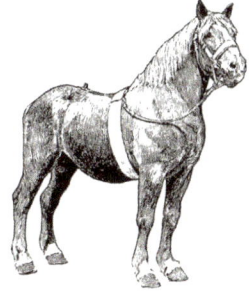

Chapter Five: Breads

Lovely Artisan Loaf

I don't know why everybody seems to be hopping on the "no-carb" bandwagon, especially if one doesn't need to; sometimes bread is just too hard to resist. Do people sometimes eat too much bread? Perhaps; but to give it up completely? That seems harsh and life is short.

When I told one of my online editors I was writing a soup/bread cookbook, he requested that I include a recipe for bread bowls. Originally I had not planned on doing that, but this loaf is suitable to adapt to a bowl conversion. I know it might seem strange, but I am constantly following a diet (which I hate, of course…). A bread bowl is—let's face it—a LOT of bread. I suppose you're not supposed to eat the bowl…? But that's a waste of good bread. And so, when it comes to food, you are often damned if you eat and damned if you don't.

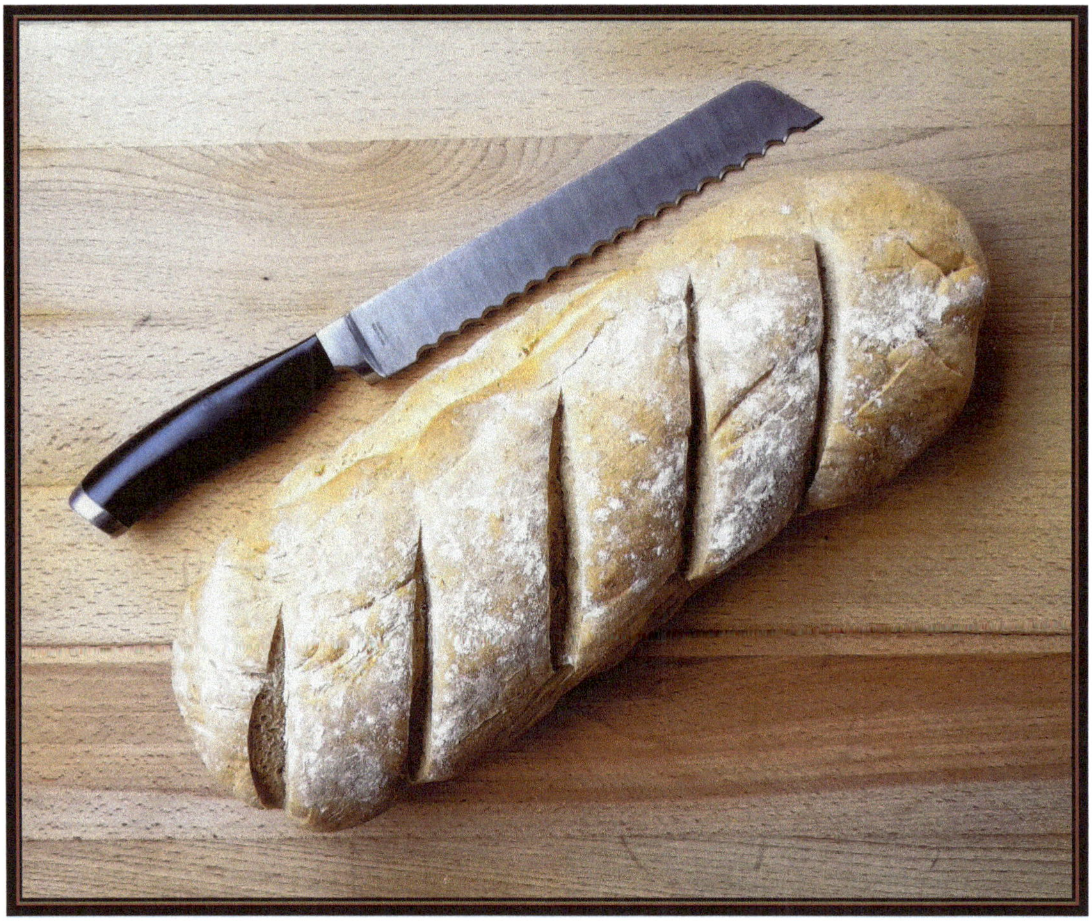

Total preparation time: approximately 3 hours and 15 minutes (or 3 hours for bread bowls)

1½ cups water
1 tablespoon coarse kosher salt
1 (¼-ounce) packet active dry yeast
    (2¼ teaspoons)
1/3 cup dark rye flour
1/3 cup semolina flour
1/3 cup whole wheat flour
1¾ cups plus 1 1/3 cups bread flour
1 tablespoon olive oil
1 tablespoon cornmeal
Additional all-purpose or bread flour

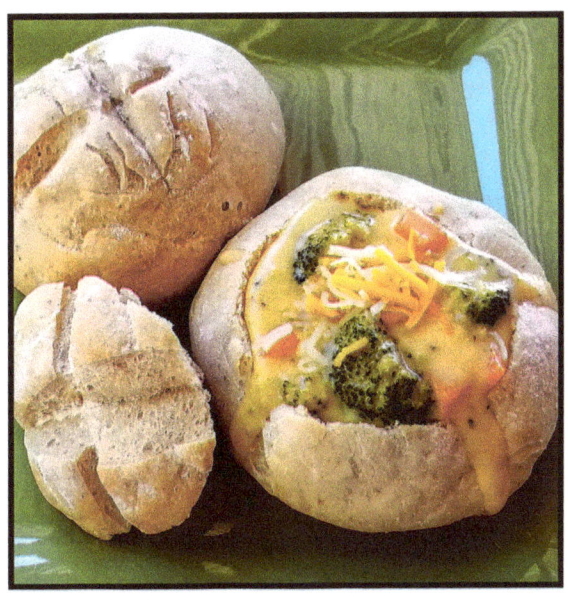

MICROWAVE the water on HIGH 1 minute, then pour into a stand mixer bowl. Add the salt and yeast and combine. Add the rye, semolina, and wheat flours, plus the 1¾ cups bread flour. Mix on low for a few seconds, then on medium speed for 1 minute. Add the remaining bread flour and mix on low another minute. Switch to a dough hook and mix 5 minutes on the lowest speed. Knead a few times on a lightly floured surface. Pour oil in the mixing bowl; place the dough back in the bowl and move it around to coat all over with oil. Cover with a towel and let rise in a relatively warm, draft-free place for 1 hour. *(See the parenthetical remarks for the bread bowl option.)*

    COAT a large (18" by 13") baking sheet with cooking spray or grease lightly. Sprinkle with the cornmeal. Press down the dough and knead a few times. Form into a loaf about 12-14" long *(divide into 6 portions; roll into balls)*. Place on the prepared sheet, cover with the towel and let rise 45 minutes.

    PREHEAT oven to 400°. With a very sharp knife, make 5 slashes in the top of the loaf, about 1" deep *(slash the top of each bowl with a large X)*. Dust the top of the loaf *(bowls)* with some extra flour. Bake 30 minutes *(20 minutes)*. Let stand on pan 15 minutes *(10 minutes)*, then place on a rack for 30 minutes. Slice diagonally *(remove the upper portion of the bowl with a sharp knife and set it next to the bowl; pull out some of the bread within and fill with your desired soup)*. Cover and keep at room temperature or refrigerate; it freezes well. 12-14 slices *(6 bowls)*.

GOOD PAIRINGS:

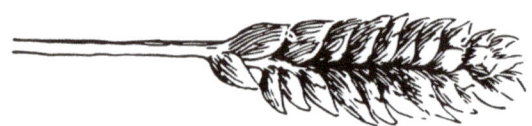

- ★ Saffron Madness Soup
- ★ Awesome Avgolemono
- ★ Oodle Noodle Soup

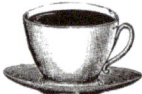 *This is one of the ways I sneak rye flour into our meals, since Bob hates rye bread. It is lovely served while still warm with butter; later on, toast it to a golden brown. It will be lovely with butter, lovely with jams. It will even make a lovely sandwich.*

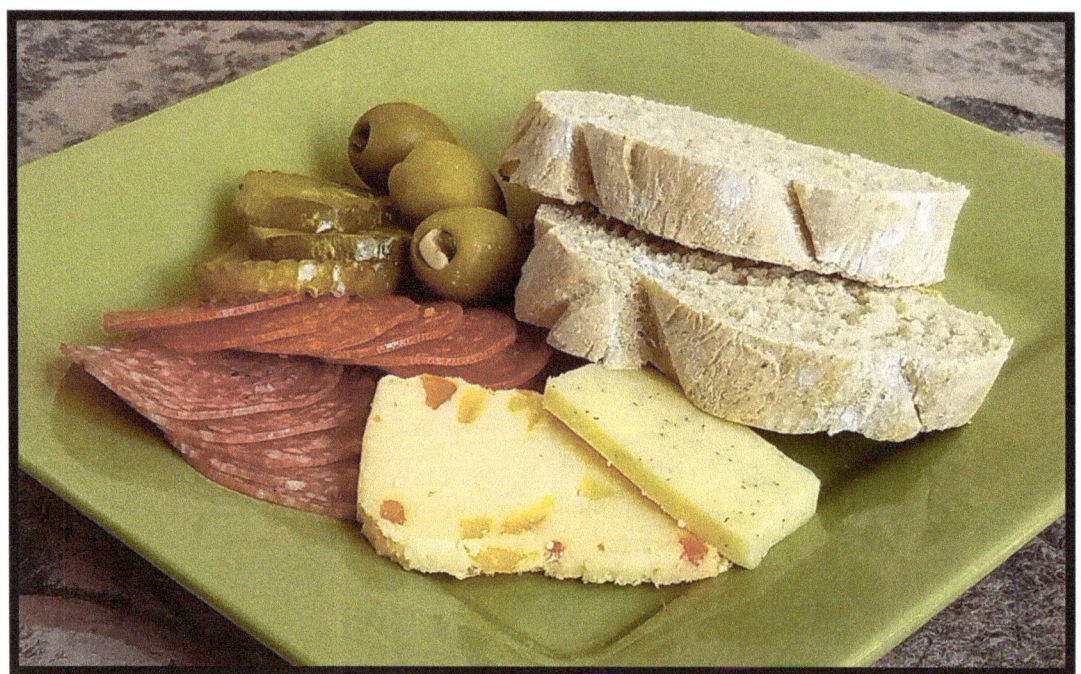

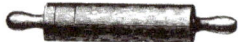

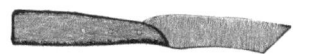

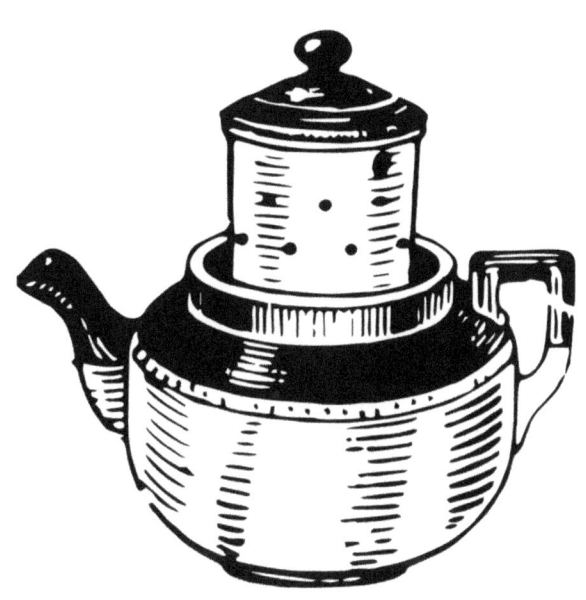

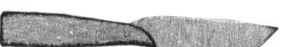

Nifty "Narnian" Biscuits

The Chronicles of Narnia often mention a sort of hard biscuit, or hardtack. This is supposed to sustain you on the road while you are running away from evil witches and other enemies. Of course, biscuit can also mean cookie, at least according to C. S. Lewis. For my Internet writing, I eventually decided to invent a nice biscuit, in the American sense, because obviously nobody really wants a recipe for hardtack.

You will see I have parenthesized the word "soft" in the ingredient list below. This is because conflicting theories about butter abound. Should it be cold and cut into small bits? Should you freeze it and then shred it? What about soft butter? I heard a famous chef once proclaim that butter should always be cold; otherwise, your product won't rise properly. With something like biscuits, I like to use soft butter, since it makes the mixing so much easier. I once conducted an experiment and tried all three butter textures. They all worked, and all produced an agreeable biscuit. The famous chef was… wrong. One advantage to soft butter, however, is not having to cut it up or shred it. Labor saved! But it is nice to know that when you get that urge to make biscuits and you only have frozen butter around, just get your box grater out and work quickly before your hands melt the butter.

Total preparation time: approximately 30 minutes

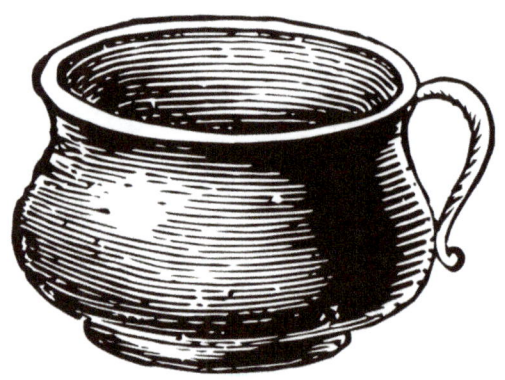

2 cups all-purpose flour
¼ cup whole wheat flour
1 tablespoon sugar
1 tablespoon baking powder
¾ teaspoon salt
¾ teaspoon cream of tartar
½ cup (soft) salted butter
1¼ cups fresh buttermilk, room temperature
Additional all-purpose flour

PREHEAT oven to 450°. Coat a medium (13" by 9") baking sheet with cooking spray or grease lightly. Combine the flours, sugar, baking powder, salt, and cream of tartar in a large bowl. Add the butter and mix in rather well with a wooden spoon, leaving some bits of butter throughout. Add the buttermilk and combine just until moistened. With floured hands, turn dough onto a floured surface. Knead a few times. Pat into a 9" by 6" rectangle, about 1" thick. Cut into 12 portions, 3 by 4. Lay on the prepared sheet (they'll be rather close together). Bake 13-15 minutes. Let stand on pan 5 minutes before serving. Keep leftovers covered at room temperature. Makes 12.

GOOD PAIRINGS:

- ★ William Said This Was His Favorite Soup
- ★ Enchanted Forest Soup
- ★ Bob's Old-Fashioned Beef Stew

These biscuits are stable and just the tiniest bit crispy. They can handle any sort of butter, jam, or honey you would like to spread on them without falling apart too much.

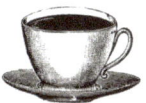

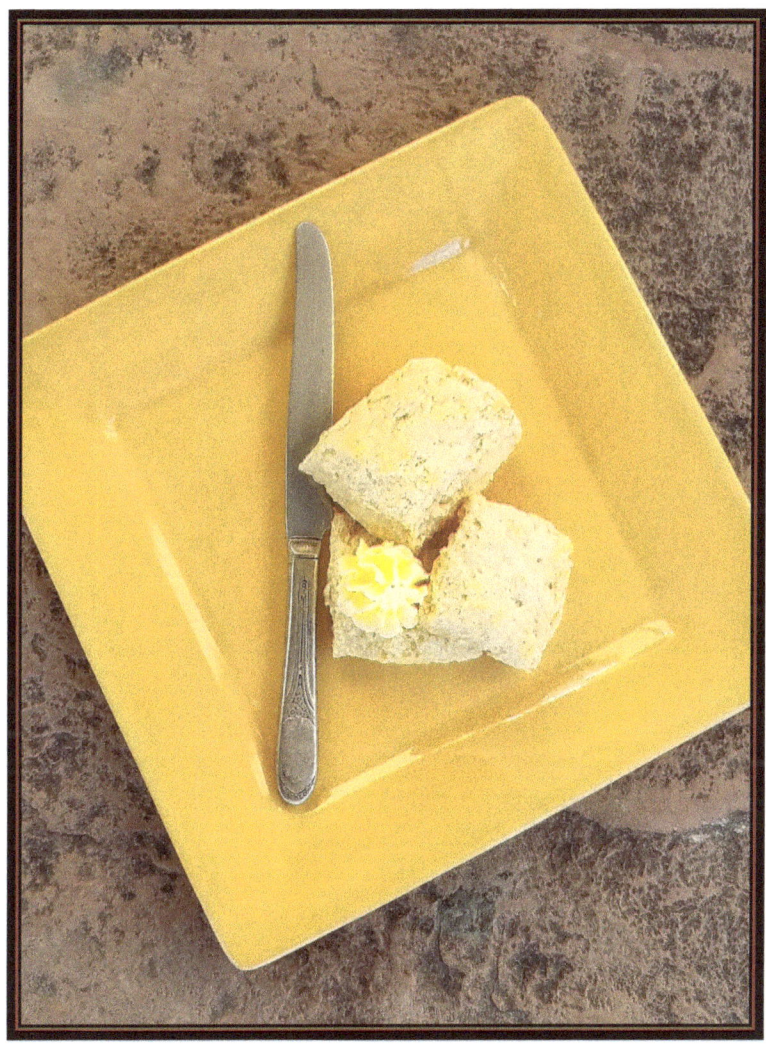

Chapter Five: Breads

Easy Focaccia

I have whipped this up in a large food processor (which makes it easy!), but you can certainly mix up your dough by hand in a large bowl (knead your dough for a few minutes, until smooth), or in a stand mixer (after mixing, use a dough hook on the lowest setting for 4-5 minutes). Other changes you might make: you could use flavored olive oils, add a teaspoon of onion and/or garlic powder, or a teaspoon of dried herbs (or a tablespoon or two of fresh minced herbs). If you're extra careful, you can slice a piece horizontally to make a sandwich the next day.

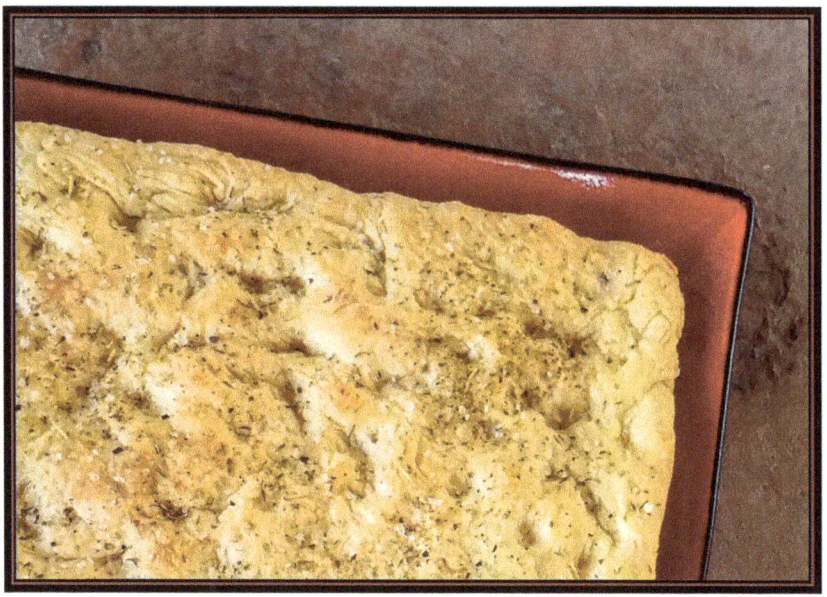

Total preparation time: approximately 2 hours and 30 minutes

2½ cups all-purpose flour (bread flour will also work out well)
1 (¼-ounce) packet active dry yeast (2¼ teaspoons)
1½ teaspoons salt
¾ cup water
¼ cup olive oil
2 tablespoons 1% milk
1 tablespoon plus 1 tablespoon olive oil
1 teaspoon dry Italian seasoning (or 2-3 tablespoons fresh, minced; your choice)
½ teaspoon coarse kosher or sea salt
Additional all-purpose flour

COMBINE the flour, yeast, and salt in a large food processor fitted with the dough blade. Process for a few seconds. Combine the water, ¼ cup olive oil, and milk in a 2-cup glass measuring cup. Microwave on HIGH 45 seconds. Pour into the processor and mix well until the dough becomes a mostly smooth ball, about 1-2 minutes. Place dough on a floured surface; cover loosely with a towel and let rise in a relatively warm, draft-free place for 1 hour.

BRUSH a medium (13" by 9") baking sheet with 1 tablespoon olive oil. Press down the dough and knead a few times on a lightly floured surface. Press dough into prepared pan evenly to the edges. Cover with the towel and let rise 45 minutes.

PREHEAT oven to 400°. Press fingers all over the dough to make dimples. Brush with the remaining olive oil. Sprinkle the Italian herbs all over evenly, then sprinkle with coarse salt evenly. Bake 20 minutes. Let stand in pan 5-10 minutes before cutting. Cover and keep at room temperature or chill. Serves 8-12, or you can cut smaller pieces to serve more.

GOOD PAIRINGS:

- ★ It's a Nice Day for a Wedding Soup
- ★ Pasta e Fagioli
- ★ Stracciatella Bella (a.k.a. "Hoth Broth")

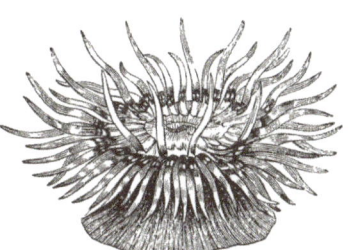

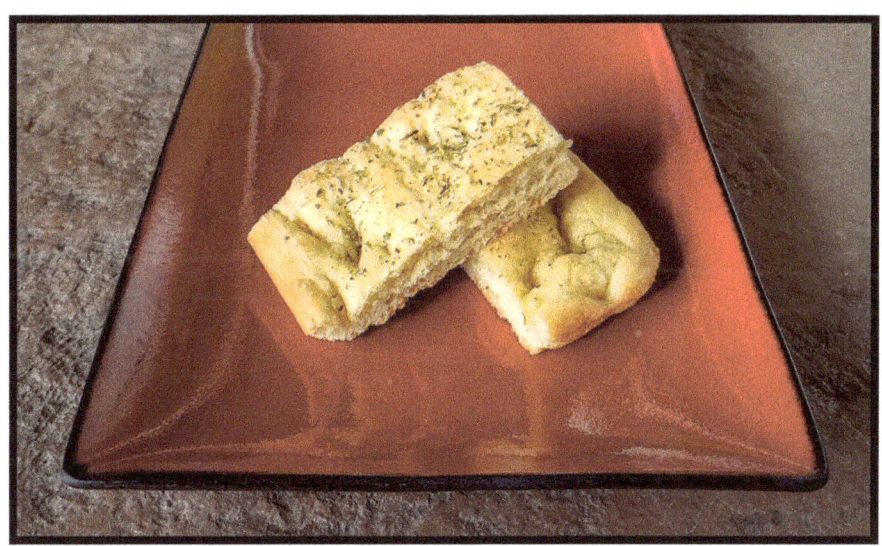

Chapter Five: Breads   175

Epic Iron Skillet Cornbread

This cornbread has a wonderfully crunchy texture inside, and its crispy, golden brown exterior is due to a liberally buttered cast iron skillet. My grandsons love this cornbread. Well, we all do.

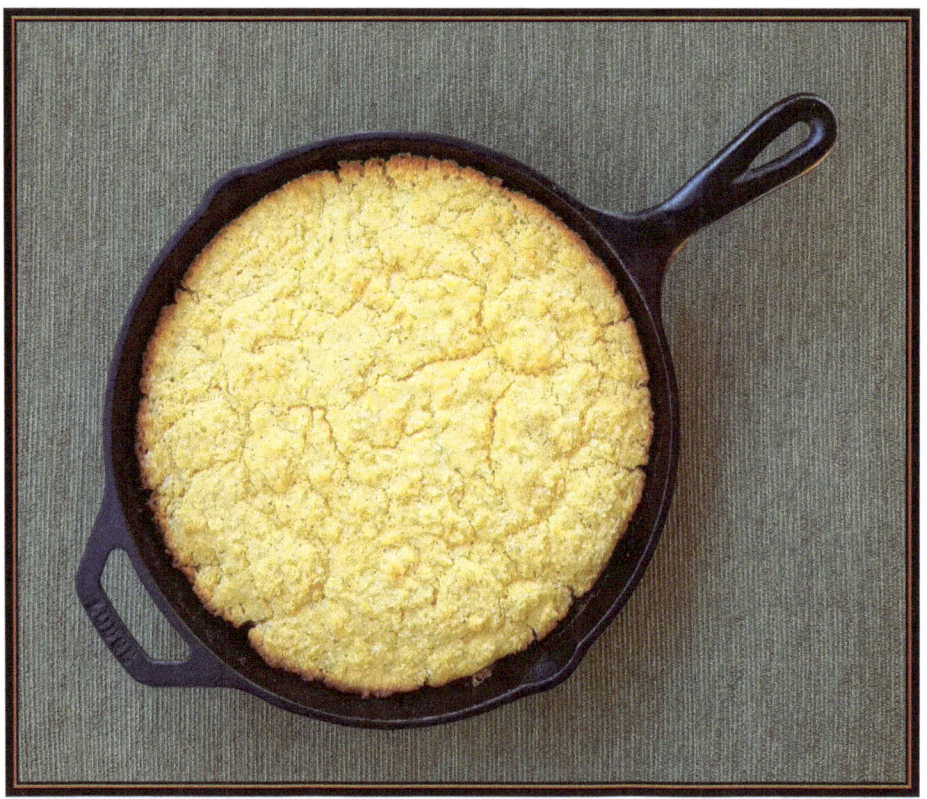

Total preparation time: approximately 40 minutes

6 tablespoons plus 2 tablespoons salted butter (1 stick)
2 (1-ounce) packages instant grits (quick grits are also fine)
1 cup yellow cornmeal
1 cup all-purpose flour
¼ cup sugar
1 tablespoon baking powder
1 teaspoon salt
1½ cups fresh buttermilk, room temperature
2 large eggs, room temperature

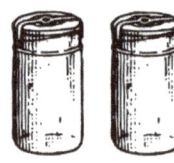

PREHEAT oven to 450°. Microwave 6 tablespoons butter in a small glass bowl on HIGH until melted; set aside. Combine the grits, cornmeal, flour, sugar, baking powder, and salt in a large bowl and set aside. Whisk the buttermilk and the eggs well in a 4-cup glass measuring cup. Whisk the melted butter into the buttermilk mixture and set aside. Melt the 2 tablespoons butter over very high heat in a 10" cast iron skillet, swirling it around to coat the bottom and sides. Mix buttermilk mixture into the flour mixture just until all is moistened. Pour into the prepared skillet. Bake 20 minutes. Let stand in skillet 5 minutes. Cut into 8 wedges. Cover and keep at room temperature or refrigerate. Serves 8.

Good Pairings:

- ★ Tecolote Chili
- ★ Bodacious Brisket Soup
- ★ Jumbo Gumbo
- ★ Any of the other chilis

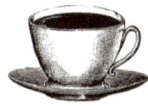

I've only used the original flavor for my grits, but the cheesy, butter, and bacon varieties should work just as well; they'll merely add different flavor profiles to your cornbread. If you need to substitute the instant grits, I found that the 2½-minute Cream of Wheat will work out fine. This leads me to think that pretty much any sort of quick or instant dry hot cereal (unsweetened and with a small texture) will also work out fine. So, Cream of Rice, Wheatena, Malt-O-Meal, etc., will work, though they might not deliver the same satisfying, yet subtle, crunch as the grits; plus, the flavor would change slightly, of course. Even quick-cooking steel cut oats will work.

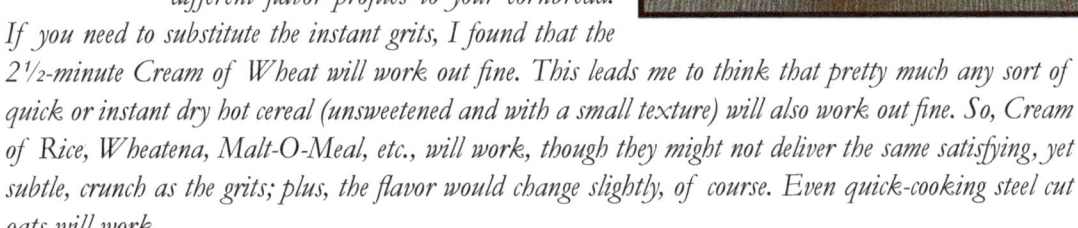

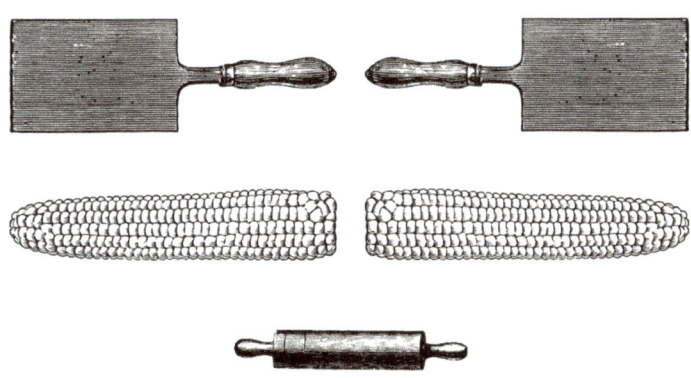

Chapter Five: Breads

Land of Enchantment "Lembas" with Spicy Honey Butter

These are deliciously savory, yet slightly sweet. They are good plain, with butter, or even with jams or jellies. Then I decided to invent a spicy/sweet butter to go with them, which will also work with most other carby products you might have around. Structurally, they resemble the "lembas" I invented for my first cookbook, which was directly inspired by Middle-earth and Narnia. I doubt that Professor Tolkien would have appreciated the smoky spice within these morsels, but I sincerely believe his mysterious elvish product was open to interpretation.

If you have trouble obtaining chipotle powder, you can use regular chili powder (or other varieties of chili powder, such as ancho) or even omit it. Chipotle is the smoked version of a red-ripe jalapeño.

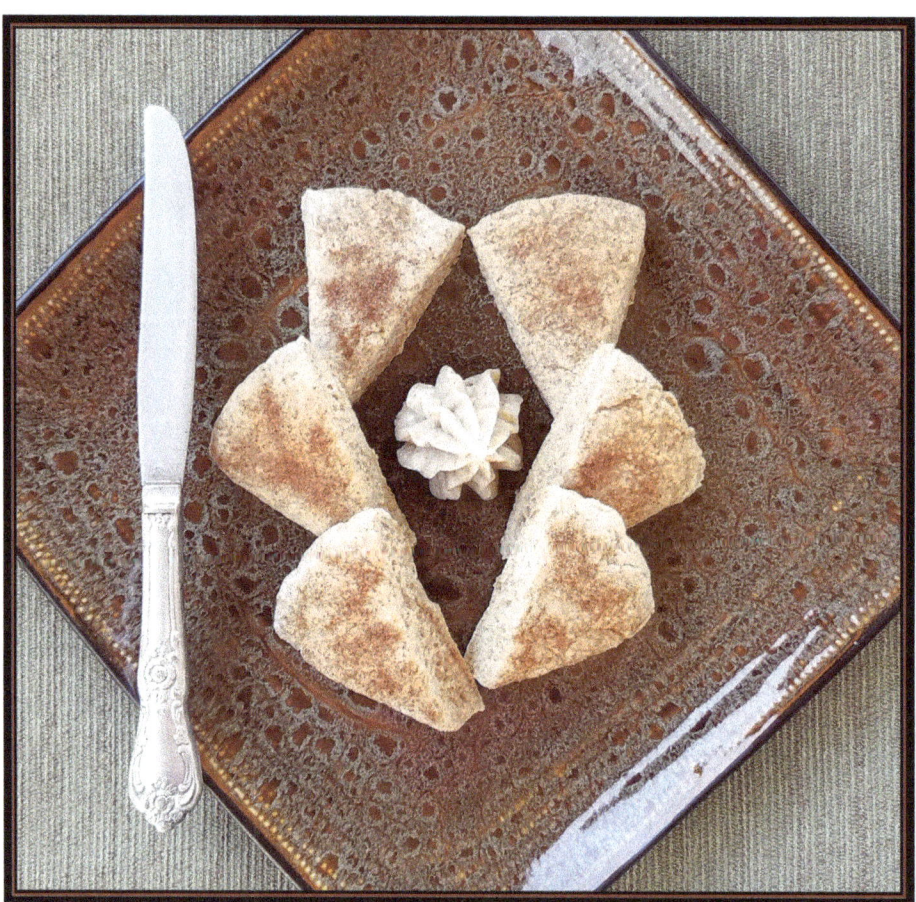

Total preparation time: approximately 35 minutes

¼ cup water
¼ cup honey
1½ cups all-purpose flour
½ cup whole wheat flour
1⅛ teaspoons salt, divided
1⅛ teaspoons chipotle powder, divided
2 tablespoons packed golden brown sugar
½ teaspoon cinnamon
½ teaspoon baking powder
½ cup soft salted butter
Additional all-purpose flour
1 teaspoon cinnamon sugar (¾ teaspoon sugar mixed with ¼ teaspoon cinnamon)
Water in a spray bottle

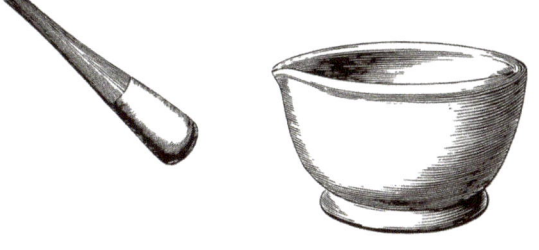

COMBINE the water and honey in a 1-cup glass measuring cup. Microwave on HIGH 20 seconds. Whisk to mix; set aside while you prepare the dough.

PREHEAT oven to 400°. Coat a large (18" by 13") baking sheet with cooking spray or grease lightly. Combine the flours, 1 teaspoon salt, 1 teaspoon chipotle powder, brown sugar, cinnamon, and baking powder in a large bowl. Mix in the soft butter with a wooden spoon, then mix with your hands until coarse crumbs form. Mix in the honey mixture with the wooden spoon until well combined. Knead a few times on a lightly floured surface until smooth. Divide in half. Roll each half into a ball. Flatten one ball to a ½" thick circle, about 6-7" in diameter. Cut into 8 wedges and carefully set on the prepared pan, ½" apart. Repeat with the other half of the dough.

COMBINE the cinnamon sugar, remaining ⅛ teaspoon salt, and ⅛ teaspoon chipotle powder in a tiny bowl. Spray the wedges lightly with water. Sprinkle the cinnamon sugar mixture evenly all over. Bake 9-11 minutes. Let stand on pan 3 minutes before serving. Serve with Spicy Honey Butter, or other spreads, if desired. Cover and store at room temperature. Makes 16.

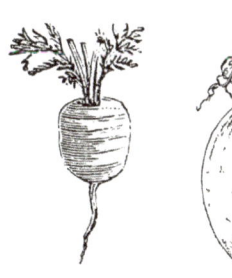
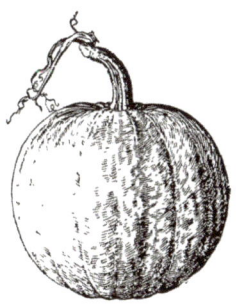
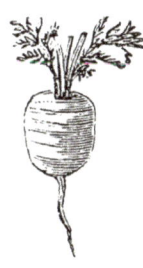

Chapter Five: Breads

Spicy Honey Butter

½ cup soft salted butter
1 tablespoon powdered sugar
1 tablespoon honey
¼ teaspoon chipotle powder
¼ teaspoon cinnamon

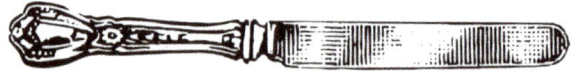

COMBINE all ingredients well in a small bowl. Cover and refrigerate leftovers; bring to room temperature to serve. Makes ½ cup.

GOOD PAIRINGS:

★ Any of the five posoles
★ Little Squash: Little Stew

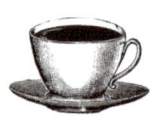

Why is New Mexico called The Land of Enchantment? Some brilliant marketer came up with the idea to put the phrase "Land of Enchantment" on New Mexico's license plates back in 1941. The phrase was meant to reflect New Mexico's rich history, which dates back to the establishment of our state capital, Santa Fe, in 1607. Santa Fe is the second oldest city in the United States. The phrase also alludes to our myriad scenic vistas, which have attracted world-renowned artists such as Georgia O'Keeffe, or photographers such as Ansel Adams. Most recently, our state has been featured beautifully, even in some exceptionally unsavory scenes, in two of my favorite television shows, Breaking Bad *and* Better Call Saul. *Will you fall under its spell if you visit? There is only one way to find out.*

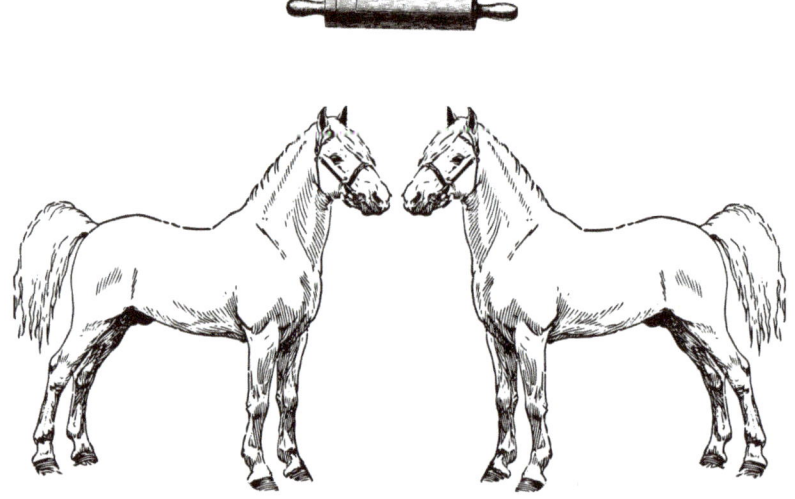

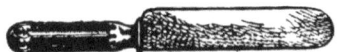

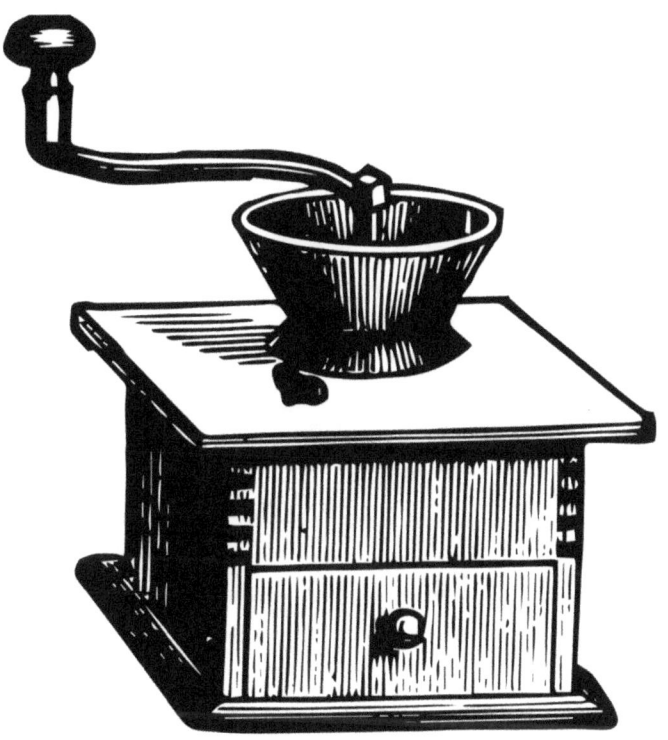

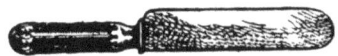

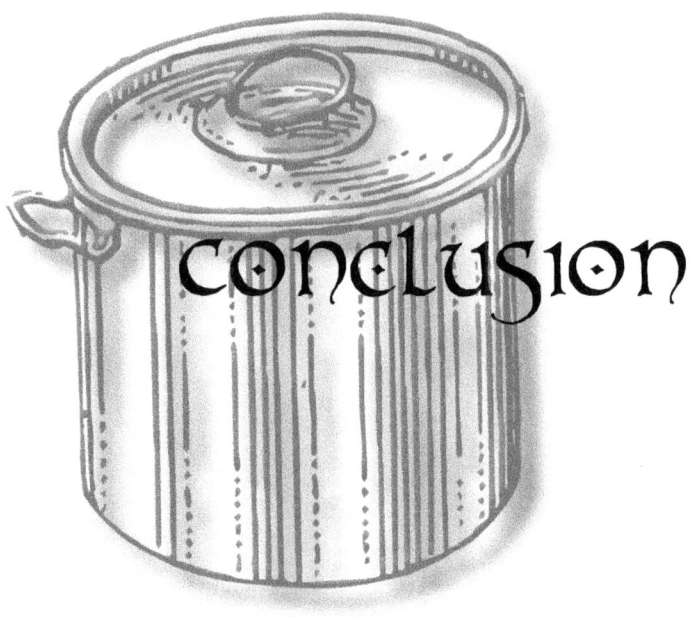

conclusion

Chloë told me she once heard (or read, she's not sure which) that somebody summed up the seasons in Albuquerque thusly (she didn't use the word *thusly*...):

Winter ★ luminarias (These are small paper bags with sand and candles inside, arranged on and around residences and businesses for the Christmas season.)
Spring ★ wind (Come on, lots of towns and cities have a lot more wind than we do...)
Summer ★ cockroaches (One could move to Antarctica to avoid bugs, right?)
Autumn ★ Balloon Fiesta (Our international, extremely busy event is held in October; book early if you plan a trip.)

I guess two of those seasons sound rather desirable. But I would like to sum up our seasons with more beauty, and more food, of course:

Winter ★ posoles, tamales, and biscochitos (You know about posoles now; will my next cookbook deal with tamales? Probably not. But it will definitely have a biscochito recipe; these are lovely anise-flavored cookies.)
Spring ★ roadrunners, robins, and roses (We have many other birds and flowers.)
Summer ★ guacamole and salsa; margaritas and beer (Well, these are year-round, actually...)
Autumn ★ green chile roasting and red chile ristras hung up to dry (Once you start to eat chile, you won't want to stop!)

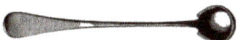

One night back in 2018, I spent a few hours at a restaurant meeting with actual, real-life people from a Facebook writers group. I happened to be seated across from a truly grumpy curmudgeon. If I had known this was to be my dinner companion, I would have stayed home with my more familiar and much more pleasant grumpy curmudgeon. Nevertheless, I persisted in foolishly attempting to have a conversation with this man who obviously hadn't wanted to accompany his wife to this get-together. He asked me why I would bother to write a cookbook when all the recipes in the world were already on the Internet. He then proceeded to inject insulin into his abdomen while I concentrated on keeping my expression neutral. I told him I was well aware that everyone and his/her mother has a peppy recipe blog, but I still felt like writing my own and putting it into book form. I felt like it was a bliss I could follow, especially since my nest had emptied. It just doesn't matter to me that a billion recipes exist on the Internet—these are MY recipes and I felt like sharing them. I'm hoping you will find some new favorites within these pages!

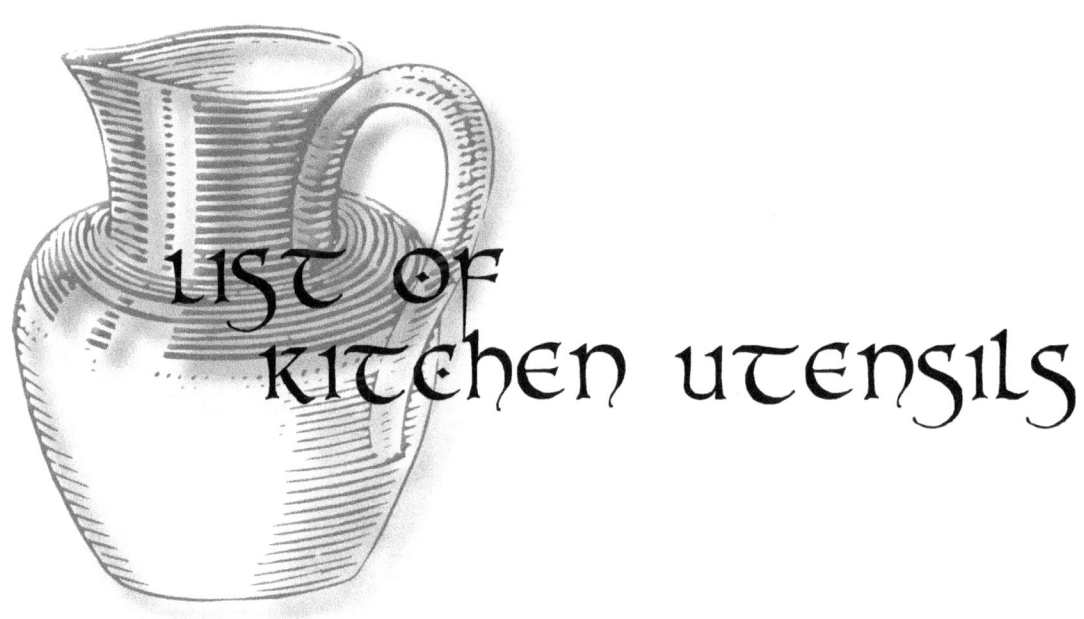

List of Kitchen Utensils

Brand names are not recommendations; they are merely what I happen to have in my kitchen, at least at the moment. You don't really need a stand mixer if you happen to have luck with a hand mixer and a large bowl, or if you are used to mixing things up completely by hand. I actually sort of miss having a 4-quart KitchenAid around; the 5½-quart I currently own sometimes seems too big for what I often do.

REGARDING BAKING DISHES AND COOKWARE: glass or metal products will be fine, though a heavy ceramic dish might require some adjustments (but maybe not). Your cookware is bound to be different from mine, but you shouldn't need to make many changes with cooking times. I've also noticed a new trend in cookware design, where pots and pans are beginning to become smaller; i.e., a 5½-quart saucepan appears to be the new 6-quart and a 7½-quart is the new 8-quart. I usually allow plenty of space in my saucepans, so if your pots are a bit smaller than what I have called for, you'll still (probably) be okay.

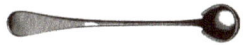

Cooking Utensils & Miscellaneous Items

- Measuring cups for dry ingredients (⅛, ¼, 1/3, ½, 2/3, ¾, and 1 cup)
- Glass measuring cups for liquid ingredients (1-, 2-, and 4-cup)
- Measuring spoons (⅛, ¼, ½, and ¾-teaspoon, ½ tablespoon, 1 tablespoon)
- Kitchen scale (a minimum of 1-pound—I have a digital 11-pound, which I love)
- Knife set (a few good, sharp knives, including a serrated one; I also use a cleaver)
- Storage containers with lids (various sizes; plastic and glass)
- Assorted mixing bowls, both glass and stainless steel (various sizes, from small to very large)
- Vegetable peeler / spatula / wooden spoon / cutting boards
- Towels / cloth napkins / potholders / box grater / pastry blender
- Whisks—various sizes / strainers and colanders—assorted sizes
- If you want to be fancy with your garnishing: pastry bag with various basic tips / plastic squirt bottle (perfect for drizzling crème fraîche)
- I use a soup ladle that measures about ½ cup; very handy for measuring, then serving
- Rolling pin / timer / spray bottle for water / pastry brush / bent spatula
- A 12-ounce microwave-safe ceramic mug that is rather open at the top
- Aluminum foil, both light and heavy duty

Small & Large Appliances

- Blender (Oster—5-cup variety)
- Optional: hand blender (Sometimes called an immersion blender—some people swear by these; I'm not completely sold, but I did cave in and buy a KitchenAid variety… and I hardly ever use it.)
- Optional: hand mixer
- Gas stove with conventional oven / microwave
- Small food processor (Cuisinart "Mini-Prep"—4-cup variety; a 3-cup is also fine)
- Large food processor (Cuisinart—12-cup variety, with standard accessories)
- 5½-quart stand mixer (KitchenAid—with the standard beater, whisk, and dough hook)

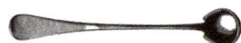

Pots & Pans

- Saucepans (pots) with lids (2-, 3-, 4-, 6-, 8-, 12-, and 16-quart—the 12- and 16-quart pots might not be necessary for all of your particular needs, so only purchase them if you plan to double recipes or make your own stock/broth)
- Medium skillet, 10" / large skillet, 12" / cast iron skillet, 10"

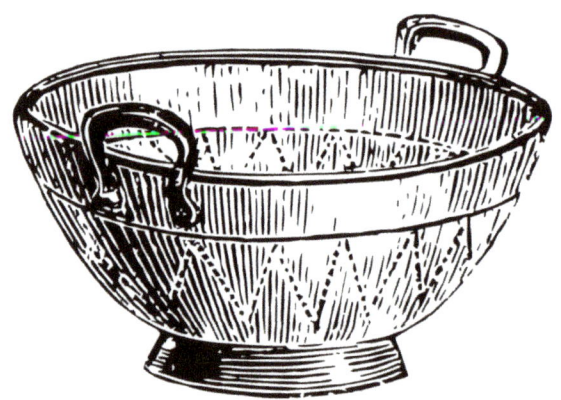

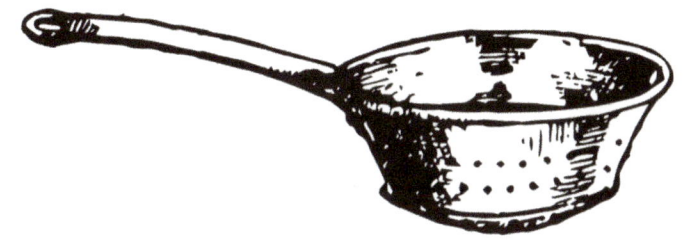

Baking Essentials

- Muffin pan—regular size (to make 12)
- Quarter sheet (medium) baking pan (13" by 9"—heavy aluminum, with 1" rim)
- Half sheet (large) baking pan (18" by 13"—heavy aluminum, with 1" rim)
- Small baking sheet (I just use the 10" square one from my toaster oven)
- Cooling racks
- Two 8½" by 4½" loaf pans (glass or metal)
- 11" by 7" baking dish (glass or metal)
- 13" by 9" baking dish (glass or metal)
- 9" springform pan (2" sides)

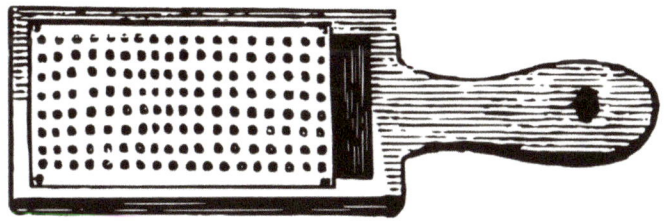

List of Kitchen Utensils

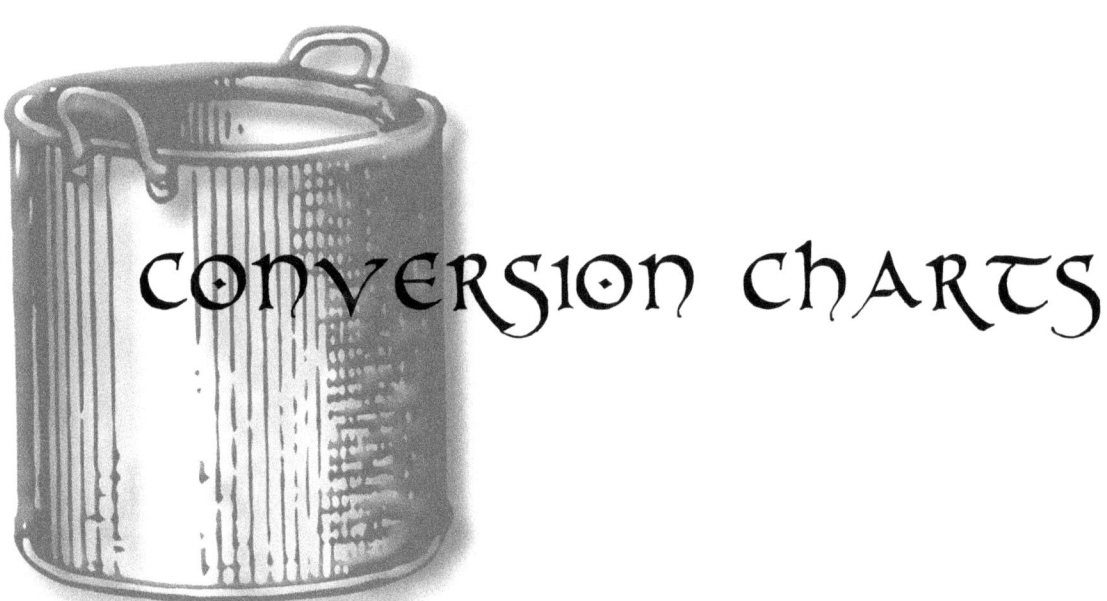

CONVERSION CHARTS

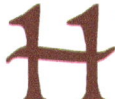ere are some basic measurement conversion charts. All equivalents are approximate.

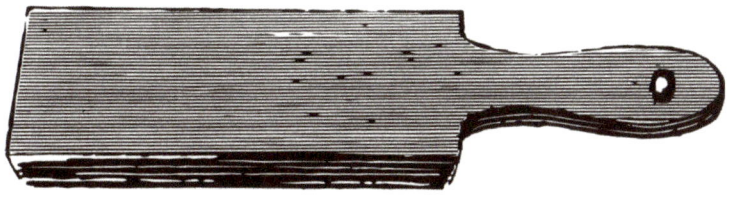

Dry Ingredients by Weight

Multiply number of ounces by 28 to convert to grams.

⅛ teaspoon	a pinch			
3 teaspoons	1 tablespoon			
⅛ cup	2 tablespoons	1 ounce		28 grams
¼ cup	4 tablespoons	2 ounces	⅛ pound	56 grams
1/3 cup	5 tablespoons plus 1 teaspoon	3 ounces		84 grams
½ cup	8 tablespoons	4 ounces	¼ pound	113 grams
2/3 cup	10 tablespoons plus 2 teaspoons	5 1/3 ounces	1/3 pound	150 grams
¾ cup	12 tablespoons	6 ounces		168 grams
1 cup	16 tablespoons	8 ounces	½ pound	230 grams
1¼ cups		10 2/3 ounces	2/3 pound	300 grams
1½ cups		12 ounces	¾ pound	340 grams
2 cups		16 ounces	1 pound	450 grams
4 cups		32 ounces	2 pounds	900 grams
			2.2 pounds	1 kilogram

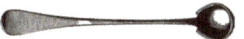

Liquid Ingredients by Volume

The column with parenthetical measurements on the right is for rounding up, if you don't need very precise conversions. Multiply number of ounces by 30 to convert to milliliters.

¼ teaspoon				
½ teaspoon				
1 teaspoon			5 ml	
1 tablespoon	3 teaspoons	½ ounce	15 ml	
1 fluid ounce	2 tablespoons	⅛ cup	30 ml	
2 ounces	¼ cup		60 ml	
3 ounces	1/3 cup		80 ml	
4 ounces	½ cup		120 ml	
5 1/3 ounces	2/3 cup		160 ml	
6 ounces	¾ cup		180 ml	
8 ounces	1 cup	half a pint	240 ml	(250 ml)
12 ounces	1½ cups		350 ml	
16 ounces	2 cups	1 pint	475 ml	(500 ml)
24 ounces	3 cups		700 ml	(750 ml)
32 ounces	4 cups	1 quart	1 liter	
128 ounces	16 cups	1 gallon	3.8 liters	(4 liters)

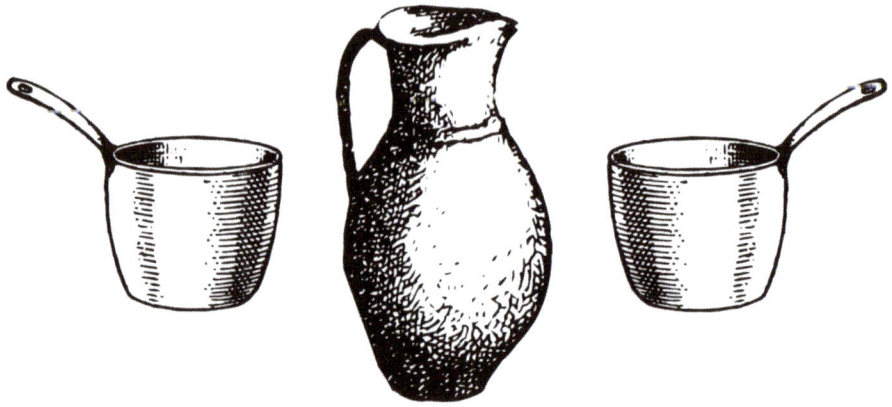

Lengths & Widths

Multiply number of inches by 2.5 to convert to centimeters.

1 inch			2.5 cm	
6 inches	½ foot		15 cm	
12 inches	1 foot		30 cm	
36 inches	3 feet	1 yard	90 cm	
40 inches			100 cm	1 meter

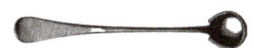

Temperatures

Fahrenheit	Celsius	Gas Mark
32°	0°	(freezes water)
212°	100°	(boils water)
225°	110°	¼
250°	130°	½
275°	140°	1
300°	150°	2
325°	160°	3
350°	180°	4
375°	190°	5
400°	200°	6
425°	220°	7
450°	230°	8
475°	240°	9

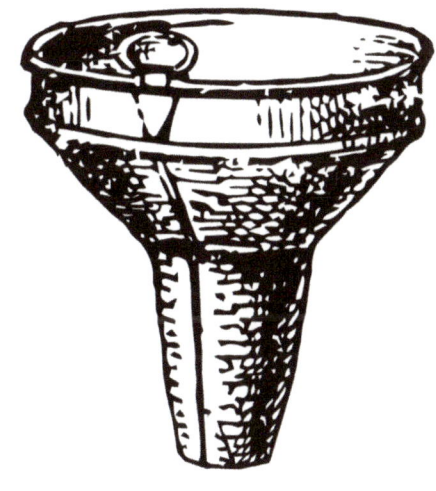

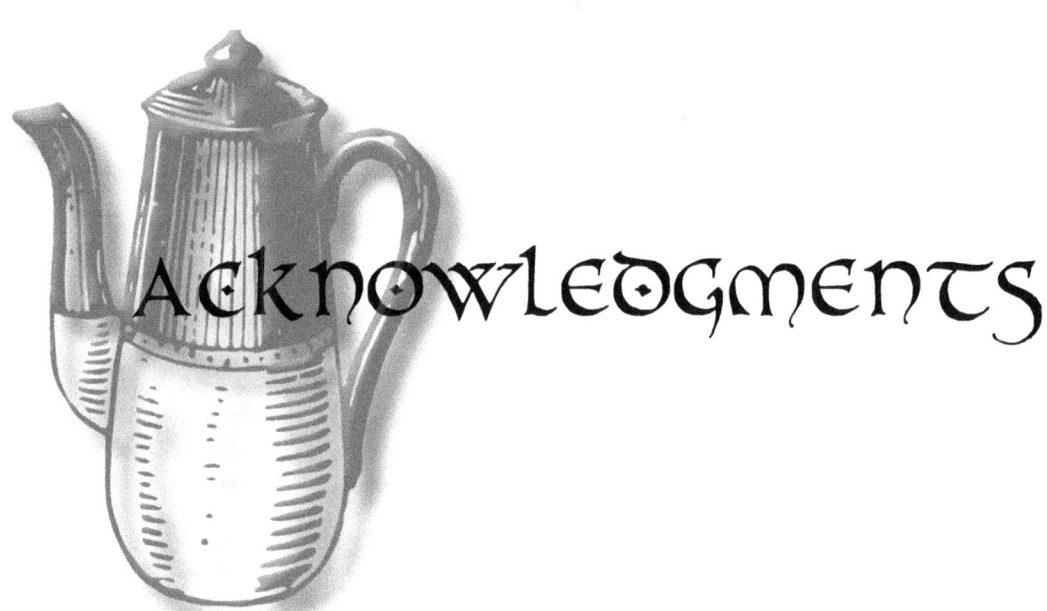

Acknowledgments

My deepest thanks go to my editor, Dawn Catanach, for her thoughtful and helpful suggestions. It is always rather daunting to hand your work over to another person, but we both survived the experience. I greatly appreciate the insights of my band of Beta Readers. Any errors that reveal themselves to me are solely my responsibility. I'm sure I'll locate them after the initial printing…

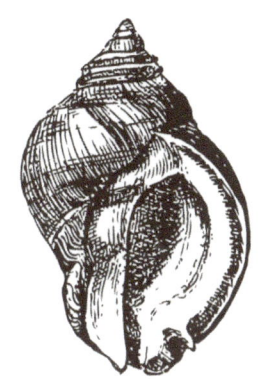

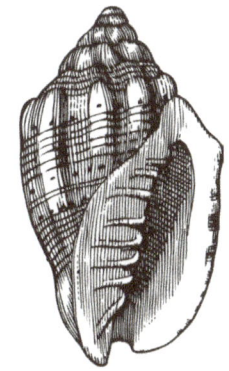

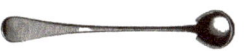

My heartfelt gratitude goes to Ellen, Chloë, and Callista. They are the best women I know and I am incredibly happy that I have them in my life.

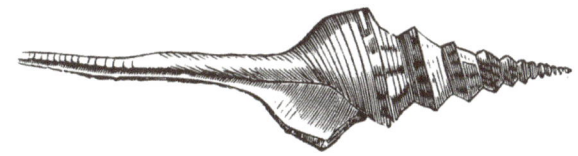

You might think it is odd that I have a dragon centerfold within this book (at least, Chloë does). My first cookbook was filled with awesome dragon artwork and I wanted this book to have a little bit of dragon in it, too. Back in 2017, I took a photo of a neighborhood sculpture on Montgomery Boulevard for a future book. I wasn't completely sure I would use it, but I figured I'd have it in reserve. Iron sculptures popped up all over the Northeast Heights of Albuquerque a few years ago, and I'm not sure who the artist was—I don't think anyone knows who the actual artist was, though I think the art was affiliated with a store that is no longer in business.

A year or so later, I noticed it had been vandalized; it was battered and practically torn out of the ground. That convinced me to go ahead and use my photo as a tribute to this enchanting work, so here it is. Just recently, however, I drove by and saw that somebody had tried to piece it together again. And even though this somebody made a valiant effort to resurrect the mythical beastie, it unfortunately now looks like some sort of mutated creature—definitely not a dragon. Ah well, sometimes art is an ephemeral thing, and only lives on in a photo or a memory.

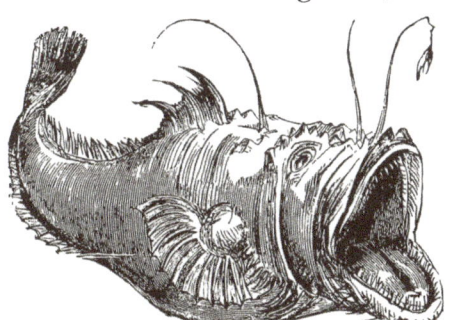

Acknowledgments 193

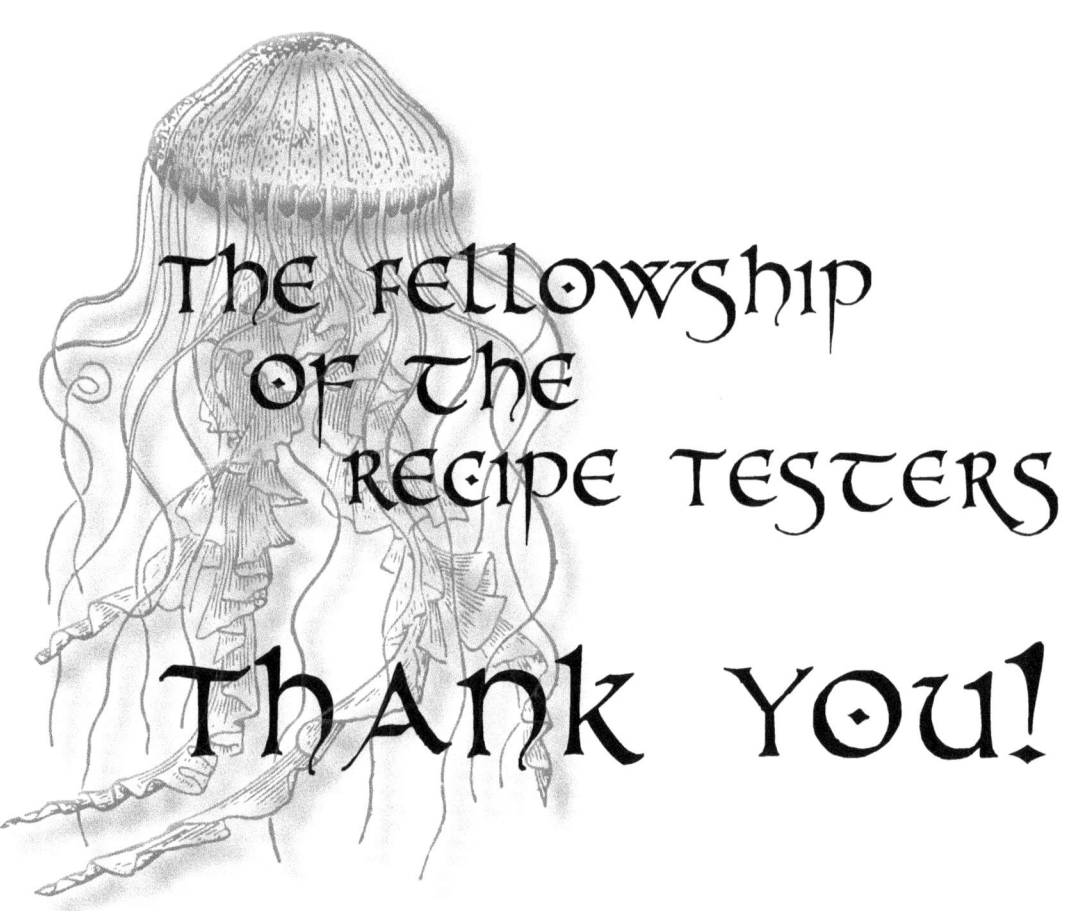

The Fellowship of the Recipe Testers
Thank You!

I had a crack squad of recipe testers for this cookbook! I am absolutely thankful for all of their constructive commentary and many of their suggestions are integrated within. Thank you all for your invaluable help.

I have found, however, that recipe testers are a bit like Goldilocks. I had a chili recipe that was tried by three different people. For one, it was way TOO spicy. For another, it was mostly good, but could have used DOUBLE the amount of chile. For the third, it was JUST RIGHT! So in the end, whatever is here is based on my particular taste. And that's why cooks sometimes write notes in margins.

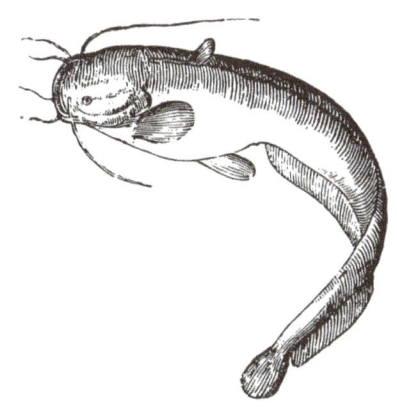

Arasiz
Elvish Black
Jody R. Boyce
Michael & Juliet Bresler
Dr. Judy Busby
Claire "Third-Breakfast" Buss
Suzan Dentry
John R. Harstine

The Johnson Family:
Keith, MaryBeth, Karl, and AnneMarie
Masato Kaida
Alistair Kraft

House Markert:
Dana, Oli, and Thaddäus
Kaci Payne

Clan Ramsey:
Tina, Yvonne, and Michelle
Mark & Ellen Sturmer
Cindy Tomamichel
The Winegar-Garrett Family
The Winegar-Valdez Family

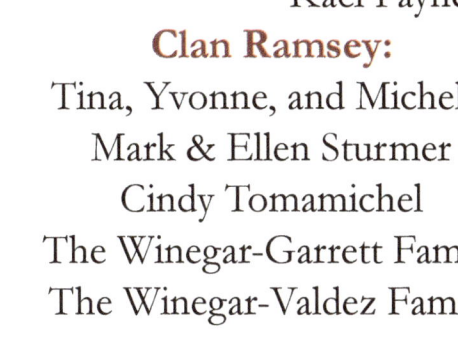

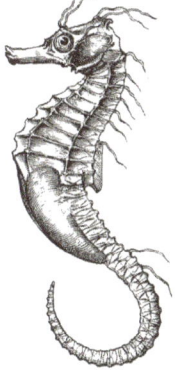

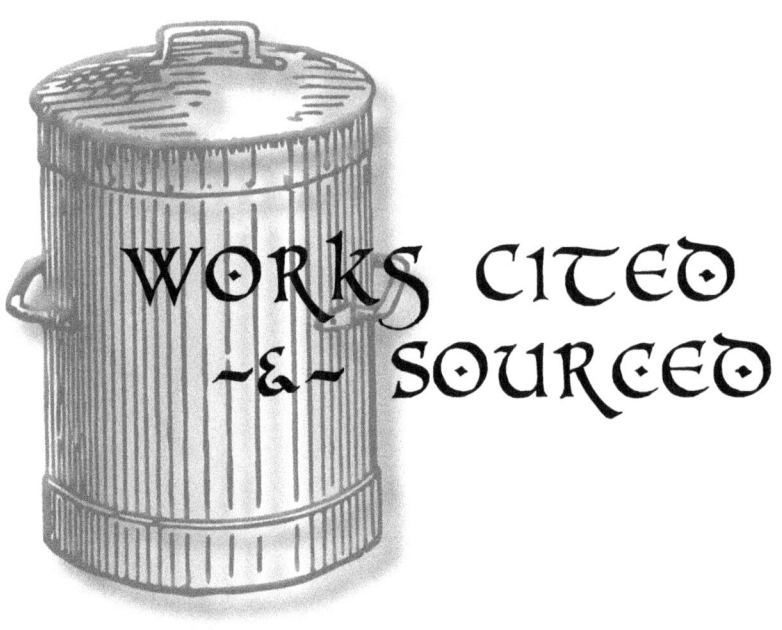

Austin Powers. Dir. Jay Roach. Screenplay by Mike Myers. Perf. Mike Myers et al. United States: New Line Cinema, 1997-2002.

Better Call Saul. Television series, created by Vince Gilligan and Peter Gould. Perf. Bob Odenkirk et al. United States: Sony Pictures Television, 2015-2022.

Breaking Bad. Television series, created by Vince Gilligan. Perf. Bryan Cranston et al. United States: Sony Pictures Television, 2008-2013.

Chang, David and Meehan, Peter. *Momofuku*. New York: Clarkson Potter/Publishers, 2009.

City Slickers. Dir. Ron Underwood. Screenplay by Lowell Ganz and Babaloo Mandel. Perf. Billy Crystal et al. United States: Castle Rock Entertainment, 1991.

Game of Thrones. Television series, created by David Benioff and D. B. Weiss. Perf. Peter Dinklage et al. Home Box Office (HBO), 2011-2019.

The LEGO Batman Movie. Dir. Chris McKay. Screenplay by Seth Grahame-Smith et al. Perf. Will Arnett et al. United States: Warner Bros. Pictures, 2017.

Leitch, Donovan. "Mellow Yellow." *Mellow Yellow*. Epic, 1967.

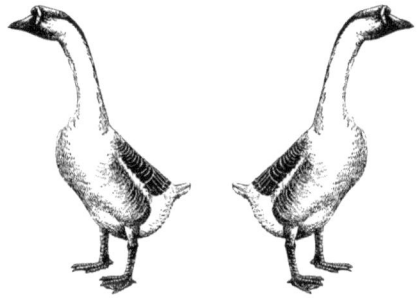

Lewis, C. S. *The Chronicles of Narnia*. Seven volumes. New York: The Macmillan Company, 1950-1956.

—. *The Lion, The Witch and The Wardrobe*. New York: The Macmillan Company, 1950.

—. *The Silver Chair*. New York: The Macmillan Company, 1953.

—. *The Voyage of the Dawn Treader*. New York: The Macmillan Company, 1952.

Works Cited & Sourced

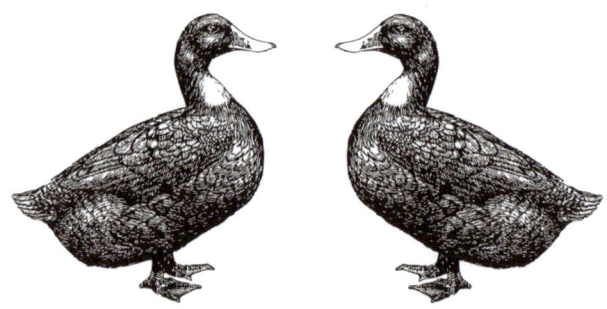

Poole, Lauren. *Shit Burqueños Say. YouTube,* uploaded by Blackoutdigital, 07 February 2012, www.youtube.com/watch?v=IucBp1yrr7A.

Seinfeld. Television series, created by Larry David and Jerry Seinfeld. Perf. Jerry Seinfeld et al. United States: National Broadcasting Company (NBC), 1989-1998.

Star Wars: The Empire Strikes Back. Dir. Irvin Kershner. Screenplay by Leigh Brackett and Lawrence Kasdan. Perf. Mark Hamill et al. United States: 20th Century Fox, 1980.

Star Wars: The Force Awakens. Dir. J. J. Abrams. Screenplay by Lawrence Kasdan et al. Perf. Harrison Ford et al. United States: Walt Disney Studios Motion Pictures, 2015.

Star Wars: The Last Jedi. Dir. Rian Johnson. Screenplay by Rian Johnson. Perf. Mark Hamill et al. United States: Walt Disney Studios Motion Pictures, 2017.

Tolkien, J. R. R. *The Hobbit*. Boston: Houghton Mifflin Company, 1966.

—. *The Lord of the Rings*. Collector's Edition. Boston: Houghton Mifflin Company, 1965.

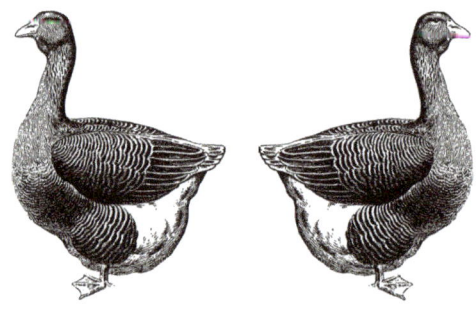

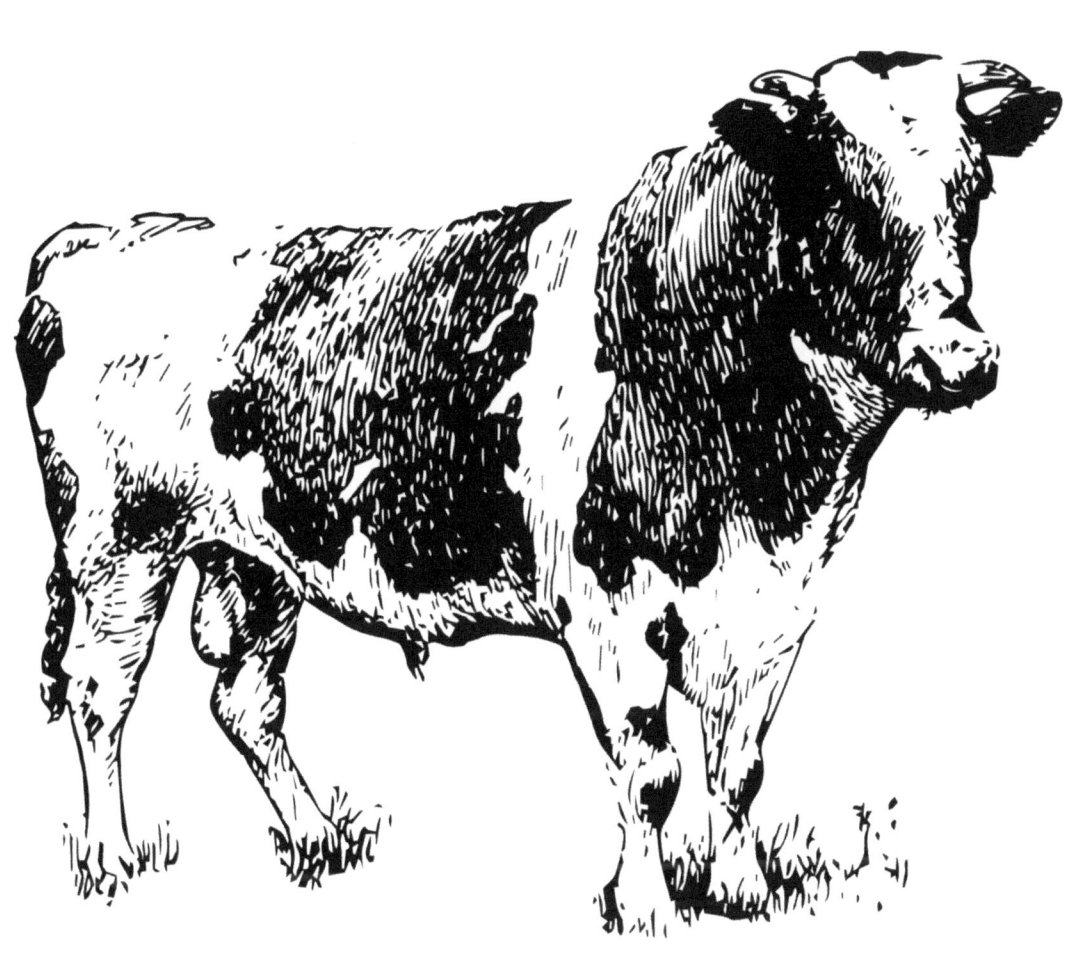

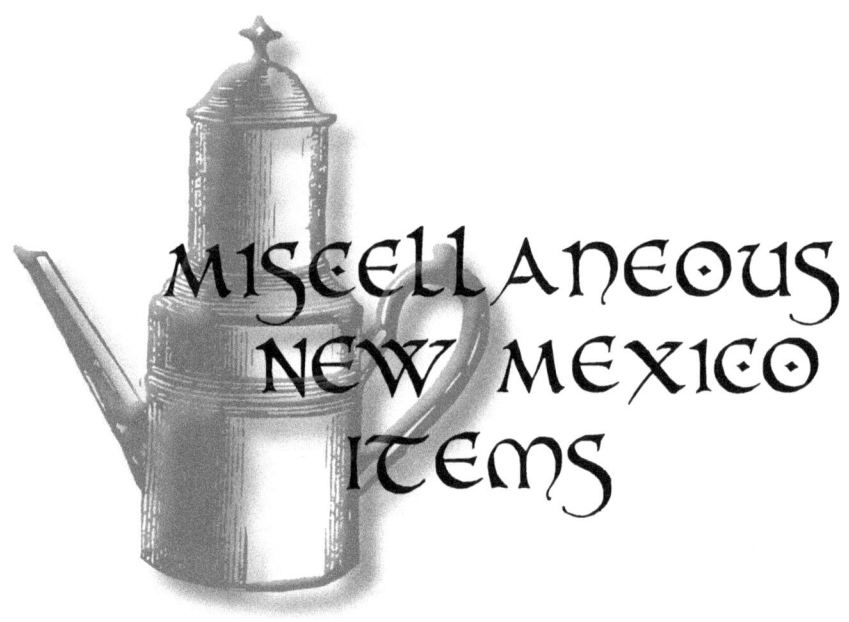

Miscellaneous New Mexico Items

These businesses were active as of October, 2023.

The Albuquerque International Balloon Fiesta is held yearly during the first two complete weekends in October. Book your accommodations early.

★ Their website is: www.balloonfiesta.com ★

Bear Mountain Lodge is located in Silver City, New Mexico; south of the Gila National Forest.

★ Their website is: www.bearmountainlodge.com ★

The Owl Café in Albuquerque is located at 800 Eubank NE.

★ Their website is: www.facebook.com/owlcafealbuquerque ★

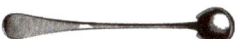

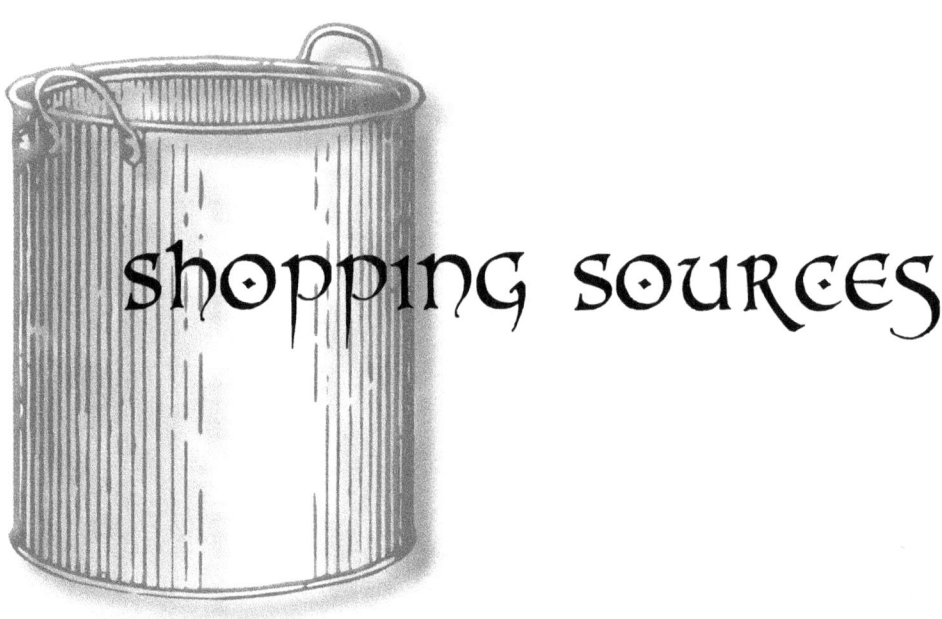

shopping sources

If you'd like to order chile supplies directly from New Mexico, here are a few sources. Some are also restaurants here, which Bob and I have frequented. These websites reflect Albuquerque-based businesses with active mail order services as of October, 2023.

505 Southwestern	www.505southwestern.com
Bueno Foods	www.buenofoods.com
Cervantes Salsa	www.cervantessalsa.com
Chile Traditions	www.chiletraditions.com
El Pinto	www.elpinto.com
La Salita	www.lasalita.com
Monroe's	www.monroeschile.com
Sadie's	www.sadiesofnewmexico.com

You can even order many ingredients from the Amazon, of course. If you buy chile, it is preferable to buy it in glass, rather than cans. But even canned chile is better than no chile at all!

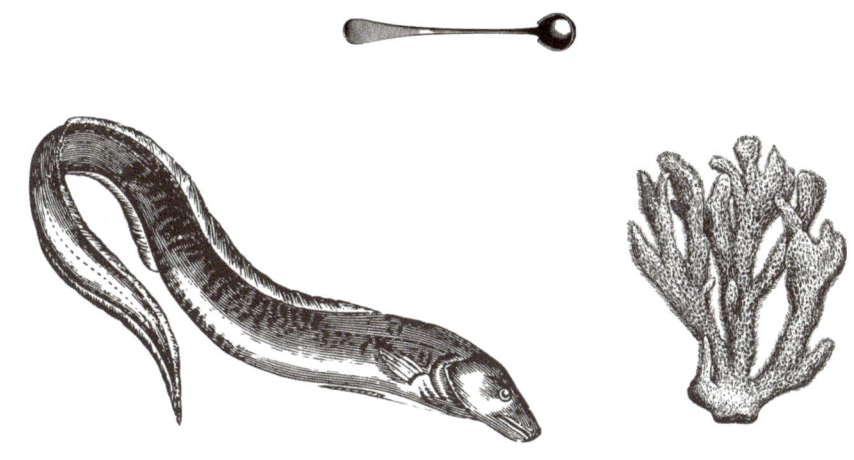

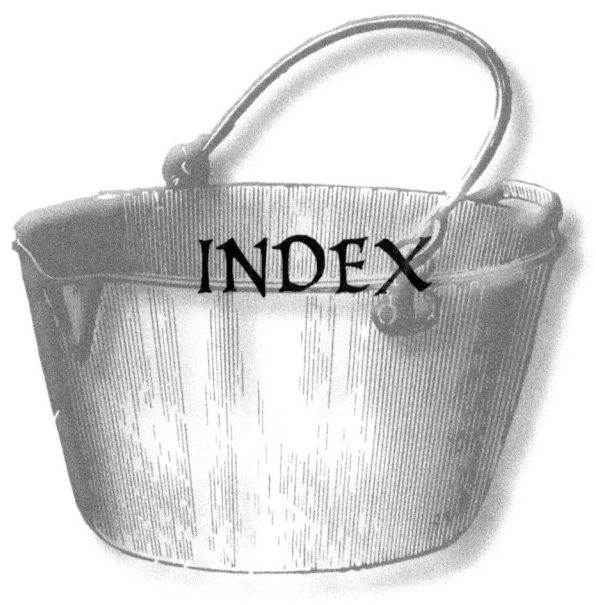

Rather than cross-listing each soup into a multitude of individual categories, I've determined a maximum of four more dominant or notable ingredients to represent each item, beyond each recipe's name and category. Therefore, most items will be listed no more than five or six times in the index. If an ingredient category ended up with only one recipe within it, I deleted the entire category. I have not assigned categories for the more ubiquitous vegetables (such as onions, carrots, and celery); otherwise, I'm afraid this index would have ended up being more like 50 pages long!

A

ALCOHOL (MEANING WINE, BEER, OR OTHER ALCOHOL IS A RATHER NOTABLE INGREDIENT)
   Bob Hates Cauliflower Soup, 104
   Bodacious Brisket Soup, 20
   Butternut Risotto Soup, 92
   Dragon Fire Chili, 26
   Onion Soup C'est Magnifique, 116
   Ten-Alarm Butternut Chicken Chili, 60

Asbjorn's New England Clam
   Chowder, 94
Awesome Avgolemono, 36

B

Baba Yaga Borscht, 128

BARLEY
   Chloë's Kale-apalooza, 108
   Robert the Bruce's Cock-a-Leekie
      Soup, 40

BEANS OF ALL KINDS
   Bob's Old Fashioned Beef Stew, 12
   Broken Tooth Soup (a.k.a. Sopa del
      Diente Quebrado), 132
   Casbah-Rockin' Chicken Stew, 48
   Dragon Fire Chili, 26
   Little Squash: Little Stew, 122
   My Darling Minestrone, 140
   Pasta e Fagioli, 22
   Pepper Pot Chili, 18
   Sopa del Diente Quebrado (a.k.a.
      Broken Tooth Soup), 132
   Tecolote Chili, 98
   Ten-Alarm Butternut Chicken Chili, 60
   Turkey Black Bean Soup, 56

BEEF (VEAL, LAMB, AND VENISON)
   Bob's Old Fashioned Beef Stew, 12
   Bodacious Brisket Soup, 20
   Cheeseburger Soup, 24
   Coconut Beef Stew, 28
   Dragon Fire Chili, 26
   Happy Medium Ramen, 6
   Holy Beef Posole, Batman!, 4
   It's a Nice Day for a Wedding Soup, 14
   Oodle Noodle Soup, 30
   Pasta e Fagioli, 22
   Pepper Pot Chili, 18

Bill's Table Tortillas, 156
Bob Hates Cauliflower Soup, 104
Bob's Old Fashioned Beef Stew, 12
Bodacious Brisket Soup, 20
Bran's Brans, 164

BREADS
- Bill's Table Tortillas, 156
- Bran's Brans, 164
- Buffins, 154
- Cottage Dill Bread, 160
- Crazy Croutons (garnish for Warren Asked for Seconds (!) Tomato Soup), 119
- Easy Focaccia, 174
- Epic Iron Skillet Cornbread, 176
- FAB Crostini (garnish for Funky Artichoke Bisque), 101
- Game of Scones, 166
- Ginormous Cheesy Toasts (garnish for Onion Soup C'est Magnifique), 116
- Land of Enchantment "Lembas" with Spicy Honey Butter, 178
- Lovely Artisan Loaf, 168
- Naughty Naans, 158
- Nifty "Narnian" Biscuits, 172
- Oaten Cake with "Narnian" Wheat, 162
- Puffy Spinach Bread (a.k.a. "Rey's Savory Quarter-Portion"), 70
- "Rey's Savory Quarter-Portion" (a.k.a. Puffy Spinach Bread), 70
- Toasty Muffin Bread, 152

Broken Tooth Soup (a.k.a. Sopa del Diente Quebrado), 132

BROTHS/STOCKS
- Roasted Beef Bone Broth, xxiv
- Roasted Chicken Stock, xxv
- Seafood Stock, xxvii
- Slow-Roasted Herbed Vegetable Stock, xxviii
- Turkey Frame Broth, xxvi

Buffins, 154

BUTTERMILK
- Bran's Brans, 164
- Buffins, 154
- Epic Iron Skillet Cornbread, 176
- Game of Scones, 166
- Nifty "Narnian" Biscuits, 172
- Oaten Cake with "Narnian" Wheat, 162
- Toasty Muffin Bread, 152

Butternut Risotto Soup, 92

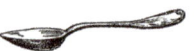

C

CABBAGE
- Baba Yaga Borscht, 128
- Chloë's Kale-apalooza, 108
- Creamy Vegetable Posole, 114
- Mmm... So Spicy Miso Soup (a.k.a. "Poe Pho"), 52
- "Poe Pho" (a.k.a. Mmm... So Spicy Miso Soup), 52
- Tater Ham Chowder, 106

Callista's Amazing Avocado Chicken Soup, 58
Carpe Caldillo, 80
Casbah-Rockin' Chicken Stew, 48

CAULIFLOWER
- Bob Hates Cauliflower Soup, 104
- Ellen's Exotic Cauliflower Bisque, 134
- Saffron Madness Soup, 138

Charming Chili Garnishes, v
Cheeseburger Soup, 24

CHEESY
- Cheeseburger Soup, 24
- Cottage Dill Bread, 160
- Enchanted Forest Soup, 126
- Funky Artichoke Bisque, 100
- Ginormous Cheesy Toasts (garnish for Onion Soup C'est Magnifique), 116
- "Hoth Broth" (a.k.a. Stracciatella Bella), 66
- Naughty Naans, 158
- Onion Soup C'est Magnifique, 116
- Stracciatella Bella (a.k.a. "Hoth Broth"), 66
- Turkey Black Bean Soup, 56
- Walter's Bitchin' Buffalo Soup, 42

CHICKEN (TURKEY & OTHER ASSORTED POULTRY)
- Awesome Avgolemono, 36
- Callista's Amazing Avocado Chicken Soup, 58
- Casbah-Rockin' Chicken Stew, 48
- Elegantly Sufficient Egg Drop Soup, 44
- "Hoth Broth" (a.k.a. Stracciatella Bella), 66
- Jumbo Gumbo, 88
- Mmm... So Spicy Miso Soup (a.k.a. "Poe Pho"), 52
- Nothing Wrong with Mulligatawny, 46
- "Poe Pho" (a.k.a. Mmm... So Spicy Miso Soup), 52
- Rev It Up Posole, 34
- Robert the Bruce's Cock-a-Leekie Soup, 40
- Sopa de los Burqueños, 62
- Stracciatella Bella (a.k.a. "Hoth Broth"), 66
- Ten-Alarm Butternut Chicken Chili, 60
- Troy's Terrific Thai Turkey Soup, 38
- Turkey Black Bean Soup, 56
- Walter's Bitchin' Buffalo Soup, 42

Chloë's Kale-apalooza, 108

COCONUT
- Coconut Beef Stew, 28
- Nothing Wrong with Mulligatawny, 46
- Troy's Terrific Thai Turkey Soup, 38

Coconut Beef Stew, 28
Cooked Hominy, xx

CORN (AND CORNMEAL)
- Broken Tooth Soup (a.k.a. Sopa del Diente Quebrado), 132
- Buffins, 154
- Epic Iron Skillet Cornbread, 176
- Game of Scones, 166
- Happy Medium Ramen, 6
- Little Squash: Little Stew, 122
- Sassy Shrimp Posole, 76
- Sopa del Diente Quebrado (a.k.a. Broken Tooth Soup), 132
- Toasty Muffin Bread, 152
- Walter's Bitchin' Buffalo Soup, 42
- William Said This Was His Favorite Soup, 124

Cottage Dill Bread, 160
Crazy Croutons (garnish for Warren Asked for Seconds (!) Tomato Soup), 119

CREAMY RECIPES
- Asbjorn's New England Clam Chowder, 94
- Bodacious Brisket Soup, 20
- Broken Tooth Soup (a.k.a. Sopa del Diente Quebrado), 132

Index   207

Butternut Risotto Soup, 92
Casbah-Rockin' Chicken Stew, 48
Creamy Vegetable Posole, 114
Crème de la Crème Fraîche, xviii
Crème Fraîche Mimic, xix
Ellen's Exotic Cauliflower Bisque, 134
Enchanted Forest Soup, 126
Funky Artichoke Bisque, 100
Mexican Crème, xix
Mom's Masher Soup, 120
Notorious CSC, 78
Saffron Madness Soup, 138
Savory Mushroom Soup, 136
Sopa de los Burqueños, 62
Sopa del Diente Quebrado (a.k.a. Broken Tooth Soup), 132
Sweet Crème Dream, xx
Ten-Alarm Butternut Chicken Chili, 60
Turkey Black Bean Soup, 56
Warren Asked for Seconds (!) Tomato Soup, 118

Creamy Vegetable Posole, 114
Crème de la Crème Fraîche, xviii
Crème Fraîche Mimic, xix

CURRY POWDER
Coconut Beef Stew, 28
Naughty Naans, 158
Nothing Wrong with Mulligatawny, 46
Notorious CSC, 78
Troy's Terrific Thai Turkey Soup, 38

D

Donna's Christmas Eve Posole, 74
Dragon Fire Chili, 26

E

Easy Focaccia, 174
Easy Herbes de Provence, xxix
Elegantly Sufficient Egg Drop Soup, 44

EGGS
Awesome Avgolemono, 36
Elegantly Sufficient Egg Drop Soup, 44
"Hoth Broth" (a.k.a. Stracciatella Bella), 66
It's a Nice Day for a Wedding Soup, 14
Stracciatella Bella (a.k.a. "Hoth Broth"), 66

Elfryda's Söt Suppe (a.k.a. Elfryda's Strawberry Soup), 142
Elfryda's Strawberry Soup (a.k.a. Elfryda's Söt Suppe), 142
Ellen's Exotic Cauliflower Bisque, 134
Enchanted Forest Soup, 126
Epic Iron Skillet Cornbread, 176
Esther's Manhattan Clam Chowder, 82

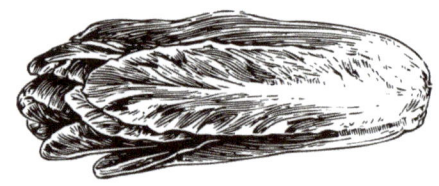

F

FAB Crostini (garnish for Funky Artichoke Bisque), 101

FRUIT
Bran's Brans, 164
Casbah-Rockin' Chicken Stew, 48

Coconut Beef Stew, 28
Elfryda's Söt Suppe (a.k.a. Elfryda's Strawberry Soup), 142
Elfryda's Strawberry Soup (a.k.a. Elfryda's Söt Suppe), 142
Nothing Wrong with Mulligatawny, 46
Robert the Bruce's Cock-a-Leekie Soup, 40

Funky Artichoke Bisque, 100

G

Game of Scones, 166
Ginormous Cheesy Toasts (garnish for Onion Soup C'est Magnifique), 116

GREEN & RED CHILE
Callista's Amazing Avocado Chicken Soup, 58
Carpe Caldillo, 80
Donna's Christmas Eve Posole, 74
Dragon Fire Chili, 26
Holy Beef Posole, Batman!, 4
Pepper Pot Chili, 18
Rev It Up Posole, 34
Sassy Shrimp Posole, 76
Sopa de los Burqueños, 62
Tecolote Chili, 98

H

Happy Medium Ramen, 6
Holy Beef Posole, Batman!, 4

HOMINY
Cooked Hominy, xx
Creamy Vegetable Posole, 114
Donna's Christmas Eve Posole, 74
Holy Beef Posole, Batman!, 4
Rev It Up Posole, 34
Sassy Shrimp Posole, 76

"Hoth Broth" (a.k.a. Stracciatella Bella), 66

I

It's a Nice Day for a Wedding Soup, 14

J

Jumbo Gumbo, 88

L

Land of Enchantment "Lembas" with Spicy Honey Butter, 178
Little Squash: Little Stew, 122
Lovely Artisan Loaf, 168

M

Mexican Crème, xix

MISCELLANEOUS
Cooked Hominy, xx
Crème de la Crème Fraîche, xviii
Crème Fraîche Mimic, xix
Easy Herbes de Provence, xxix
Mexican Crème, xix
Spicy Honey Butter, 180
Sweet Crème Dream, xx

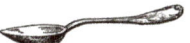

Mmm... So Spicy Miso Soup (a.k.a. "Poe Pho"), 52
Mom's Masher Soup, 120

MUSHROOMS
Elegantly Sufficient Egg Drop Soup, 44
Happy Medium Ramen, 6
Mmm... So Spicy Miso Soup (a.k.a. "Poe Pho"), 52
"Poe Pho" (a.k.a. Mmm... So Spicy Miso Soup), 52
Savory Mushroom Soup, 136

My Darling Minestrone, 140

N

Naughty Naans, 158
Nice New Mexican & Mexican Garnishes, iv
Nifty "Narnian" Biscuits, 172
Nothing Wrong with Mulligatawny, 46
Notorious CSC, 78

O

Oaten Cake with "Narnian" Wheat, 162
Onion Soup C'est Magnifique, 116
Oodle Noodle Soup, 30

P

Pasta e Fagioli, 22

PASTA (NOODLES, MACARONI)
Bob Hates Cauliflower Soup, 104
Happy Medium Ramen, 6
It's a Nice Day for a Wedding Soup, 14

Mmm... So Spicy Miso Soup (a.k.a. "Poe Pho"), 52
My Darling Minestrone, 140
Oodle Noodle Soup, 30
Pasta e Fagioli, 22
"Poe Pho" (a.k.a. Mmm... So Spicy Miso Soup), 52

Pepper Pot Chili, 18
"Poe Pho" (a.k.a. Mmm... So Spicy Miso Soup), 52

PORK (HAM, BACON, AND SAUSAGE)
Bob Hates Cauliflower Soup, 104
Butternut Risotto Soup, 92
Carpe Caldillo, 80
Chloë's Kale-apalooza, 108
Donna's Christmas Eve Posole, 74
Esther's Manhattan Clam Chowder, 82
It's a Nice Day for a Wedding Soup, 14
Jumbo Gumbo, 88
Tater Ham Chowder, 106
Tecolote Chili, 98

POTATOES AND/OR SWEET POTATOES
Asbjorn's New England Clam Chowder, 94
Baba Yaga Borscht, 128
Bob's Old Fashioned Beef Stew, 12
Bodacious Brisket Soup, 20
Carpe Caldillo, 80
Cheeseburger Soup, 24
Coconut Beef Stew, 28
Esther's Manhattan Clam Chowder, 82
Mom's Masher Soup, 120
My Darling Minestrone, 140
Notorious CSC, 78
Robert the Bruce's Cock-a-Leekie Soup, 40

Saffron Madness Soup, 138
Tater Ham Chowder, 106
William Said This Was His Favorite Soup, 124

Puffy Spinach Bread (a.k.a. "Rey's Savory Quarter-Portion"), 70

R

Rev It Up Posole, 34
"Rey's Savory Quarter-Portion" (a.k.a. Puffy Spinach Bread), 70

RICE
Awesome Avgolemono, 36
Butternut Risotto Soup, 92
Callista's Amazing Avocado Chicken Soup, 58
Holy Beef Posole, Batman!, 4
Jumbo Gumbo, 88
Troy's Terrific Thai Turkey Soup, 38

Roasted Beef Bone Broth, xxiv
Roasted Chicken Stock, xxv
Robert the Bruce's Cock-a-Leekie Soup, 40

S

Saffron Madness Soup, 138
Sassy Shrimp Posole, 76
Savory Mushroom Soup, 136

SEAFOOD
Asbjorn's New England Clam Chowder, 94
Esther's Manhattan Clam Chowder, 82
Funky Artichoke Bisque, 100
Jumbo Gumbo, 88
Notorious CSC, 78
Sassy Shrimp Posole, 76

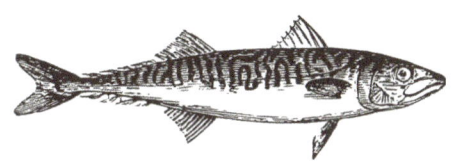

Seafood Stock, xxvii
Slow-Roasted Herbed Vegetable Stock, xxviii
Sopa de los Burqueños, 62
Sopa del Diente Quebrado (a.k.a. Broken Tooth Soup), 132
Spicy Honey Butter, 180

SPINACH AND/OR KALE
Callista's Amazing Avocado Chicken Soup, 58
Chloë's Kale-apalooza, 108
Elegantly Sufficient Egg Drop Soup, 44
"Hoth Broth" (a.k.a. Stracciatella Bella), 66
It's a Nice Day for a Wedding Soup, 14
Puffy Spinach Bread (a.k.a. "Rey's Savory Quarter-Portion"), 70
"Rey's Savory Quarter-Portion" (a.k.a. Puffy Spinach Bread), 70
Stracciatella Bella (a.k.a. "Hoth Broth"), 66

SQUASH
Butternut Risotto Soup, 92
Coconut Beef Stew, 28
Little Squash: Little Stew, 122
My Darling Minestrone, 140
Ten-Alarm Butternut Chicken Chili, 60

Stracciatella Bella (a.k.a. "Hoth Broth"), 66
Sweet Crème Dream, xx

T

Tater Ham Chowder, 106
Tecolote Chili, 98
Ten-Alarm Butternut Chicken Chili, 60
Toasty Muffin Bread, 152

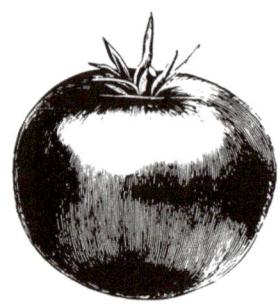

TOMATOES (IN MANY FORMS)
Carpe Caldillo, 80
Casbah-Rockin' Chicken Stew, 48
Chloë's Kale-apalooza, 108
Donna's Christmas Eve Posole, 74
Ellen's Exotic Cauliflower Bisque, 134
Esther's Manhattan Clam Chowder, 82
Nothing Wrong with Mulligatawny, 46
Oodle Noodle Soup, 30
Pasta e Fagioli, 22
Rev It Up Posole, 34
Warren Asked for Seconds (!) Tomato Soup, 118
William Said This Was His Favorite Soup, 124

Troy's Terrific Thai Turkey Soup, 38
Turkey Black Bean Soup, 56
Turkey Frame Broth, xxvi

V

VEGETARIAN
Baba Yaga Borscht, 128
Broken Tooth Soup (a.k.a. Sopa del Diente Quebrado), 132
Creamy Vegetable Posole, 114
Elfryda's Söt Suppe (a.k.a. Elfryda's Strawberry Soup), 142
Elfryda's Strawberry Soup (a.k.a. Elfryda's Söt Suppe), 142
Ellen's Exotic Cauliflower Bisque, 134
Enchanted Forest Soup, 126
Little Squash: Little Stew, 122
Mom's Masher Soup, 120
My Darling Minestrone, 140
Onion Soup C'est Magnifique, 116
Saffron Madness Soup, 138
Savory Mushroom Soup, 136
Sopa del Diente Quebrado (a.k.a. Broken Tooth Soup), 132
Warren Asked for Seconds (!) Tomato Soup, 118
William Said This Was His Favorite Soup, 124

W

Walter's Bitchin' Buffalo Soup, 42
Warren Asked for Seconds (!) Tomato Soup, 118
William Said This Was His Favorite Soup, 124

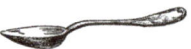

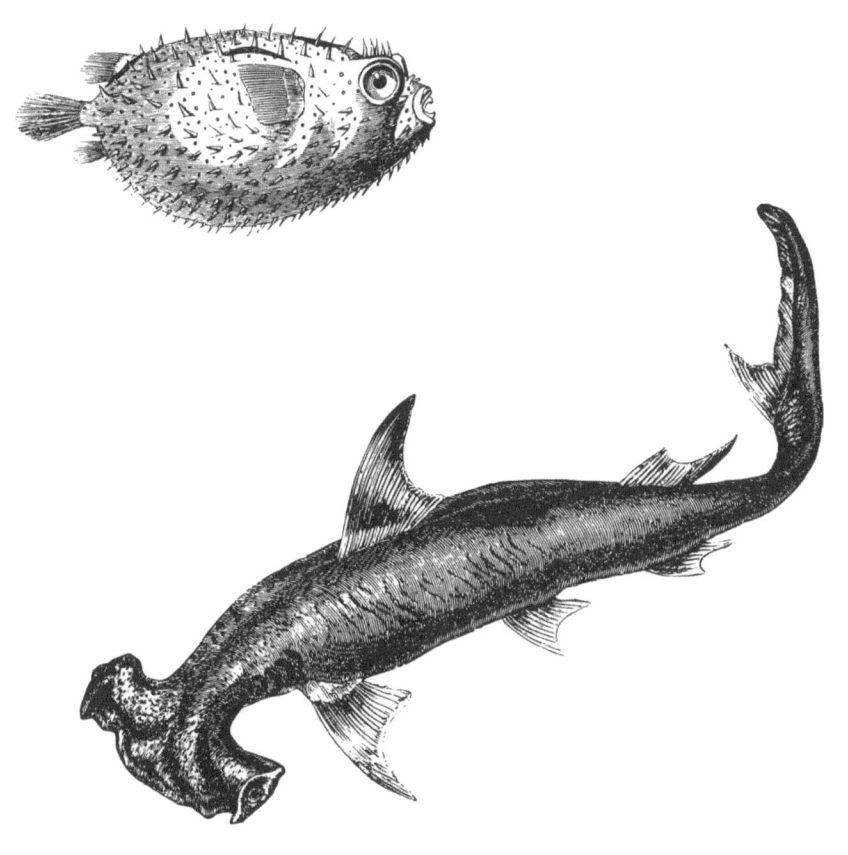
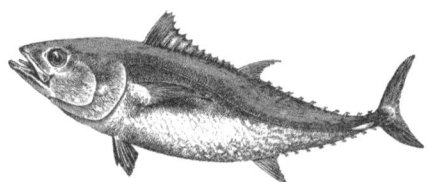

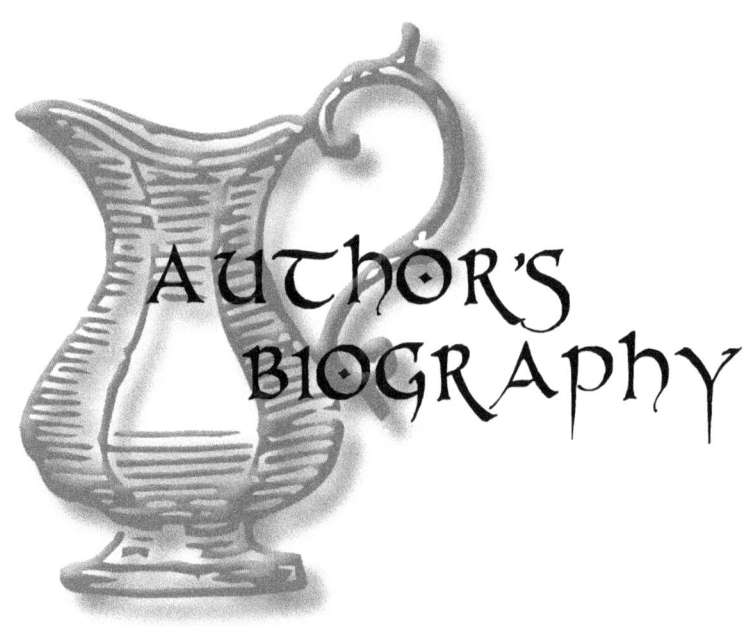

Author's Biography

Astrid Tuttle Winegar is the author of *Cooking for Halflings & Monsters: 111 Comfy, Cozy Recipes for Fantasy-Loving Souls*, which was a finalist in the 2018 New Mexico/Arizona Book Awards. Astrid has been cooking, baking, and reading fantasy (and plenty of other literature!) for over 40 years. She has a bachelor's degree in English and Latin and a master's degree in Comparative Literature and Cultural Studies from the University of New Mexico. She has loved C. S. Lewis since childhood and J. R. R. Tolkien since middle and high school. She also loves all Star things, both Trek and Wars, all things Whedon, and many other things besides… She lives in the enchanted city of Albuquerque, New Mexico, with her husband; she is also a mother and a grandmother. For more information, go to www.astridwinegar.com.

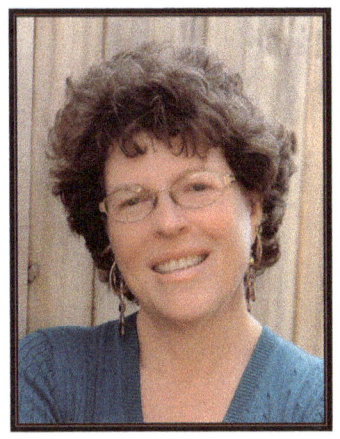

Etsy shop: Elegant Sufficiencies
Facebook: Astrid Tuttle Winegar
Look for her on other social media platforms, which will remain in place until retirement (in theory); all will usually be some sort of iteration of the name Astrid (Tuttle) Winegar.

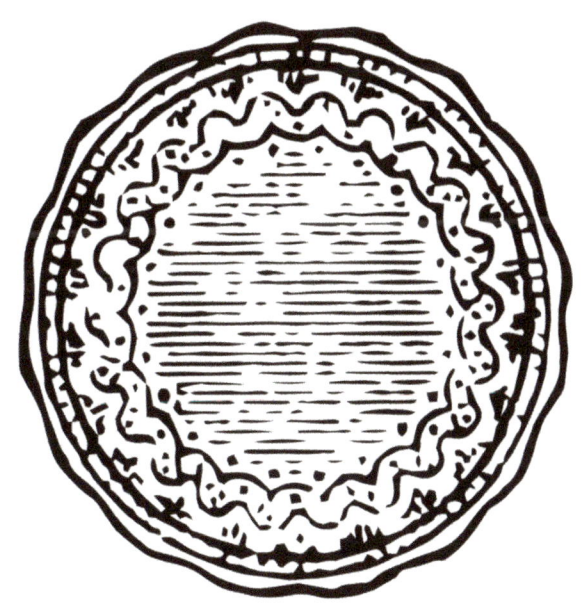

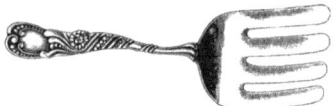
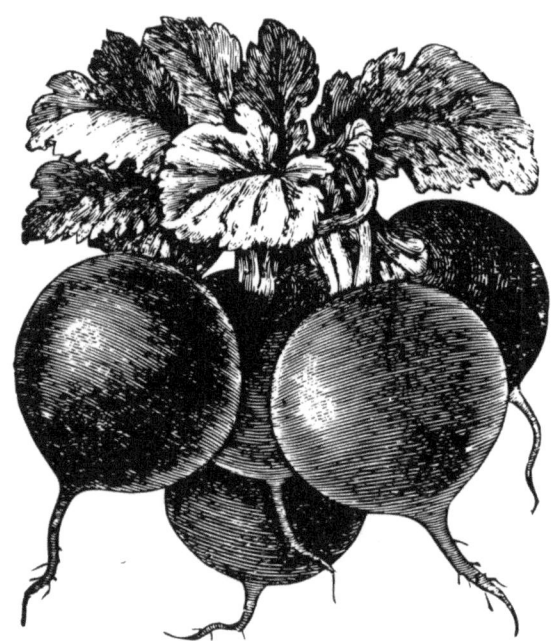
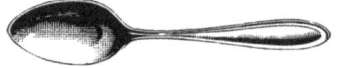

www.ingramcontent.com/pod-product-compliance
Lightning Source LLC
Chambersburg PA
CBHW061153010526
44118CB00027B/2955